Your
Perfectly
Pampered
Menopause

Health, Beauty,

and Lifestyle Advice

for the Best Years

of Your Life

Your
Perfectly
Pampered
Menopause

Colette Bouchez

BROADWAY BOOKS
New York

Broadway Books titles may be purchased for business or promotional use or for special sales. For information, please write to: Special Markets Department, Broadway Books, specialmarkets@randomhouse.com

This book is not intended as a substitute for medical advice from your physician. The reader should regularly consult with a physician in matters relating to her health, particularly in respect to any symptoms that may require medical attention.

PRINTED IN THE UNITED STATES OF AMERICA

BROADWAY BOOKS and its logo, a letter B bisected on the diagonal, are trademarks of Random House, Inc.

Visit our Web site at www.broadwaybooks.com

First edition published 2005

Library of Congress Cataloging-in-Publication Data

Your perfectly pampered menopause : health, beauty, and lifestyle advice for the best years of your life / Colette Bouchez.
p. cm.
1. Menopause—Popular works. 2. Middle-aged women—Health and hygiene.
I. Bouchez, Colette, 1960–

RG186.Y68 2005
618.1'75—dc22   2004048875

ISBN 0-7679-1756-1

10 9 8 7 6 5 4 3 2 1

To my mom and dad—who gave me not only the gift of life, but all the gifts of life. My dream is to always make you proud—in heaven and on earth.

And to Uncle "Rick"—I will never stop missing you. You made me your little star—and I will never shine as brightly as I did in your eyes.

To St. Jude—thank you for my soul. You have never let me down—and my prayer and my praise are never ending.

And to "Mr. Right"—who happened upon my heart just in the nick of time. Thank you for being someone I can believe in—and thank you for believing in me.

Contents

Acknowledgments

~~~~~~

I would like to express my gratitude and appreciation to all the physicians and researchers who contributed to this book, either directly, by so generously sharing their time and expertise, or indirectly, through their tireless efforts to improve the quality of women's health care, not only at midlife, but throughout life.

I would especially like to thank Dr. Steven Goldstein, clinical professor of obstetrics and gynecology at New York University Medical Center, for his efforts in bringing the problems of menopause to the world's stage, and for never being too tired or too busy to answer my questions or teach me something new, or be my friend.

My gratitude also goes to Dr. Julia Smith, codirector of the Lynn Cohen High Risk Program for Breast and Ovarian Cancer at Bellevue Medical Center and the NYU Cancer Center. Thank you for your unwavering dedication to women's health care—and for your kind heart and your friendship.

My thanks also go out to NYU's Dr. Shari Lusskin, director of reproductive psychiatry, and endocrinologist Dr. Loren Wissner Greene for her expertise in all things hormonal. A special thank-you to Dr. Ted Daly of Garden City Dermatology and Dr. Michael Reed of NYU Medical Center for sharing their expertise on hair loss. To Dr. James Dillard, of Columbia College of Physicians and Surgeons, my gratitude for teaching me so much about natural medicine. To my dear friend Andrew Lessman, my gratitude for not only sharing your time and knowledge about vitamins, herbs, and other natural treatments—but for teaching me the true meaning of integrity with everything you do.

To Dr. Patricia Saunders of the Graham Windham Services to Families and Children in New York City, NYU nutritionist Samantha Heller, and Lenox Hill Hospital's Dr. Reginald Puckett, thank you for never letting me down—your expertise is an invaluable part of this book. To some of the world's best dermatologists: Dr. Zoe Diana Draelos, Dr. Amy Newburger, Dr. Daryl Rigel, Dr. Robin Ashinoff—I can't thank you enough for always having all the answers.

There are also several medical organizations that went the distance to help in the preparation of this manuscript, and I would be sorely remiss if I did not thank them now: the American College of Obstetricians and Gynecologists, the Harvard Medical School, the *Harvard Women's Health Newsletter* editorial staff, the American Diabetes Association, the American Academy of Dermatology, the American Society of Dermatologic Surgeons, the American Academy of Plastic Surgeons, and the North American Menopause Society. Thank you all for sharing your expertise in countless ways.

And to my very favorite ladies of substance and style: the incomparable Adrienne Arpel, the all-knowing Laura Geller, the fountain of beauty Holly Mordini, the stylishly clever Toni Brattin, and the "it girl" of all things cool, Valerie Sarnelle. You taught me the secrets of beauty and style and you let me share them, and I can't thank you all enough.

And to hair-care experts Peter Lamas, and Juan Juan of J Beverly Hills Salon—thank you for sharing your secrets and your style!

I am deeply grateful to Lynn Odell, vice president of NYU Medical Center, and her entire staff—I would not "be" if it were not for you all. My most sincere thanks to Nadine Woloshin, Renee Baer, and Howard Rubenstein Associates: Every day I am reminded how lucky I am to have you in my life.

To Bryan Dodson of Columbia Presbyterian Medical Center—you have been my friend and my colleague for so long I don't know how to live without you! To Myrna Manners and the staff of New York Hospital-Cornell Medical Center, your expertise has never failed me. To Joanne Nicholas of Memorial Sloan Kettering Medical Center: How lucky can a journalist get to have you on her side? To Lucia Lee at the Mount Sinai Medical Center: You are simply the best—and you prove it every time I call! And to Sandy Van and Kelly Staunning of the Cedar Sinai Medical Center in Los Angeles, you make me feel like New York and California are right next door: Thank you for welcoming me to the "left coast" with your warmth, your kindness, and, especially, your help. And to my dear friend Greg Philips—how could I survive without your daily e-mails and your smiles? Your help, your caring, your support, and your friendship mean the world to me.

A special thank-you to Eleanor Rawson, the first lady of publishing, who taught me life lessons—and writing skills—beyond what I ever knew existed. And please indulge me while I take a moment to give a heartfelt salute to my "day job" editors. To Tim Hilchey, managing editor of the New York Times Syndicate: Thank you for your friendship, your integrity, and your standards of excellence.

To Sean Swint, Dr. Michael Smith, Dr. Charlotte Grayson, Dr. Brunilda Nazario, Jayne Garrison, Marjorie Martin, Lisa Habib, Robert Allen, and Sylvia Davis of the incomparable WebMD staff: Your support and encouragement has meant more to me than I can ever say. Thank you, from my heart, for welcoming me onto the team, and for setting new and higher standards of medical reporting excellence for us all. And to Bill Boyle, managing editor of the *New York Daily News*—thank you, for not forgetting.

To my legal adviser and friend Gerald Shargel: My utmost respect and thanks for all you have taught me. You are, quite simply, a genius!

And to the group that matters the most in my heart—the world's best girlfriends, whose stories appear throughout this book and who would tie me to a stake if I dared to even mention their names. You know who you are—so thank you for sharing your highs and your lows, your laughter and your tears, your hormones and your mood swings and your temper tantrums . . . and mine . . . and through it all making certain we remained the best of pals.

And to all of you I met in menopause chat rooms and support groups online—thank you for sharing your stories and especially for asking the

questions. You will no doubt find your voices, and your answers, throughout this book. It was an honor to get to know you all.

And to Princess Darcie and the Pinkland Brain Trust: You mean the
world to me!

And I save my best and most heartfelt thanks for last: My deepest appreciation to Broadway Books for taking yet another chance on me. To
Stacy Creamer, deputy editorial director, my gratitude for launching this
idea, and for helping everyone see my vision. To Bill Thomas, thank you
for saying "Yes." And to senior editor Tricia Medved—I couldn't ask for a
better partner on this or any book: You made me laugh, you made me cry,
and you made me the very best writer I can be. To Beth Datlowe—your
comments, your insights, and especially your warmth and kindness are
simply irreplaceable, and I appreciate every way in which you have made
writing this book a sheer joy.

My continued respect and admiration to physician and healer Dr.
Niels Lauersen: Your voice will never be silenced.

Thank you all again.

COLETTE BOUCHEZ
www.ColetteBouchez.com

Your
Perfectly
Pampered
Menopause

Once Upon a Time . . .

Cinderella, Hormone Replacement Therapy,
and Other Fairy Tales of Modern Life

My good friend Martha just turned fifty—but regardless of her age, I will always lovingly think of her as a kind of displaced feminist hippie who never quite found her way out of Woodstock. A warm and gentle soul, she still believes that everything we eat should be organically grown, that Birkenstocks and Levi's are the only clothes anyone ever really needs, and that those of us who put sugar in our cranberry juice—or saccharine in our coffee—are just a lost cause. To say the least, Martha is one of the original "Nature Girls," and, bless her kind heart, nothing about her has changed in thirty-five years. That's one of the reasons I was so surprised when she called one day to ask me about, of all things, *hormone replacement therapy.*

"I need to pick your brain," she said, excusing herself for chewing on a piece of wheatgrass while we talked. "I need to know about hormone therapy."

"Hormones? You mean like . . . natural hormones—like from soy?" I knew that she had been feeling the "burn" of menopause symptoms for quite some time now, but knowing her background I just assumed she would turn to natural treatments for help. Surprisingly, I was wrong.

"No, I mean unnatural hormones—like the kind from horse urine, or whatever it is they are making this stuff out of. I just heard it's really dangerous—and I don't know what to do," she said in a somewhat bewildered tone.

Unbeknownst to me, Martha had actually become one of the millions of women who turned to traditional HRT (hormone replacement therapy) to relieve her midlife symptoms. She had, I found out that day, been wearing an estrogen patch and supplementing that with progestin, a popular chemical form of the hormone progesterone. And she was, she said, perfectly content with that choice. However, it was the summer of 2002 and Martha had just heard the news that rocked her world: Like Cinderella and Snow White, hormone therapy, it seems, was nothing more than a fairy tale with promises that were destined never to come true.

Indeed, the bombshell dropped that summer on all womankind— the announcement by the federal government that they were prematurely halting what should have been a fifteen-year, 160,000+-woman study designed to examine, among other things, the risks and benefits of HRT. The project, known as the Women's Health Initiative (WHI), had run into what experts were calling unforeseen negative results. In reality, much to everyone's surprise, preliminary findings indicated that not only was hormone therapy *not* going to be our personal fountain of youth, bending over to take a drink could very well kill us.

More specifically it was reported that daily dosing with 2.5 milligrams of progestin (medroxyprogesterone acetate), together with 0.625 milligrams of conjugated equine estrogen (known as Prempro), yielded the following result:

- A 26 percent increase in the risk of invasive breast cancer

- A 20 percent increase in the risk of heart attacks

- A 41 percent higher rate of stroke

- A 100 percent increase in blood clots in the lung

Wow. This realization shook an entire generation of women—and my friend Martha was no exception. In fact, from almost the moment the news went public all hell broke loose in my little circle of friends. My home phone nearly went up in smoke.

"Did you know about this ahead of time—if you did, I will kill you for not sharing," my friend Natalie screamed into my ear.

"This has got to be a mistake—oh-my-God, this can't be right—

what the heck is going on—call me RIGHT NOW," my friend Robyn defiantly blasted into my home answering machine.

"You! You told me to listen to my doctor and take the hormones—that they would help me feel better—now, now look what's happened." That was Laura, the "guilt mother" of the crowd.

Indeed, the problems on *Sex and the City* were nothing compared to what my little group was facing now. Could, in fact, this hormonally induced fairy tale of life after estrogen really *be* just another Cinderella lie we all bought into—like Prince Charming and the glass shoe? Had they hoodwinked us once again, with their promises of eternal youth—or at least moist vaginas? As time went on, it seemed as if they had.

In the months that followed, we also learned that using HRT could make it harder to detect tumors in the breast, causing dangerous, even life-threatening diagnostic delays. When tumors were found in hormone users they were larger and more deadly, causing women to die of breast cancer up to 25 percent more often. In late 2003, a large Swedish study looking at HRT in breast cancer survivors was also halted when doctors found an overwhelming number of cancers recurring in women who used hormones. This finding, reported in the journal *Lancet* in early 2004, prompted the head of the American Cancer Society to issue a statement saying it would be "unwise" to prescribe HRT to any woman with a history of breast cancer.

And while it was once presumed that the estrogen component of this formulation had at least the potential to protect our mind—mostly by warding off the risk of Alzheimer's disease—studies published in 2003 squelched that dream as well. Here we learned that women who used hormone replacement therapy had roughly *twice* the risk of developing dementia. More research was brought forward in October 2003 to reveal an increase in ovarian cancer among hormone users as well.

As more study results began to pour in we also learned HRT could increase the risk of urinary incontinence—with urge incontinence up by 50 percent and a fourfold increase in stress incontinence compared to what was experienced by women who were not using hormones. What's more, a study reported in June 2003 by Ob.Gyn. News revealed that the longer a woman uses HRT, the higher her risk of incontinence—up to five times higher by the fourth year of therapy.

Finally, in February 2004, the NIH announced that it was also stopping the final leg of the WHI trial—the portion of the study that was analyzing the safety of estrogen-only therapy in women who had undergone a hysterectomy. Ostensibly the point of this trial was to see if, in fact, estrogen could protect against heart disease in these women. After seven years of research the doctors concluded that not only was estrogen not protecting these women's hearts, it was increasing their risk of stroke by about 8 percent—nearly the same rate as when estrogen and progestins were used together. Clearly, an even more dismal picture was continuing to emerge for HRT, and you can be sure women were not taking the news lightly.

"So you're telling me here that not only will HRT *not* protect my heart and breasts, but if I use it to battle my hot flashes, it's also going to make me pee in my pants? Well this really sucks," said my most outspoken friend, Dee.

"Well I guess we're just going to have to cope the way men cope with midlife—buy a red sports car, and find a lover half our age." That was Tina, the "optimist" of the group.

Even politically minded Martha weighed in with an opinion on this one: "I think this whole HRT controversy is just one great big conspiracy designed to gaslight us all back to prefeminist times!"

I, on the other hand, was just simply outraged. Not so much because I no longer had the promises of HRT to ensure my future, but because that promise was made to all of us without there ever being any solid science to back it up! Talk about your Monday morning quarterbacking—this had to define the concept for an entire generation of women.

So, Where Do We Go from Here?

Fortunately, the news that summer—and in the summers to come—wasn't all bad. As it turns out, for some women hormone therapy might still hold some future promise—and for some, it might even be an answer right now. And you'll discover how HRT fits into *your* life—or if it fits at all—later in this book.

At the same time, however, if you're anything like my little circle of friends, you're also asking yourself: "If not hormones, *then what?*" Well,

I'm happy to tell you there is a "what"!—which is really the reason I decided to write this book. As a reporter and journalist covering medicine for some twenty years, I have been afforded a unique peek into the world of midlife health—with more than a passing glance in all directions. What I have found: From hot flashes to night sweats, memory lapses to mood swings, erratic periods to round-the-clock PMS and more, there *is* a light at the end of the tunnel—and HRT is not the only torch in town! From alternative medicine to bioidentical "natural" hormones, to traditional medications *and* some exciting cutting-edge treatments as well, I have found there is a treasure chest of potential treatments that can really help. Indeed, whether you ultimately decide to use hormone therapy or not, by using the information in this book you can work with your doctor and other health-care professionals to not only feel better today but also set the stage for a healthier tomorrow—including learning what to do right now to gain future protection from heart disease, osteoporosis, even cancer.

And while it's clear your doctor will play an important role in all of this, so will you. While it might not feel this way now, I can tell you without hesitation that much of what you are experiencing in the way of symptoms is under *your control*. From the foods you eat to the exercises you do, to the ways in which you manage stress—even how you relax—all these things can play a huge role in how easily your time of change unfolds. As you begin to take control in each of these areas—and you'll learn how as this book unfolds—I know you'll be amazed at the huge difference you can make not only in how you feel, but in how you feel about this time of life. I think one of the most important personal discoveries I have made over the last several years is that how you treat *yourself* during these middle years can sometimes make the biggest difference of all. In fact, if there was ever a time when a little self-indulgence goes a l-o-o-o-o-n-g way, that time is now! Which is why I've also devoted a good portion of this book to out-and-out, unabashed midlife pampering! From making the most of your changing skin to filling up that makeup bag with the newest cosmetic advances, to stemming the tide of wrinkles, thinning hair, and *just about everything else that may sag, droop, or drop*— you'll soon discover that not only are you worth the extra time and care, you can have a ball heaping some of this much-deserved pampering attention on yourself! You'll even learn how to harness the newest form of "girl power" so that you and your friends can *help pamper each other*—as you all land feetfirst in the second half of your lives!

In fact, regardless of how you feel today, I know you will feel better tomorrow as you come to see that *yes you can* move forward with your life—perhaps in ways that might have never have possible before. In the encouraging words of journalist Diane Sawyer—who was wishing the amazing Oprah Winfrey a happy fiftieth birthday—"If you're over the hill, girl, you just gotta pick up speed!" And this is the book that can show you how to put the pedal to the metal—and help you know and *believe* you have the power to do just that!

But before our journey begins, I also want to take a moment to remind you that you are not going through this time of change alone. Besides you and me, there are millions in our generation who share our concerns, our fears, and even some of our hopes and dreams for the future. Indeed, this time of life can—and should—be a shared experience, and one that allows us not only to renew our feelings of sisterhood but to experience the sense of camaraderie many of us have not felt since we were pregnant. Or burning our bras!

So, whether you're hooked on the idea that without hormones you just can't survive, or convinced the "white knuckle–no hormones" approach is the only way *to* survive—and especially if you're one of millions who are perched on the fence wondering just *how* you're *going to* survive—I invite you to read on. I promise you'll discover not only a world of midlife health-care options but also the opportunity to know, understand, and yes, pamper your body, mind, and spirit in a way you never have before.

So, buckle up that seat belt, crank up those old Beach Boys tapes, and get ready for the ride of your life! The best part is about to begin . . .

Understanding This
Thing Called Menopause

What You Need to Know
Right from the Start

My good friend Nadine hit me with a sobering thought this morning. We were headed to our local gym to meet Laura, Robyn, Tina, and few other friends for our regular "We're-not-getting-older-we're-getting-better" workouts when she decided to fill me in on the morning's news.

"I read in the paper today that between the year 2005 and 2030 there will be 1 billion women going through menopause . . . all at the same time," she said almost innocently. I wasn't quite sure if she thought this was a good thing or a bad thing. But I know what I thought: That's *waaay* too many of us having hot flashes and mood swings all at the exact same moment. Talk about your weapons of mass destruction . . .

The funny part is, though, that despite what we have all been conditioned to believe or expect, it's not really this *thing called menopause* that's going to change our lives in any kind of dramatic way. Because—and I'm speaking strictly in medical terms here—menopause is now clinically defined as not having had a menstrual period for twelve months or more. It is considered the official *end* to your reproductive years—and for many women that also means an end to some of the most troubling symptoms associated with this time of life, including hot flashes, night sweats, moods swings, and those "touch me and I'll kill you" temper outbursts. And, in fact, as lots of women who have already passed through this transition will likely tell you, reaching menopause can seem more like a beginning than an end anyway—the start of the second phase of your life. If you look at gals who have already opened the door for us—incredible, talented, *and, yes, gorgeous* women like Diane Sawyer, Oprah Winfrey, Diane Keaton, Tina Turner, Cher, Suzanne Somers, Hillary Clinton—then you know that what's on the other side can be pretty spectacular.

But the getting there—ahhh, now that's a *different* story. Doctors use the word *perimenopause,* which technically means the years leading up to menopause—a period that can begin as young as thirty-five or as late as fifty, be as short as one year or as long as ten or more. My friends and I— well, we have coined an entirely different term to describe *this* time zone. And if you've just rounded the bend past forty—and particularly if you are heading toward age fifty—it's likely you've got a few terms of your own to describe this particular time of life. (Does the word *yikes!* come to mind?) As you no doubt already know, it's the perimenopause years that can leave you wondering if anything about life is ever going to seem normal again.

- You pick up the phone to call a client—and while it's ringing, you've completely forgotten whom you've called.

- You wake up in the middle of the night warm and flushed and breathing heavy—and sex is the *furthest thing from your mind.*

- The bakery is out of rye bread—and you cry for forty minutes. In the store.

- You begin to wonder if it's possible to have PMS for forty-seven days in a row.

- You are convinced beyond any reasonable doubt that global warming has arrived—and it's hovering over your house 24/7.

- You go on vacation and without warning your period arrives—
ten days early and heavier than you've ever experienced before.

If this all sounds a bit too familiar, then you probably know this can be a time that tries a woman's soul, tests her patience, challenges her resolve, and in many instances leaves her wondering why, after going through labor, giving birth, raising a family—and breaking through a glass ceiling or two along the way—she now has to put up with *this*! Not to mention a partner whose testosterone levels have been dropping since *he* hit thirty-five!

Before you get too discouraged, remember, there is an upside. With just a little bit of knowledge—and some patience and resolve—you can discover how to put that "kick" back in your engine, pick up speed, and head into the second half of your life, raring to go! How do you begin? For me, the best place to start was in discovering my new body—what's changed, what's different, and, overall, what I can come to expect from myself and my own slightly used biology, now and in the years to come.

It's Not Your Mother's Menopause— But Nobody's Told Your Ovaries

One of the really great things about being in perimenopause today—as compared to when your mom or grandmother went through it—is that it really doesn't signify much, except an aging of your ovaries. Indeed, thirty or forty years ago "middle-aged" was considered "elderly"—with women resigned to living out the second half of life in frumpy print dresses and low-heeled shoes. Well, it's not your mother's menopause! Today turning fifty comes with a whole new attitude—not to mention a whole new look—with high-achieving, high-energy gals from all walks of life proving that the face of aging is definitely changing. And, with a few shots of Botox and a bottle of moisturizer, the future can look pretty darned good! Unfortunately, your ovaries don't quite share in that same youthful enthusiasm. No matter how young you look or feel or act, when it comes to your reproductive system . . . well, let's just say you're lucky your ovaries are on the inside of your body. Because the truth is, they are aging, and that fact is pretty much responsible for most, if not all, of the perimenopause symptoms you are or will soon be experiencing—including the common symptoms like hot flashes and night sweats and mood swings, but also the less discussed problems such as dysfunctional bleeding, memory loss, insomnia, and more.

Before you can fully appreciate all that changes as your ovaries age, it's important to understand a little something about how they work in general—and how they control hormonal activity during all the phases of your life. In this respect, much of their activity revolves around the production of estrogen and progesterone. During your peak reproductive years—from your teens to your mid-thirties—the vast majority of the estrogen in your body, and pretty much all of your progesterone, is the direct result of what's going on in your ovaries. The other two hormones that matter most are FSH, short for follicle-stimulating hormone, and LH, short for luteinizing hormone. While both are manufactured in the brain, their primary activity is to stimulate the ovaries.

The other key players on your reproductive team are your follicles—tiny sacs within each ovary that contain the biological makings of an egg. At birth you have several million follicles already in place, just waiting for puberty to jump-start your hormones and allow the reproductive process to begin. When it does, a tightly wound network of action and reaction begins, and it all plays out something like this:

- As each monthly cycle starts, estrogen levels are relatively low—something which your brain readily senses. When it does, it begins to producing the chemical FSH. As the name (follicle-stimulating hormone) suggests, a rise in FSH stimulates the follicles inside your ovary to grow and eggs to begin developing, which makes estrogen levels rise.

- As this occurs, your ovaries send another message to your brain to initiate the production of LH, a hormone that encourages the release of your developing egg—a process known as ovulation. The sac in which the egg developed—known as the *corpus luteum*—is left behind, and it begins producing progesterone. Together, estrogen and progesterone help create a thick, spongy lining inside your uterus in anticipation of a newly fertilized egg.

• If that egg isn't fertilized and no pregnancy occurs, levels of estrogen and progesterone drop sharply. This, in turn, causes the newly thickened uterine lining to shed, leaving your body in the form of menstrual blood. After it does the whole cycle begins again—and a month later, you get another period.

That's the way it goes, month in and month out, for pretty much most of your reproductive life. As you begin to age, however, some of these steps begin to change. As early as age thirty-five, for example, your cycle may go from the average twenty-eight-day schedule to twenty-four or twenty-five days. While doctors don't understand why, older women seem to ovulate within ten or twelve days of their last period, instead of the customary fourteen, thus shortening their cycle. Eventually—usually between age thirty-five and forty—you will stop ovulating every month. Although it sounds like the several million follicles you are born with should last well into your nineties, they don't. As you age many begin to die off. The follicles that do remain are getting "older"—and they don't respond to hormonal stimulation quite as readily. So, while in your peak reproductive years you were probably ovulating every twenty-eight days, and doing so ten or twelve times a year, once you hit age forty, you are probably ovulating just six to eight times a year—and the older you get, the fewer eggs you "hatch," so the less frequently you ovulate. The end result here: Your estrogen levels begin to fluctuate, sometimes dramatically.

This is even more true if you are overweight, since fat cells can convert other hormones into estrogen—causing your levels to be double or even triple that of a thin woman. While holding on to more estrogen may seem like a good thing, here's the glitch: When you are not ovulating, your body fails to produce progesterone—and without this hormone your estrogen levels become dominant. This not only leads to a whopping case of PMS (one reason you have so many mood swings and crying jags and may even experience depression during perimenopause), it also causes another, potentially more serious problem to occur—a condition that doctors call "dysfunctional bleeding." You probably know it as "irregular periods"—you miss one cycle, or even several, and then you're hit with an exceptionally heavy bleed. Or your periods may come closer together or further apart, or your bleeding can sometimes be a lot lighter than you experienced in the past, or much heavier. Regardless of the form it takes, doctors report that up to 90 percent of all women experience some form of dysfunctional bleeding during perimenopause (see Chapter 3 for more on this subject).

In addition, the same hormone imbalance that is causing your bleeding irregularities—particularly the up-and-down action of estrogen—is also setting the stage for a number of other malfunctions, bodywide. That's because estrogen receptors—cells that need estrogen to function— are distributed throughout much of your body. They are found not only in your female organs, such as your breasts, ovaries, and uterus, but also in your brain, liver, digestive tract, urinary system, blood vessels, skin, bones, and even your central nervous system. In fact, estrogen stimulates the production of proteins that help maintain the healthy function of a good number of organs and systems.

What's more, these hormone receptors also act like little "docking stations"—welcoming in and accepting the estrogen that floats through your bloodstream. When the receptors in any system of your body receive the proper amount of this hormone, they can direct that system to work as it should. The end result is that you feel great. But what happens when, as hormones levels get wonky, there just isn't enough estrogen to go around? Some of those receptors are left "empty"—and that means many systems in your body don't work as they should. And you can begin to feel the effects bodywide. Not only can you experience the classic hot flashes, night sweats, and mood swings, there can also be headaches, joint aches and pains, fatigue, sexual dysfunction, even memory loss—all the result of hormones that have run amok. Later in this book you'll learn even more about how your "dancing hormones" affect the way you feel— and bring on a variety of symptoms.

1, 2, 3, Testing . . . For Menopause: What You Should Know

Since it's clear that the basis for menopause is changes in various hormone levels, many women wonder if a simple blood or urine test could validate their reproductive status and, at the very least, help verify where they are in the menopause process. For many years doctors believed that blood tests for either estrogen or, more importantly, FSH (follicle-stimulating hormone) *could* reveal a woman's current reproductive status. This, however, is not the current line of thinking. Why?

While an elevation of FSH around the third day in any menstrual cycle can be a predictor of *fertility*, doctors now know that unless you're trying to get pregnant, this test is not likely to tell you much. That's because hormone levels continue to rise and fall so dramatically during the entire course of perimenopause, getting a clear and accurate reading is almost impossible. Medical studies that have attempted to do so found that levels fluctuate dramatically from day to day—and sometimes even hour to hour—making it nearly impossible to draw any kind of solid conclusion. In fact, the older a woman gets, the less reliable an FSH test is.

The same is true for estrogen and progesterone tests. Levels, in fact, can fluctuate so widely, even during a normal cycle, that the tests won't really tell you much. Needless to say, most experts agree that this caveat also applies to home hormone tests, many of which are available on the Internet, and in drugstores nationwide. What's more, there is another caution to consider if you do decide to try a home test kit—particularly if you are using it to nail down the reason behind your dysfunctional bleeding.

While a self-administered test might give you *some* clue to your hormonal status, it can't tell you *anything* about other possible causes for your symptoms, particularly dysfunctional bleeding. It won't, for example, give you even a hint if fibroid tumors or polyps are part of your health picture or if you are experiencing a potentially dangerous buildup of uterine tissue cells (see Chapter 3). For this reason it's important that you check out any abnormal symptoms—but particularly dysfunctional bleeding—with your doctor before spending your money on a home test or jumping to any perimenopausal conclusions about your health. And for heaven's sake, *don't* stop using your normal method of birth control—regardless of what your drugstore test tells you. The truth is, unless you have not had a menstrual period for one full year, you can still get pregnant!

The bottom line: Regardless of what is available in the way of testing, most doctors believe that the most reliable information about your menopause status comes directly from you—one reason why so many

From the "M" File

SALIVA AND HORMONES:
DOES THIS NEW TEST REALLY WORK?

Q: I've been on the Internet and I see all these menopause tests being sold that use saliva to measure hormone levels. This sounds almost impossible—is there a way this can be done, and if so, are the tests reliable? I'm forty-six but hardly ever get a period anymore—and I'd like to know if I'm in menopause.

A: In addition to whatever tests your doctor might decide to give you, there are, as you pointed out, many home menopause tests available as well. And while some use urine specimens to measure FSH, others rely on saliva samples to determine your hormone status. Although it sounds a bit strange, research has shown that, much like your blood and urine, saliva is a body fluid that contains a variety of natural chemicals, including hormones such as estrogen, progesterone, DHEA, cortisol, melatonin, and testosterone. What's more, the structure of the hormones found in saliva is slightly different from that found in blood—and may be more indicative of what is truly available to be used by your body. In fact, most hormones that circulate through your bloodstream are

physicians now rely heavily on the self-reporting of symptoms to make a diagnosis. This includes not only cycle irregularity but also hot flashes, memory problems, fatigue, mood swings, night sweats—even the condition of skin and hair can help predict your true perimenopause status.

Your Personal Perimenopause: What You Must Know

While sooner or later every woman passes through a series of symptoms and physiologic changes on her way to menopause, certain variables can make that road trip somewhat unique for each of us. The age at which we develop symptoms, how long they last, and even the severity with which

attached to a protein. This is a molecule that acts like a little wagon, ferrying the hormone wherever it needs to go. It's only when it finally reaches its destination—usually an organ such as your uterus—that it jumps off the protein wagon and is considered useful. When you use a blood test to measure hormone levels you are getting the "total sum" of the hormones that are available to be "loaded off" the protein wagon. By comparison, when you measure hormone levels in saliva you get the percentage of what has already been transported and is ready for immediate use by the body. So, in this respect, testing saliva levels might give you a truer, more accurate picture of the amount of hormones capable of being used by your body at any given moment. The unfortunate part of this idea is that hormone levels found in saliva are extremely volatile—ranging from very high to very low in just hours, with the time factor changing almost every day. In addition, studies show that saliva samples that are not frozen soon after collection can degrade, sometimes to the point where an accurate reading may not be possible. Most conventional medical researchers agree that unless saliva testing is done professionally, and involves multiple samples taken over a twenty-four-hour period, it's difficult to ascertain an accurate enough reading of hormonal levels to determine menopause status.

we experience them can be as varied as out taste in shoes and handbags. In fact, while your hormonal ups and downs may form the backdrop against which many of your symptoms will play out, how you actually experience their effects—or if you do at all—can be influenced to a large degree by a number of other, highly personal factors. Until fairly recently, doctors had only small, population-based studies and limited research to help guide them in terms of what each of us can expect. Now, that has changed—thanks to a landmark study by the National Institutes of Health. The fifteen-year project, begun in 1994, is known as the SWAN study (short for Study of Women's Health Across the Nation), and it was designed specifically to help us understand what factors other than hormones can influence the course of menopause transition. Although the research is still ongoing, it has now hit the ten-year mark, and some of the findings have been released. What has been learned thus far: Your weight, level of body fat, diet, lifestyle, and overall health status, and even your personality can all influence your menopause experience. What really sets this research project apart is that it is the very first study to consider the role of ethnicity in the menopause experience. In short, SWAN researchers discovered that different women experience menopause in different ways according to their ethnic and cultural background. To this end the project included over three thousand women from five ethnic groups, including Caucasian, African-American, Chinese-American, Japanese-American, and Hispanic.

How We Cope: Who We Are Matters Most

My friend Jeannie always likes to make a point of letting us all know that she's really coping very well with her perimenopause symptoms. And every time she does, my highly realistic friend Tina rolls her eyes in disbelief, snorts, and gives a loud chuckle. Once it almost came to a fistfight between them.

"I heard that," Jeannie snapped, referring to Tina's snort/chuckle following her statement that she wasn't experiencing *any* more mood swings. Tina, not one to sit idly by, was quick to respond.

"Well, *I'm glad* you heard it—because that means you're at least listening," she said defiantly.

"And what does *that* mean?" Jeannie was just as quick to respond. But Tina came right back at her. "It means that you must *not* be listening to yourself, for heaven's sake, because if you were you'd know that you are definitely *not* escaping mood swings as often as you think you are!"

Wow. Take away some estrogen and things can get *mighty nasty* at the quilting bee. But the truth is, whether or not we recognize our symptoms matters a lot less than how we choose to cope—even if coping itself requires some denial (Not so great for your friends, maybe, but if it works for you—hey, who are we to say it's wrong!) Indeed, one of the things that really jumped out at researchers during the SWAN study was just how differently each of us deals with our midlife symptoms. Wondering how you fit into the statistical profile? Here's what the SWAN folks found:

- One in five of us between the ages of forty and fifty-five used hormone replacement therapy, including not just traditional HRT, but also birth control pills. Keep in mind, however, that this research was done prior to the Women's Health Initiative, or WHI, study— before the new information on the dangers of hormone use was known.

- Caucasian women were the most likely to choose hormone therapy (24 percent usage among this group), while Hispanic women were the least likely to turn in this direction for help—only 10 percent chose hormones.

- Nearly half of all women aged forty-two to fifty-two used *some* type of complementary or alternative treatment for symptoms. Those who did generally had a higher level of education, higher incomes, and better health practices overall (they didn't smoke, for example, and most were involved in formal exercise regimens).

- African-American women embraced the change of life with the most positive attitude of all the ethnic groups studied, while Chinese and Japanese women were the least positive about this time of their lives.

The bottom line: While it's true that menopause symptoms do run in families—moms and daughters often have similar patterns—don't be surprised if you seem to be on a desert island during this time of your life. It's entirely possible that you could fall well within the "normal" range of symptoms and still be experiencing your changes differently from everyone you know—even your own family members.

At the same time, take some comfort in knowing that we are all sisters in more ways than one, and that those within our ethnic family may share our hormonal ups and downs a little more closely than other women. So, don't be afraid or ashamed to share how you are feeling with others in your personal and extended family. There is strength in numbers—and in sisterhood—and it's there when you need it!

Also know that as you read further, you will learn much more about yourself and your body—information that can help you to better understand and *cope with* your symptoms. From hot flashes to night sweats, mood swings to temper tantrums, heart palpitations to heartbreak and more, you will come to see that there are reasons for *everything*—and in most cases, solutions as well. At the same time, it's important to realize that, as the SWAN study shows, no one answer is right for every woman. The only thing you can really count on about the "change of life" is that it's constantly changing! And while it may seem as if there's *always* something going on with your body, the good news is that no one problem will last so long as to cause any kind of permanent damage to your health, or even your state of mind. So, in this respect you shouldn't be alarmed by any one symptom you experience—because it's very likely that it's going to pass in not too long a time. At the same time, it's important to not automatically blame everything that goes wrong in your body on your change of life. Too often I have seen women, and even some doctors, overlook important health symptoms simply because perimenopause happened to be going on at the same time. While certainly this transition is behind an awful lot of wacky symptoms, it's definitely not behind *everything* you will experience. So, if at any time a symptom is troubling you, listen to your intuition and push your doctor for a more complete diagnosis, or tests if you need them. Don't routinely accept perimenopause as the reason behind all that ails you.

You should employ this same line of thinking in your personal relationships, particularly with your mate. If there are problems within the relationship—be it sexual dysfunction or emotional communication—don't automatically blame your hormones, and don't let *him* do so either. Certainly, hormones can play a role in how we feel and how we act and react. But problems can develop within a relationship at any time, regardless of what your hormones are doing.

At the same time, it's also important to recognize that how you react to the people and events in your life during this time may be somewhat mediated by your physiology at any given moment. Some of what you may experience—like sexual dysfunction or even severe hot flashes—can have a tangible effect on your life. Just as often, the effects of your "dancing hormones" will be vague and hard to pin down—and sometimes influence how you react to certain events and situations without your even realizing this is the case. At least some of the time, you can expect your reactions to be overblown or exaggerated, out of proportion to what is really going on, and probably very different from what you would experience when your hormones aren't on a rampage. During the times when you are calmer and your physiology is more stable, its likely your feelings will change, as you home in on a truer pricture of any given situation. The best advice I can give you here is to step back and take a "time-out" for yourself as often as you can. Later in this book I'll offer you some concrete ways to reduce the stress in your life and make coping with perimenopause easier. In the meantime it may be helpful to remember that almost nothing in life has to be decided immediately. And, what may seem like a hurtful or painful situation for you at one moment might look entirely different when you take a step back and leave a day or two between feeling and reacting.

So, when your mate seems unbearable, your kids are driving you to distraction, and your best friend seems to be acting like a complete b**ch, take a deep breath, put those negative thoughts on the back burner, and do something nice for yourself. Later on that day—or perhaps in a few days—revisit how you feel about the person or situation, and see if you still feel the same way. Chances are you won't—and your crisis will have passed, with your family and your friendships still intact.

In the end, remember that perimenopause is *your* transition time—a period in your life when yes, your body is changing, but not necessarily for the worst. It's not bad, it's just different. If you can embrace this time with *that* spirit, you middle years can be an exciting, adventurous time, filled with the kind of self-discovery you may have forgotten is possible.

2

Warming Up to Midlife Changes . . . Or, Open the Window or I'll Scream!

Hot Flashes, Night Sweats, and Other Fun Ways to Know You're Over Forty!

I will never forget the time my friend Sheila had her first hot flash. We were window-shopping on Madison Avenue and had just stepped inside this tiny shoe boutique to look around. While I was trying on this great pair of red patent leather stilettos, I glanced across the small store to notice Sheila grabbing the counter and nearly toppling an artful display of sandals. I immediately hobbled over to her (the stilettos were *killing* me!).

"Oh my God," she whispered in that hushed tone that is a prerequisite for shopping on Madison. "I am so dizzy—and I think my hair is on fire," she said, clutching the back of her head with a kind of reckless panic that told me she was convinced it really was. I watched as her face turned from a light, just-back-from-the-Bahamas tan to a bright pink and then a crimson stayed-out-in-the-sun-way-too-long red.

"I think I'm having one of those medical Twilight Zone episodes where people spontaneously combust from a rapid rise in body temperature," Sheila said, trying to keep her equilibrium as her dizziness seemed to get worse. "We've got to get out of here," she almost bellowed, more than an edge of panic now in her voice. I quickly kicked off my red heels and jumped into my clogs, and as Sheila clung to my arm for dear life, we headed out the door. Once outside I propped her against a parked car as I went out into the street to hail a cab.

"It's a stroke—I know it's a stroke—get me to NYU Medical," she told the cabbie in a loud, defiant voice as we piled into the backseat. While I was pretty sure that someone having a stroke couldn't yell instructions at a New York City cabdriver, I didn't want to argue with my friend. So I motioned to the driver to go, and we headed downtown to NYU.

Well, I probably don't have to tell you that by the time we actually got to the hospital, Sheila was feeling fine—and a little silly, I might add. Ultimately, we just told the cabbie to turn around and head for my friend's Upper East Side apartment. The next day she did visit her gynecologist, and his diagnosis was something I had guessed back there in the shop on Madison. Although she was only forty-three, Sheila was having her first hot flash—and perimenopause had officially begun.

While it's true that the path that cuts through the middle of our life is literally strewn with crazy symptoms (and you'll learn more about all of them throughout this book), perhaps none marks the bend in the road more than the veritable "hot flash." As we slowly morph our way from Reproductive Goddess to, well, simply Goddess, that undeniable rush of body heat can't help but be a familiar companion. And while the National Institute on Aging estimates that 60 percent of all women approaching menopause have hot flashes, judging by the women in my world, I'm figuring the "real" number has got to be closer to something like 99 percent. Quite honestly, I don't know a single gal who hasn't reached age fifty without having at least one uncontrollable urge to run naked into a blinding snowstorm seeking hot flash relief.

Yes, It's Hot in Here!

As irritating and exasperating an experience as a hot flash can be, traditionally doctors didn't pay a whole lot of attention to this mostly female phenomenon. In fact, it wasn't so very long ago that medical science barely acknowledged the existence of hot flashes, let alone made any efforts toward understanding why they occur. In fact, I was stunned to discover that the first medical paper exploring the physiology of what happens during a hot flash wasn't even published until 1975. That's when a little-known publication called the *Journal of Applied Physiology* first documented what actually happens to a woman's body during one of these events—besides the desire to tear off your clothes, that is. Of course, if a man's pants were on fire the same way our face and neck burn during a flash, I can't imagine that medical science wouldn't have put a move on finding out why, but I try not to be bitter. At least we finally had some information as to what was going on and why.

What the *Journal* documented back in 1975 was that during a hot flash your skin temperature goes up, then down; you begin sweating, and your heart rate increases by about 13 percent at the start of each flash. According to NYU professor Dr. Steve Goldstein, it's not uncommon for your pulse to reach 150 beats per minute when a flash is coming on.

What all this amounts to is something called "vasomotor instability"—or blood vessels that contract and expand without any real rhyme or reason. The cause of all this commotion is, as far as anyone can tell, the result of a snafu in our body thermostat—a system that is nestled securely in an area of the brain called the hypothalamus.

Normally, when we are overheated—from exercise, for example, or, heaven help us, great sex—it is the thermostat in our brain that sends the "cool down" message to our body. This, in turn, dilates or widens the blood vessels in the skin, which then allows heat from the blood coursing through our inner core to escape. The end result is that we cool down. When our body once again reaches the ideal temperature, the thermostat directs the blood vessels to constrict or tighten to keep heat in. In this way, we maintain a pretty even body temperature 24/7. Except, of course, during perimenopause. This is when our thermostat goes completely wacky, jumping up and falling down with absolutely no regard for what we are doing—or wearing, as the case may be—at the time.

In this instance, the thermostat in our brain erroneously gets the message that we're hot. We could be sitting comfortably under a shade tree sipping a frozen margarita with our feet up as a cool breeze whistles through our hair—no matter. When you're in perimenopause, at any given time your inner thermostat can simply decide "Yikes, this woman is burning up—cool her down!" When it does, your brain sends the message to dilate those vessels—and fast! And this, in turn, causes a sudden rush of heat to leave your body through your skin—which is also why you feel that sudden "spreading" of warmth. While you can feel the "flash" pretty much anywhere on your body, for most women it's the upper torso, particularly the hands, arms, trunk, neck, and face, where you feel it the most. In fact, so much heat can leave your body so quickly that your skin may actually turn beet red and feel warm to the touch as if it's burning. Or as Sheila now says, "You can fry an egg on my chest every time I flash."

The ironic part here is that your internal thermostat doesn't take long to figure out "Ooops, I made a mistake—she's not really overheated." So, usually within about five minutes or less, it sends another message to shut down those blood vessels and stop the heat from pouring out. And, when this occurs, the flash stops. And while three to five minutes is thought to be the average length of a hot flash (and when your mate says, "Oh, five minutes is not so bad," remind him how it might feel if you held a blow-torch between his legs for five minutes), sometimes it can go on longer. In some women a hot flash can last up to thirty minutes—or flashes can come and go so rapidly over a period of thirty to sixty minutes that it can seem like one long flash. In addition, because you have lost a great deal of body heat quickly—if you weren't overheated to begin with—at least some women feel a shivering cold just minutes after a hot flash ends. Others, however, simply return to a normal body temperature.

While researchers may know what's happening in our body when a flash occurs, they're still not certain about what puts all this strange activity in motion. Among the first conclusions was that low estrogen was to blame. Pretty soon, however, they began to reason that before puberty all girls have low estrogen levels and no hot flashes occur. Conversely, during the third trimester of pregnancy, when estrogen levels are soaring, women frequently *do* have hot flashes. Ultimately, many experts have come to believe the culprit is not the hormone, but its activity. Specifically, it's the "fluctuation" of estrogen—the continual up-and-down motion that sets our little perimenopausal thermostat on fire. Because the hypothalamus gland is thought to be "estrogen sensitive," as levels become unstable, it struggles to regain its footing. As it does, your body thermostat is affected.

Still another theory pegs the whole event to levels of another brain chemical known as norepinephrine, which studies show is higher in women who have hot flashes compared to those who don't. Hot flash researcher Dr. Robert R. Freedman of Wayne State University in Detroit, Michigan, says that estrogen withdrawal has been linked to elevated levels of norepinephrine in both animal and human studies. But how does norepinephrine affect us? According to Freedman we all have a "natural range" of temperatures that go from high (which causes us to sweat) to low (which causes us to shiver). In women who don't get flashes, Freedman says the "neutral" zone is wider, allowing more room for body temperature to fluctuate before the effects are felt. In women who get hot flashes, he says, the range between high and low is a lot smaller—meaning even *slight* changes in body temperature can kick off a flash. Norepinephrine, he says, may be one brain chemical that narrows down the range between high and low and in that way sets the stage for hot flashes to occur.

While sometimes outside forces can exacerbate flashes—like stress, warm temperatures, spicy foods, anxiety, or even exercise—just as often they can come on without rhyme or reason, in a cool room with a cold drink in your hand.

In the Heat of the Night— Hot Flashes in Your Sleep

When you're twenty-five and you roll over and whisper to your partner that you're too hot to sleep . . . well, let's just say they're the words men live to hear. Say that same thing once you're past forty, however, and it takes on a *whole* different meaning. I'm talking about night sweats—those exasperating changes in body temperature that appear in the middle of sleep, often waking you up soaked in what they used to call "glow" but is now clearly dripping, construction-worker-caliber "sweat."

WHAT ELSE CAUSES THE BURN

While most women associate hot flashes with menopause, there are a number of other situations or conditions that can cause you to get that "burning feeling." Some may even cause men to experience a hot flash. According to a report in the journal *Alternative Medicine Review*, factors able to cause a hot flash include medications such as calcium channel blockers (for high blood pressure); SSRIs (antidepressants); cephalosporin; some SERMs (drugs like Tamoxifen); Niacin (B vitamin); and aromatase inhibitors (cancer drugs). Also capable of causing a flash are food additives such as monosodium glutamate (preservative/flavor enhancer), sodium nitrate (preservative), and sulfites (preservative). Migraine headaches, as well as stress and anxiety, can also get your cheeks burning.

Although for many years it was believed that night sweats occurred independent of any other symptoms, the current line of thinking is that they are actually the result of a series of hot flashes that occur while you sleep. Although the flashes may not wake you initially, they are believed to interfere with your sleep—acting as a kind of gentle nudge that keeps you from falling into a deep slumber. Think of it as someone lightly shaking you each time you are drifting off to sleep, and you'll have an idea of how these night flashes are affecting you. When enough "nudges" occur, you do wake up—usually drenched in sweat. Even if you don't wake until the morning, the disturbance caused by the night flashes can keep you from getting a deep, restful night's sleep. This can cause you to feel not only fatigued by morning, but also irritable and short tempered. Some doctors even believe that by simply controlling the depth of sleep you get every night you can decrease some of the quick-tempered moodiness that is associated with perimenopause. Later in this book you'll find some ways to encourage a deeper, healthier sleep, despite night flashes and sweats. And, in fact, many of the same treatments that will quell your daytime flashes (and you'll learn more about those in the following section) can also help your night sweats—and help you get a better night's sleep.

Four Hot Flash Fixes:
How Your Doctor Can Help

Although for most women, really dramatic episodes of day or night flashes usually last less than a year, for some they can continue on for much longer, sometimes five to seven years or more. Indeed, while they usually do abate as time goes on (decreasing in both frequency and severity), they can also continue for as long as it takes for your hormones to stabilize. While many women turn to natural therapies to alleviate this and many other symptoms of perimenopause (and you'll learn more about what can help in Chapter 10), for others, traditional hormone replacement therapy (HRT) can still be the most effective way to control this symptom—even in light of the recent reports about the dangers. And later on in this book you'll learn how to assess your personal risk factors and find out if this treatment approach is a possible solution for you.

But if you're not completely sold on either Mother Nature or Father Hormone, you might be interested to know that more recently a few additional treatment options have come on the scene. In the event that your flashes become intolerable you can talk to your doctor about prescribing any one of the following four medications. In many instances they can be at least as helpful as HRT, without most of the disturbing side effects.

HOT FLASH FIX ONE: ANTIDEPRESSANTS, INCLUDING ZOLOFT, EFFEXOR, AND PAXIL

No, it doesn't mean that hot flashes are all in your head! This group of medications, known as serotonin and norepinephrine reuptake inhibitors, work a special kind of "magic" on the estrogen receptors involved in controlling temperature mechanisms. Independent of any antidepressant activity—and usually given in a much smaller dose than what is used to treat depression—these medications generally kick in with relief after anywhere from one to three weeks, about the same amount of time it would take for hormone therapy to work. According to studies, the most effective of the group is Effexor. In a study of 180 women, a starting dose of 37.5 milligrams once daily brought some relief in about a week; building up to 75 milligrams once a day ultimately resulted in a 61 percent decrease in hot flashes in about four weeks. Paxil was found to be almost equally effective, with a starting dose of 10 milligrams for three days, then building to 20 milligrams, with the full effect, close to that of Effexor, seen in about three weeks. The least effective—though still worth a try—is fluoxetine, or Zoloft. In clinical trials conducted at the Mayo Clinic and Foundation in Rochester, Minnesota, women saw about a 50 percent decrease in hot flashes after several weeks—compared to 36 percent taking a placebo.

One word of caution: You may have to remain on the pills indefinitely in order to control hot flashes. Also, treatment is not problem-free. At least in the beginning, many women can experience fatigue, dry mouth, sexual dysfunction, and nausea.

HOT FLASH FIX TWO: CLONIDINE

Traditionally a blood pressure medication, this drug is thought to work by relaxing blood vessels, which may in turn have some localized effect on the release of body heat linked to hot flashes. In clinical trials a dosage of 0.1 milligrams daily reduced hot flashes by some 37 percent in four weeks—about 17 percent more effective than a placebo. After eight weeks, it jumped up just one more point—to 38 percent, compared to 24 percent for the placebo. Like antidepressants, however, this drug has some side effects, including dry mouth and sleep disturbances. However, most women reported that problems faded within the first few weeks of treatment. Clonidine is also available in a patch form known as Catapres. For those of you who may not find relief on the 0.1 milligrams, studies show oral dosing can safely increase to 0.2 milligrams daily (or in patch form, Catapres TTS-2) or even 0.3 milligrams daily (Catapres TTS-3). However, don't try to make the increase on your own by increasing dosages, and always check with your doctor before changing any medication regimen.

HOT FLASH FIX THREE: GABAPENTIN (NEURONTIN)

This antiseizure medication used to treat some forms of epilepsy, remarkably, also appears to help hot flashes. While no one is certain how it works, in a study published in 2003 in the *Journal of Family Practice* doc-

Hot Flash

WHAT WORKS—AT A GLANCE

Here's a quick look at the various therapies for hot flashes and the percentage of women who get relief when they try them, according to the American College of Obstetricians and Gynecologists. You can read more about all of these treatments throughout this book.

- HRT (hormone replacement therapy)—90 percent

- Progestin (alone)—50–80 percent

- Clonidine (blood pressure medication)—50 percent

- Deep breathing—50 percent

- Soy protein—0–45 percent

- Placebo—up to 30 percent

- Natural progesterone—unknown

- Vitamin E—unknown

tors found that 900 milligrams of gabapentin daily reduced hot flashes by some 54 percent. Many women find the best regimen begins with 300 milligrams daily for three days, slowly increasing the dosage to 900 milligrams, or even as high as 1,200 milligrams for optimum relief.

HOT FLASH FIX FOUR:
NATURAL PROGESTERONE CREAM

Because it is believed that a drop in estrogen is primarily what triggers hot flashes, traditionally it was believed that supplementing the body with estrogen would naturally bring this symptom under control. A slightly different take on the theory, however, tells us that it may also be change in the ratio of estrogen to progesterone during perimenopause that could be behind hot flashes. As a result, there are at least some doctors who believe that a condition known as "estrogen dominance" actually triggers the flashes—times when estrogen levels climb high and are not balanced by progesterone. When this is the case, a supplement of natural progesterone might help. (See Chapter 11 for more complete information on natural progesterone therapy.)

Although the therapy is a simple one, there is a word of caution. Even though some forms of natural progesterone are available without a prescription, don't try it without your doctor's okay. Because it is a hormone, it can have a variety of systemic effects, as well as uterine effects, and could impact or mask dysfunctional bleeding. Bottom line: Your doctor needs to know about *any* treatment, for hot flashes or for any other menopause symptom, you are taking.

Coping with Hot Flashes: Ten Things You Can Try Right Now

In addition to whatever help your doctor can provide, there are also a few things you can try on your own to reduce hot flashes—or at least control them when they do occur. Here are ten time-honored and Goddess-tested solutions that can help get you through the day and the night!

1. KEEP A HOT FLASH DIARY—AND DISCOVER YOUR TRIGGERS.

Yes, it's true, those jumping estrogen beans are what's behind all the sweating and pulsing and overheating. However, there are also a number of individual "hot flash triggers"—situations or conditions that are unique to you. By keeping a diary of your environmental factors at the time you get your flashes, you can sometimes discover what's heating you. Pay attention to what you are wearing, particularly the fabrics (nylon, polyester, and acrylic are big overheaters); what you are doing (exercising, cooking in a hot kitchen, taking a hot bath); how you are feeling (angry, anxious, depressed); what you ate just prior to the flash (spicy, sweet, hot, protein, high carb); and fragrances (your own perfume or any other scents in your environment). In about a week you should see at least some patterns emerge—and avoiding those situations or conditions could make a significant difference in coping with your flash.

2. WATCH WHAT YOU EAT.

Foods can trigger hot flashes—or make those that are already occurring last longer or feel worse. The most obvious are, of course, hot beverages, particularly anything with caffeine, which can naturally make your heart race and increase body temperature. But some women find that drinking a very cold caffeinated beverage can also kick off a hot flash, so don't be surprised if you feel warm after a cool glass of cola. Other foods that trigger flashes include hot spicy dishes and any very warm foods—such as hot soup or a very hot meal. Alcohol is another big offender, often bringing on a hot flash even when you're not in perimenopause. Limit alcohol consumption and you might eliminate all but a few hot flashes. (Be sure to check out Chapter 7 for the anti–hot flash diet.)

3. WATCH YOUR TEMPER.

The term "blood boiling mad" didn't come out of thin air—it's true that when we get angry our blood pressure goes up and our body chemistry changes. While your blood doesn't actually *boil,* some of the physiological changes that do occur can make you feel warm—and in the process, kick off or exacerbate a hot flash. If you feel a bout of anger or stress coming on, walk away, and if possible get outside (if it's cool). Or, you can go to the ladies' room or your own bathroom and put a cold compress on the back of your neck or the insides of your wrists or elbows. This can help head off a hot flash—or even stop one in progress. At the very least it will get you out of the room and away from the source of your anger—which in turn might just save your job, your marriage, or your sanity.

4. AVOID HOT BATHS, HOT SHOWERS, HOT TUBS, WHIRLPOOLS, AND JACUZZIS.

Anything that combines skin stimulation with hot water can kick off a hot flash. Cool showers can have the opposite effect, calming your body down and helping to head off a hot flash brought on by other factors, including when *it really is "hot in here."*

5. RELAX—AND MEDITATE.

When you feel calm and relaxed your body is less likely to react even to stressful hormonal changes. Plus, the more you remain calm, particularly when you are having a flash, the more quickly it will pass and the less likely it is to recur soon. By comparison, getting excited by the fact that you are getting a flash will only make you feel warmer, and make the flash and the sweating worse. In addition, try to breathe through your nose and not your mouth. Mouth breathing can cause you to hyperventilate, which in turn can make you feel warmer or even bring on a hot flash. Check out Chapter 9 for more ideas on stress reduction during menopause.

6. DRESS IN LAYERS . . .

. . . with the bottom layer always being a camisole or sleeveless tank top. As you feel a flash coming on, remove as many layers as you can—if necessary getting down to the camisole. If you feel self-conscious doing this in your office or place of business, then go to the ladies' room and remove as much of your clothing as possible. If you also carry a package of baby wipes with you, you can quickly swipe off after the flash is over, which in turn will make you feel cooler and drier.

7. CARRY A PAPER FAN.

Yes it's coy and even a bit old-fashioned. But a sturdy, handheld bamboo and paper fan that you can whip out of a handbag or desk drawer can go a long way in helping you feel instantly cooler—not to mention a little flirty. You can also invest in a handheld battery-operated fan to keep in your desk or even your handbag for the same purpose. It works, but it's not nearly as romantic.

8. KEEP EXERCISING.

There is good evidence to show that regular exercise can help to deter hot flashes—and women who work out generally report fewer episodes than sedentary women. One theory says it's because exercise raises levels of endorphins, the natural body chemical that makes us feel good. Not coincidentally, there is some evidence to show that endorphins are involved in the regulation of body temperature. So the higher the levels, the more reliable your internal "thermostat" may be.

9. RESET YOUR BODY THERMOSTAT.

Running your wrists under cold water or putting an ice pack or even a can of cold soda on your wrist, the inside of your elbow, or any pulse point will send a message to your brain that your body needs to conserve heat—and your thermostat should reset almost immediately. You can also invest a few dollars in a product known as Cooldana (see the resource section at the back of this book). This is a gel-filled scarf that you run under cold water and let air dry a few minutes. The gel absorbs the water and keeps it cool—and if you tie the scarf around your neck you can remain ultra cool for hours. Many women report this can actually keep hot flashes from coming on by offering some measure of control over the inner thermostat.

10. STOP SMOKING.

There is some evidence to show that smoking can exacerbate hot flashes, particularly in thin women. Stopping or cutting down on the number of cigarettes you smoke may help reduce your number of hot flashes or their intensity.

The "Other" Midlife Burn: When the Hot Flash Is in Your Mouth

Oh, I know what you're thinking . . . so get your mind off those daytime soaps! The burning *I'm* referring to is a seldom discussed but surprisingly common symptom of perimenopause called "burning mouth syndrome," or BMS. According to experts at the Yale University School of Medicine Taste Laboratory, the problem is often characterized by a sudden onset of pain and burning that usually builds in intensity over the course of a day. It often begins on the tip of the tongue—and many women describe it as the kind of feeling you get when you taste a scorching hot spoon of soup—but the sensation can quickly spread to other parts of the mouth. This includes the insides of the cheeks, the roof of the mouth, or the back of the throat. While you might wake up feeling just fine, by mid-morning you notice the burning sensation starting. The feelings generally increase as the day goes on and you might also begin feeling a "dry" sensation in your mouth.

According to the Yale experts, you may also be plagued with what they call "taste phantoms"—bitter or other strange taste sensations not linked to anything tangible. Once the syndrome begins, it's usually ongoing, with the worst symptoms felt in the evening. Often, they calm down during the night, so that by morning there is significantly less pain. By mid-afternoon, however, the burning and other problems—including dry mouth and taste sensations—can be in full swing again.

Although no one is certain what causes BMS, according to a recent report in the journal *American Family Physician,* it affects up to 40 percent of all women seeking treatment for menopause-related symptoms. According to some reports, 90 percent of all cases of BMS are found in women of menopausal or postmenopausal age—with the greatest frequency beginning three years prior to menopause, and up to twelve years afterward. You would think this meant a clear-cut indication that hormones are the cause—but no such justification can be found. In fact, at least one study published as early as 1992 found that taking HRT has no impact on burning mouth syndrome, even when other symptoms, like hot flashes, subside.

Although BMS has not been positively linked to any other single medical condition, it often appears when certain other problems are present. These include headaches, type 2 diabetes, chronic anxiety or depression, nutritional deficiencies, oral yeast infections, a cranial nerve injury, and changes in salivary gland function. However, doctors are quick to caution that just as often there is no link to any of these conditions. Additionally, many women report their first episode of BMS follows a dental procedure or an illness of some sort—particularly after antibiotic use—but there is currently no direct link to any of these factors either.

According to the Yale researchers, BMS may also be linked to a virus in the central nervous system—possibly the inner ear—that temporarily affects the sense of taste, which in turn exacerbates the burning mouth symptoms. Ironically, researchers report that often women with BMS feel better when they taste anything—even water.

TREATING YOUR BURNING MOUTH: WHAT YOU CAN DO

Regardless of what is causing the problem, once the burning starts, it can persist for many years. If this is the case, drugs traditionally used to treat nerve-related pain have been found helpful. To date, most studies report that low doses of medications such as clonazepam (Klonopin), chlordiazepoxide (Librium), and tricyclic antidepressants like Elavil can be helpful. Perhaps not coincidentally, some research has also shown that the antiseizure drug gabapentin (Neurontin)—mentioned earlier as a treatment for hot flashes—can also be helpful in burning mouth syndrome. Frequently there will be a partial or full spontaneous remission of all symptoms within six to seven years—even when no treatment is administered.

Hot Hormones and Cold Chocolate Bars: When Your Taste Is More Than a Matter of Style

When my best friend Dee was muddling through her perimenopause, she was convinced she had discovered an entirely new and yet unchartered treatment approach.

"Who needs HRT—and who really needs all these icky, fertilizer-ridden plant cures—the only treatment for perimenopause is Dove chocolates," she said triumphantly, as she tore the flashy blue foil wrapper from yet another piece of her "prescription."

"I mean it," she said, her mouthful of chocolate somewhat muffling the earnest tone in her voice. "I used to like them before, but boy, ever since my hormones started going wild, I can't get enough of these little darlings—and they do make me feel better. Quite frankly I think we should go into business packaging them for gynecologists' offices," she said with such conviction I almost wrote a check.

Of course there is all that research showing how chemicals in chocolate are similar to those found in the brain when we fall in love—so why wouldn't we want to wolf down these goodies without coming up for air?

But still, I suspected it was more than just *that* feeling that was driving Dee—because I could see that the older I was getting the more I too seemed to crave *handfuls* of these chocolate goodies. After checking with a few other gal pals I soon discovered this need for *more chocolate* with each passing birthday seems somewhat of a universal craving. Not only that, but those of us willing to admit things like this also frequently admit that the older we get, the more chocolate we need to quell those cravings! A little bit of research revealed some interesting reasons.

In studies conducted at Ankara University in Turkey, doctors discovered that hormones affect more than just our body temperature and our mood. They also affect our palate, with all those sneaky little estrogen curveballs causing us to have less of an ability to taste sweet foods. While that may intuitively seem as if it would cause us to turn away from that bag of Halloween goodies we have stashed in the glove compartment for traffic tie-ups (I *know* you do!), they found just the opposite is true. It seems the more our hormones dance and jive, the more we crave the sweet tastes of life and, ultimately, the more chocolate (and other sugar-laden goodies) we actually need to satisfy our cravings.

Adding more fuel to the fire (or more chocolate to the fondue, as they say) researchers at the National Institutes of Health report that girls in prepuberty as well as women who have passed through menopause (both with a minimum of estrogenic activity) have a similar reaction to taste-test chemicals—one that ultimately reflects back to a more active "sweet tooth." Interestingly, when women in their childbearing years (with high estrogen levels) are given this same taste test, they exhibit a decreased desire for sweets—thus indicating that hormonal status can play a role in taste perceptions. One reason, say experts, is that certain components of taste may be estrogen-sensitive—and in that way our taste buds change as our estrogen levels take a dive. At last—a truly scientific reason to never feel guilty wiping chocolate smudges off my mouth again!

On the not-so-good side of things, clearly, these hormone-related cravings can find many of us loading up on sweets just at a time when we should be watching not only our waistlines, but also our sugar levels. Indeed, the Turkish researchers found that nearly half the women in the study admitted that their dietary habits had changed in midlife to include a lot more sweets in their daily diet—and a lot more pounds on their hips.

So, if you're starting to realize that it takes more chocolate to satisfy your sweet tooth, you're probably right. And sometimes, just knowing what's behind your craving can help you to control it. If not, you can always fall back on what my French grandmother always believed, which is that "Chocolate is love." And who can argue with a little self-love now and again to get you through the night!

3

Your Intimate Menopause

~~~~~~

The V Zone Changes Every Woman
Must Know

I t wasn't more than a week or so ago that my friend Megan called about what she described—in hushed tones, I might add—as "an unbelievable burning—down there."

"What do you mean 'down there'? Like in Tampa–St. Pete? Are you talking weather?" I answered rather nonchalantly.

"You *know* what I mean," she said, whispering into the phone from her job at a large New York City design house. "So stop being difficult and tell me what you think is wrong!" She sounded *very* agitated, even for Megan, always a bit of a drama queen.

Now I was getting it. "Oh, you mean your vagina is burning?"

"Shhh, do you have to use that graphic word—I'm on the company phone!" she said, whispering again.

"Megan, vaginas are not graphic—it's a body part like arms or legs, or hands or fingers." I tried to get my friend to relax about whatever it was that was bothering her.

"Yes, well it's not my arms or legs or hands or fingers that feel like they are on fire—so what the heck is going on *down there?*"

For starters I ran down the list of "usual suspects"—the everyday factors that can cause vaginal irritation and lead to burning. Was she using any new bath products, powders, perfumes? Was she wearing any new or different underwear? Using different laundry detergent? How about panty liners, sanitary pads, tampons? She answered "no" to all of the above.

"Well, then I hate to be the bearer of bad news, but I think it's your hormones," I said, quite certain that, at forty-six, Megan had been showing more than a few signs of perimenopause for quite some time now.

"But my period still comes pretty regularly—I thought that would be the first clue that I'm, you know, becoming an 'M' girl," she said, lowering her voice back down to a whisper again. It was definitely not easy for Megan to accept that she was, indeed, approaching menopause.

And while she was right that irregular cycles are often an early sign that the "M" experience is just around the corner, what my friend didn't realize was that menopause-related changes can occur in many areas of the V zone, even when periods are still very regular. On the off chance that she was suffering with an intimate infection of some sort—which is also more common during this time (and you'll read more about that in a little bit)—I urged my friend to see her gynecologist. But when she reported back that her doctor had found nothing wrong, I knew my initial reaction had been right: Megan's "burning" was likely hormone related, a simple fact of life in the forties.

If, like my friend, you too are experiencing any number of what seem like odd or unusual happenings "down there," you shouldn't be surprised. In reality, among the first places that midlife changes of all kinds do occur is in your V zone–including not only your vulva and vagina, but also your cervix, and even your urinary tract. That's because all these regions contain large amounts of estrogen-dependent tissue, areas that rely on hormone stimulation in order to not only function at peak capacity but also remain in good health. That's one reason why you may also find you are prone to more vaginal infections and even irritations during your peri-menopause.

While most of us are prepared for some changes "down there," like irregular cycles or even vaginal dryness, others can take us by surprise—when your doctor diagnoses fibroid tumors or polyps, for example. Still other times you may even feel a sense of shock or disbelief when you discover you might need surgery or some other invasive procedure to solve the problem.

The good news is that today, more than ever, there are simple and even easy ways to deal with *most* midlife V zone problems—simple ones like Megan was experiencing, or even complex ones that take you by surprise. The key lies in knowing what you can expect and when you can expect it, and being prepared for the totally unexpected! In fact, while I am going to do my best to let you know the kinds of intimate changes your body will be going through, the one thing I can't predict is when they will happen, or to what extent you will experience them. Like puberty and pregnancy and all things biologically feminine, menopause is a unique and different experience for every woman. While there are frequently threads of continuity woven among family members—mothers and daughters, as well as sisters, can be remarkably similar in their menopause experiences—for the most part your personal midlife changes will be as individual as you are. Still, knowing what your body *might* do, and around what time it *might* happen can go a long way in helping you to cope with whatever V zone problems do come your way.

Understanding Your V Zone Changes

Among the places most women find the earliest and sometimes the most noticeable indication that hormone levels have started to decline is within the vagina itself, particularly in terms of comfort. What happens and why?

While you are in the prime of your reproductive life, a regular supply of estrogen promotes the production of vaginal cells rich in a substance known as glycogen—a metabolic sugar that interacts with other natural chemicals found in your vagina. As your monthly cycle ebbs and flows and estrogen levels shimmy up and down, cells lining your vaginal wall go through a natural exfoliation process—in much the same way as the skin cells on your face and body. As these glycogen-rich cells shed, they interact with natural bacteria that are present in your vagina. This little biochemical dance results in the production of still another natural chemical known as lactic acid. And this, in turn, maintains a very comfortable pH or acid level, between 3.5 and 4.5, in your vagina. For you, this means a comfortable level of natural secretions or "wetness"—so your vagina feels moist and comfortable all day long. It also means that when you are "turned on" and engaged in sexual activity, you become even more "moist," not only allowing for easier penetration by your partner, but also ensuring that making love is physically pleasurable for you.

When, however, estrogen levels begin doing the hormone "tango"— dipping up and down at highly irregular intervals—the glycogen content of your vaginal cells begins to decrease, sometimes dramatically so. When this occurs lactic acid levels also fall—and the pH or acid level of your vagina can dramatically change. This can result in a number of conditions doctors loosely classify as atrophic vaginitis. Often you will experience one or more of the following V zone symptoms:

- Dryness

- Itching

- Burning

- Painful sex

- A burning discharge

- Feelings of pressure within the vagina

- A yellow, slightly odorous discharge

- Loss of pubic hair

All of these symptoms can be further exacerbated by a subsequent increase in your risk of certain V zone infections. As the acid level in your vagina changes, suddenly all those "friendly" bacteria residing in your V zone take on the characteristics of that nasty ex-boyfriend—turning from a friendly protector of your health into a "hostile invader" that actually promotes infection. That's one reason why your risk of even simple vaginal problems like BV (bacterial vaginosis), yeast infections, or trichomonas becomes much more common in your forties, fifties, and sixties.

In addition, if you are having sex with multiple partners—or if your partner is—then you may also be at greater risk for contracting a sexually transmitted infection during your midlife transition. The reason: As the cells lining your vaginal walls decrease and the tissue becomes thinner, it also becomes a less effective barrier to any infecting organisms that may be introduced into your body during intimate contact. That means that unless you—and your partner—are in a totally monogamous relationship, you should be extra certain that he uses a condom.

As time goes on and you actually begin your menopause—remember, that means no menstrual bleeding for twelve months or more—you will likely experience even more dramatic V zone changes. As estrogen deprivation continues, the collagen and elastic fibers that also line your vaginal walls will begin to swell and fuse together, resulting in a loss of strength of the vaginal wall itself. This can make your vagina subject to painful tears and injury—sometimes from very little stimulation. Some women find it extremely difficult to even endure an internal gynecological exam after menopause due to the increased sensitivity of these tissues. It's also one reason that sex can become extremely painful during this time—or even during perimenopause. And you can read a lot more about that in Chapter 8—which devotes an entire section to what you can do to alleviate this problem, including why keeping your sex life active has terrific V zone benefits! In fact, the more sexually active you are in your middle years, and the more intimate activity you engage in, the less likely you are to experience extreme V zone problems. And since sexual activity increases blood flow to the vagina you might even find that the more sex you have, the better your V zone symptoms are overall. The phrase "use it or lose it" *really* applies here.

DON'T PLAY DOCTOR

While it's important to remain aware of your body and any problems that might develop, at the same time it's not a good idea to routinely tie every

V zone problem to wonky hormones. In fact, Dr. Gloria Bachman, chief of obstetrics and gynecology at Robert Wood Johnson Medical School, believes that neither women nor their doctors should ever automatically assume a V zone complaint *is* related to perimenopause without taking responsible diagnostic steps.

Thus, she believes every woman should bring any sign of V zone trouble to the attention of her doctor—who should, in turn, perform the following tests:

- A Pap smear, and a full cytologic exam

- A vaginal ultrasound to assess the thickness of the uterine lining

- A pH test to determine the acid level of the vagina

In addition, experts say that if there are any obvious symptoms of infection—particularly an odorous or oddly colored discharge, or itching or extreme burning—additional testing, including a sampling of vaginal fluids, and, when necessary, blood tests, should also be part of your exam.

TLC for Your Midlife V Zone

For many women, nothing more than the occasional use of a vaginal lubricant (products like AstroGlide or KY Jelly) may be necessary to resume a reasonable comfort level. While some of you may find the lubricants necessary only during sexual activity, for others, daily use can alleviate much of the common itching and burning that can come at this time of life. How much or how little you will need these products depends largely on your estrogen level, how fast it's declining, and your basic tolerance for discomfort. The one lubricant you should always avoid: petroleum jelly. While it may temporarily ease painful sex, this oil-based product *does not* dissolve in the vagina so it might increase the growth of bacteria that ultimately leads to infection.

In addition, you may find that eliminating the use of scented V zone products cuts down on irritation and, in turn, may alleviate some of your symptoms. This includes washing gels, dusting powder, and any perfumed feminine deodorants. While sometimes you may simply react to chemical compounds—even when no scent is present—studies show that more often it is the fragrance used in V zone products that holds the most potential for problems.

You may also want to avoid panty liners, particularly if your symptoms include vulvar pain. In at least one study conducted by Milwaukee, Wisconsin, gynecologist Dr. Jessica Thomason, continuous use of sanitary pads or panty liners could contribute to this problem. While there is no clear-cut reason, at least some experts suspect that chemicals found in the pads, or even the continuous pressure as they press against your vulva, may play a role.

In the event that your V zone irritation turns to real pain, particularly if sex seems impossible even with lubrication, then you may benefit from one of several topical estrogen preparations designed to put hormones back into vaginal tissue, with minimal and sometimes even no exposure in the rest of your body. And because so little of the hormone makes its way into your bloodstream, or even to your uterus or breast, there is generally no need to counter the effects of estrogen cream with progesterone, as is the case with traditional oral hormone therapy.

Some types of estrogen products that can help include prescription cream formulations of Premarin or Estrace; custom-blended hormone creams created by special "compounding pharmacies" (those that custom create medications from scratch—the way you would bake a cake without a mix) using a much less potent form of estrogen; nonprescription vaginal estrogen tablets like Vagifem; and prescription devices that release hormones when inserted into the vagina, such as Femring or Estring. Because all of these treatments are also used as remedies for sexual dysfunction during perimenopause, you'll find more information about them in Chapter 8, Sex in Menopause City.

Finally, don't overlook help from Mother Nature—particularly certain herbs and plants that many women swear by when it comes to vaginal health and comfort. Among those found most helpful include oral preparations of black cohosh, licorice, and Vitex (chasteberry). For more on all these and other herbs that might help you, check out Chapter 10, Mother Nature Never Had a Hot Flash.

Changes in Your Life Cycles:
What to Expect from Your Periods

Unlike Megan, who has a tendency to catastrophize *everything*, my friend Andrea is a well-grounded earth mamma who rarely gets thrown by anything—which is probably a good thing since her life, it seems, has become a living, breathing example of the unexpected. Whatever Andrea thinks is going to happen never does—and what she's sure won't occur always does. To put it mildly, Andrea's life is *always* full of surprises, and her menopause experience was no exception.

Because her periods were always pretty regular and never caused her much of a problem, she expected (there's that word again!) that her perimenopause transition time would be pretty uneventful as well. Not! From almost the moment it began, nothing about Andrea's experience seemed normal *to her*.

"I cannot believe this is happening to me—I've read all the books and nowhere, nowhere does it say that I should expect this kind of crazy bleeding or that I'd feel like I'm flipping out every time it happens," she said one day on the telephone, during one of her particularly frustrating perimenopause moments.

"Well, you know the books say to expect an irregular period—you do know that's part of the picture, don't you?" I was sounding only a little bit sarcastic, knowing full well that Andrea did know something of what to expect. But by this time I don't think she even heard what I was saying. She continued on.

"And what the heck does 'irregular' mean anyway—do they mean more blood, less blood, more blood more often, less blood less often—nobody gives you any specifics," she said, her voice escalating in both pitch and volume.

And, mood swings aside, I can't say I blame her. Because the truth is, you probably already know that "irregular periods" is pretty much the generic description that almost everybody uses to describe the cycle changes of perimenopause. Medically, the problem is known as dysfunctional uterine bleeding, or DUB. But regardless of the terminology, it can be difficult and frustrating trying to figure out what it all means—and what you really can expect. What can help: Taking just a few minutes to learn a little something about what your body is going through at this time, the ways in which your intimate anatomy is changing, and the way those changes are reflected in various bleeding patterns and cycle irregularities.

Understanding Dysfunctional Bleeding (DUB)

As you read in Chapter 1, through most of your reproductive life your menstrual cycle works on a kind of inner timetable—one that usually results in a period somewhere around every twenty-eight days. To review, the cycle begins when your brain sends out the hormonal messenger known as FSH (follicle-stimulating hormone), which signals your ovaries to begin "hatching" the follicles it holds into eggs. All this causes your estrogen levels to rise—and your uterine lining to build, in anticipation of receiving a *fertilized* egg. Meanwhile, one of the eggs your ovary has been hatching pulls ahead of the others in size and stature and eventually pushes itself through the outer shell in a process known as ovulation. The remnants of the shell it leaves behind begin manufacturing another hormone—progesterone. This helps stabilize your uterus and further prepare you for pregnancy. It also helps keep the growth of your lining under control. If conception occurs, both estrogen and progesterone levels remain high—so your uterus remains thick, soft, and spongy. If you don't get pregnant, then both estrogen and progesterone levels drop sharply. This, in turn, causes the lining that has been temporarily building inside your uterus to shed in the form of menstrual blood.

As neat a package as this whole process is, once you turn the bend round forty, things begin to change. First, as your ovaries "age" there are fewer follicles ready to be "hatched." So, ovulation may not occur every month. Of course your brain hasn't quite gotten that message yet, so it continues to pump out FSH like mad, trying desperately to stimulate your ovaries into production one more time. All that FSH means lots more estrogen production—which in turn means your uterine lining is building up extra cells like crazy! However, because you aren't ovulating, there is no progesterone to balance the estrogen—and consequently, nothing to stimulate a menstrual "bleed." The end result: You don't get a period that month—and, sometimes, for a second month as well.

By the time another month rolls around, however, your ovaries may decide to kick in and do a little hatching, and an egg is made. You ovulate, progesterone is manufactured, and, providing you don't get pregnant, your body initiates a period. However, because you didn't have a menstrual cycle for a month or two before, all that extra uterine lining that's been building is going to be shed all at once, right along with whatever built up during the current cycle. The end result here: You can experience an extremely heavy, sometimes even clot-filled period that, for some women, can be quite frightening, particularly if you are used to a fairly light flow.

In another scenario, small bits of this extra lining can break loose unexpectedly and begin to shed on their own. Since without progesterone the uterus lacks structural support, the lining "sloughs off" in an irregular fashion, causing "periods" to arrive at odd times. It's what also accounts for bleeding between periods, or what can cause a period to last longer than normal.

Indeed, most experts say that almost any bleeding pattern can occur during perimenopause. What's more, your "new" pattern—if you can even discern one—can be different from year to year or sometimes even month to month. This is why it's called "dysfunctional" uterine bleeding.

In general, however, doctors *do* have a way of categorizing your cycle experiences, with most changes falling into one of the following categories:

- *Polymenorrhea:* Frequent, regular periods less than every twenty-one days apart but on a regular schedule.

- *Hypermenorrhea:* Excessive, heavy bleeding during a normal-length cycle.

- *Menorrhagia:* Prolonged or excessive bleeding, longer than one week but occurring at regular intervals. This also encompasses those who lose more than 80 milliliters of blood per cycle. (Soaking one maxi pad or supersized tampon every thirty minutes for four hours, or every hour for eight hours, is considered very heavy episodic bleeding.)

- *Metrorrhagia:* Bleeding or spotting that occurs between periods and is usually not very heavy.

- *Menometrorraghia:* Frequent, excessive, and prolonged bleeding occurring at irregular intervals.

In addition, your doctor may also use the following terms to further describe your cycle changes:

- *Dysmenorrhea:* Pain during your bleeding cycles.

- *Oligomenorrhea:* Decreased frequency of your cycles.

- *Hypomenorrhea:* Decreasing amount of menstrual flow.

- *Amenorrhea:* When all bleeding stops and there is no cycle.

According to the North American Menopause Society (NAMS), a chart review of five hundred perimenopausal women found that the majority—some 70 percent—experienced either oligomenorrhea and/or hypomenorrhea as their major cycle change. Far fewer women—about 18 percent—experienced various forms of prolonged or excessive bleeding, while just 12 percent had a sudden stop to their menstrual cycle. More importantly, remember that cycle changes are uniquely personal—so don't become alarmed or even upset if what's happening to you is not the same as what happened to your mother, or is happening to your sister or even your best friend right now.

DYSFUNCTIONAL VS. ABNORMAL BLEEDING: AN IMPORTANT DISTINCTION

While most midlife cycle changes are a normal and natural part of the transition, there are also a number of other problems that can sometimes occur *around this same time,* and that may be responsible, at least in part, for some of the bleeding symptoms you experience. According to NAMS experts, the earmarks that something *else* might be wrong are:

- Blood loss greater than 80 milliliters, particularly when blood clots occur. (Bleeding is considered heavy if you soak through a maxi pad or super-tampon every thirty minutes for four hours, or one pad or tampon per hour for eight hours. You should contact your doctor anytime this level of bleeding occurs).

- Anemia (a decrease in the number of red blood cells).

- Abnormal cycles (lasting longer than seven days, or occurring closer together than every twenty-one days).

- Continual bleeding or spotting between cycles or after intercourse.

Certainly any one of these conditions can be part of a normal peri-menopause picture—and the closer you get to approaching complete menopause the more normal these "abnormalities" are. That said, when these conditions do exist, or particularly if your bleeding patterns seem ultradramatic—such as blood loss that goes on for weeks or even months—it's important that your doctor rule out any underlying conditions that might be contributing to your bleeding problems.

For a very small number of women, excessive bleeding can be the result of systemic disease—that is, a problem unrelated to your reproductive system, such as a thyroid disorder, a problem related to blood coagulation (such as Willebrand's disease), leukemia, or even a liver ailment.

For others, abnormal bleeding can be the direct result of problems within the reproductive tract but not necessarily related to the hormonal imbalances of perimenopause. These include:

- Fibroid tumors—round "knots" of uterine muscle tissue that grow in and around the uterus (see "If You Have Fibroid Tumors," later in this chapter).

- Polyps—growths of soft uterine lining tissue that has bonded together; they usually dangle from a stalk into the center of your uterus (see "If You Have Uterine Polyps," later in this chapter).

- Endometrial hyperplasia—an abnormal buildup of slightly irregular uterine cells (see "From the 'M' File: Will This Be Cancer?" later in this chapter).

- Adenomyosis—a condition where endometrial cells grow into the muscle wall, resulting in a soft, spongy enlarged uterus (see "From the 'M' File: The Uterus That Ate Cleveland," later in this chapter).

- Damage from an IUD.

- Pelvic Inflammatory Disease (PID), usually resulting from an undiagnosed and untreated sexually transmitted disease.

- An ectopic pregnancy—or the remnants of one.

- A miscarriage.

- Endometritis—a bacterial infection of the uterus.

In addition, in a small number of women the underlying cause of abnormal bleeding can be the result of an early uterine cancer. While it can occur in women during perimenopause, in most instances it develops after menopause and is normally associated with bleeding that develops after at least one year with no menstruation.

DIAGNOSING YOUR DUB: WHAT YOUR DOCTOR MUST DO

In addition to your normal pelvic exam and any routine testing, there are also several diagnostic tools that can help rule out certain specific problems. So, don't be surprised if your doctor recommends one of the following:

- *Endometrial biopsy:* An in-office procedure that requires no anesthesia, a biopsy involves removing a tiny sample of your uterine lining that is then examined in a laboratory for cell irregularities. The test is performed by inserting a thin catheter-like tube through your vagina and cervix and up into your uterus, where a tiny bit of suction is used to pull off a piece of the lining. It can cause cramping similar to menstrual pains but usually lasts just a few minutes.

- *Transvaginal ultrasound:* This involves inserting a thin wandlike probe into your vagina, sending harmless radio waves into your uterus. The probe, which is connected to a computer screen via a

From the "M" File

FLOODING, HEAVY BLEEDING, AND THE CINNAMON LINK

Q: Can you tell me what "flooding" is? I'm forty-seven and have begun experiencing extremely heavy bleeding that my doctor calls "flooding." What causes this? Is it dangerous? Sometimes I feel as if I am hemorrhaging and it's very frightening.

A: Yes, it can be scary—because "flooding" is actually the extreme end of the menstrual bleeding spectrum, an experience that can cause you to lose large amounts of blood in a very short period of time. Some women describe it as a "gush" that seems to flow without warning and is often accompanied by blood clots that you can continue to "pass" for several hours, along with more bleeding. As frightening as this sounds, most women find that the intense bleeding usually does stop within a few hours—sometimes just as you are becoming convinced you need to head to a hospital, it can quickly begin to taper off to almost nothing. While the experience itself is not generally harmful, it's important to find out what's behind the bleeding—a fibroid tumor, a polyp, or simply a buildup of endometrial cells. This is one reason you should always report all bleeding irregularities, but especially flooding, to your doctor— which clearly you have already done. Since he or she does not seem overly concerned, it's likely more serious problems have already been ruled out. And that likely means your bleeding is hormone related. If this is not the case, and you feel that you have not been adequately tested or examined, seek a second opinion and at least have a vaginal sonogram, if not more complete testing (see above).

long lead wire, relays back the image. This screening is used to measure the thickness of your uterine lining (which can be an indication of why you are bleeding) and can also capture a picture of a fibroid tumor, or sometimes even a polyp, as well as any other "mass" that may be present.

Assuming, however, you have been checked and your problems are hormone related, there is little to fear. However, you should know that biochemical reactions that occur during heavy bleeding can make some women feel panicky and extremely anxious—even if they are not necessarily frightened by the amount of blood they see—so that may be part of the reason why you feel so upset during these episodes.

You should also know that there are several medications and other treatments that can help (see below). In addition, an old folk remedy for controlling heavy bleeding is cinnamon—about half a teaspoon twice daily beginning as soon as you start to bleed and continuing as long as you like. You can sprinkle it on cereal or use it in tea, or—my personal favorite—on waffles or whole-wheat toast, with a touch of powdered sugar to reduce acidity. If you choose the Saigon cinnamon variety, the flavor is milder and less likely to irritate sensitive nerve endings in the mouth. While experts aren't certain how it works, many believe it helps to stabilize the uterus much the way progesterone does (and some doctors prescribe progesterone suppositories for this as well). The end result is that heavy bleeding is less likely to occur.

Of course, if your flooding continues to recur frequently, you should consult your doctor again. In addition, the general medical rule of thumb on this is that if you are soaking through a menstrual pad or tampon every thirty minutes for more than a few hours, or soaking a pad every hour for more than six or eight hours, you need to at least call your doctor. Heavy bleeding that continues for twenty-four hours is considered an emergency requiring medical attention.

• *Sonohysterogram:* Similar to a vaginal ultrasound, but the big difference here is that prior to imaging the uterus is filled with a harmless saline solution. The solution helps to "lift up" and more easily identify certain abnormalities, particularly polyps. Although the procedure lasts less than twenty minutes, it can cause some cramping during and afterward.

- *Endoscopy:* In this procedure—also known as *diagnostic hysteroscopy*—your doctor will insert a thin telescoping wand through your vagina and cervix, directly into your uterus. Attached to the wand are a microcamera and a light source, through which your doctor can take a firsthand look at the inside of your uterus. This can often be done in the doctor's office, using a local anesthetic, or sometimes sedation.

If any of these diagnostic procedures uncover a problem, then specific surgical treatments might be necessary. Later in this chapter you'll learn a bit more about what they are, and when they are necessary.

TREATING DUB: WHAT YOUR DOCTOR CAN DO

If you are like the vast majority of women reading this book, your perimenopausal bleeding problems will be the result of your "wild and crazy" hormones. As you read earlier, when levels begin to fluctuate and ovulation becomes highly irregular, the lining of your uterus reacts in unexpected ways—including shedding at irregular intervals and bleeding at unexpected times. This is the case for up to 75 percent of all women who see their doctor for perimenopausal bleeding irregularities. How you respond to those irregularities, both emotionally and, especially, physically, can play a big part in how your symptoms are treated—or if you need any treatment at all. Remember, "doing nothing" during your perimenopause time *is* a perfectly acceptable approach, providing no other problems are diagnosed. Known in my little circle of friends as the "white knuckle" approach to menopause, this may be the best option for many of you, particularly if your bleeding problems are not particularly troubling.

If, however, you are bothered by your irregular cycles—and particularly if your bleeding problems are causing you great emotional or physical distress, or even interfering with your ability to live your professional or personal life—then it's important to realize there are treatment options available. While some are clearly more dramatic than others, what you will require is largely determined by your personal health profile and your specific needs at the moment. So, it's important that you become familiar with all the options and make certain to discuss each of them with your doctor before deciding on what's right for you.

MEDICATION: YOUR FIRST LINE OF DEFENSE

Often, dysfunctional bleeding problems can be quickly and easily controlled via the use of certain medications. While some act directly on the uterus to stabilize the lining and control bleeding, others have a more systemic approach, reducing inflammation or even contractions that also exacerbate bleeding. If DUB has become a significant problem for you, talk to your doctor about whether or not any of the following treatments can help.

Nonsteroidal Anti-Inflammatory Drugs

If your problem is isolated events of heavy bleeding you may find some significant help in medications known as NSAIDs or nonsteroidal anti-inflammatory drugs. You probably know them as common pain medications such as Advil, Motrin, Aleve, Naprosyn, or even simple aspirin. The prescription pain reliever Ponstel (mefenamic acid) has also been shown in studies to decrease the amount of menstrual bleeding by up to 50 percent, but an analysis done in 2000 showed that naproxen was almost equally as effective. In the same study, NSAIDs were found to be more effective than either birth control pills or progesterone supplements in reducing bleeding. Many women use these medications to help control heavy bleeding during their peak reproductive years as well.

While no one is certain exactly how they work, most doctors believe they help to control the production of prostaglandins, hormones that can increase uterine contractions. Other research has shown they may also help reduce interuterine inflammation, which is also associated with excessive bleeding.

The downside: When used over a long period of time NSAIDs can increase your risk of serious gastrointestinal problems, including internal bleeding and ulcers, and they may also contribute to anemia. Another potential problem: To be most effective treatment should begin about ten days prior to the expected onset of your period. If you don't know when to expect bleeding, they may be less effective.

From the "M" File

THE UTERUS THAT ATE CLEVELAND

Q: My doctor just diagnosed me as having "adene-myosis," which he describes as an enlarged uterus. He thinks it may be the reason why I am experiencing such heavy bleeding episodes, sometimes for months on end. I'm forty-eight and figured it was all hormonal, but he says possibly not—and is suggesting a hysterectomy. I don't want this operation and want to seek a second opin-ion, but my doctor says there are no other treatment op-tions for this problem. Is he right? This seems like such a drastic solution for an enlarged uterus.

A: First off, you should always, ALWAYS seek a second, and possibly a third, opinion when treatment involves a life-altering operation such as a hysterectomy (see "Should You Say No?" later in this chapter). Whether or not any other treatment options exist is not nearly as impor-tant as making certain that you have the correct diagnosis. In terms of the specific problem your current doctor is suggesting—adenomyosis—it's a bit more complex than just an enlarged uterus. In this condition, the cells lining the soft, spongy surface of your uterus (called the en-dometrium) begin growing into the uterine muscle wall (called the my-ometrium). Other biochemical events happen simultaneously, often creating inflammation in the uterus itself. This, in turn, can result in ex-treme cramping, particularly when bleeding occurs. Although most doc-

Hormone Therapy

When your bleeding irregularities are in fact determined to be hormone related, the first line of defense is almost always hormone therapy—in-cluding birth control pills or progesterone supplements, particularly nat-ural progesterone. Unlike HRT, which is generally prescribed only after you reach menopause, the hormone options available during peri-menopause are quite different. While neither birth control pills or, par-ticularly, natural progesterone supplements carry the same types of risks

tors believed that adenomyosis occurred primarily during peri-menopause or menopause, new imaging studies reveal it may be present as early as the twenties or thirties, with symptoms appearing much later in life. And while doctors don't know why it occurs, they do know it is more likely to develop when women have had one or more children—ostensibly because of specific hormonal and other effects on the uterus that occur during pregnancy. In fact, only 6 percent of women who never had a baby develop this condition. Although hysterectomy is considered the ultimate treatment, unless the pain is severe, many women choose to do nothing at all. And in fact, if you are nearing menopause many doctors advocate doing nothing at all, since in many instances adenomyosis disappears on its own as soon as your menstruation stops. In the meantime, anti-inflammatory pain medications can be helpful. Also be aware, however, that birth control pills can aggravate adenomyosis, so if you are taking oral contraceptives to either prevent pregnancy or to cope with perimenopausal symptoms, you may want to rethink this approach. You should also know that adenomyosis is a difficult diagnosis to make. The problem is often confused with other conditions that can sometimes cause the uterus to enlarge, such as fibroid tumors. While a CA 125 blood test can help narrow down the diagnostic picture (a test result over 35 units per milliliter, together with certain symptoms, can indicate adenomyosis exists), the only real way to know for certain is via an MRI imaging exam. If, in fact, you do opt for a hysterectomy, it may be wise to have your diagnosis confirmed with this screening first.

associated with traditional hormone replacement therapy, they are clearly not the right choice for every woman. For a complete rundown of what's available in this area, see Chapter 11, HRT, Natural Hormones, and Beyond. In addition, don't forget that very often hormones can be balanced using a combination of natural herbs like black cohosh, dietary intervention, particularly soy-based foods, and even certain vitamins and minerals—all of which are fully explored in Chapter 10, Mother Nature Never Had a Hot Flash. In many instances, balancing your hormones naturally can help control bleeding irregularities—or at least make them slightly more predictable.

Tranexamic Acid

This is a synthetic form of an amino acid known as lysine, and it works to enhance blood clotting, thus reducing some bleeding. In one large-scale analysis, it was found more effective in reducing blood flow than oral progestins (a synthetic form of progesterone) or mefenamic acid (Ponstel). However, there are some downsides, including side effects like headache, nausea, and dizziness. In addition, if you are at any risk for blood clots, this is not the drug for you. Currently, tranexamic acid is recommended in the United States only when fibroids, endometriosis, or other uterine lesions have been ruled out, and when oral contraceptives are ineffective.

YOUR SURGICAL OPTIONS FOR DUB

If either fibroid tumors or polyps are causing your irregular bleeding, there are some specific surgical procedures that can help, and you'll read more about those in the next section of this chapter. However, if your doctor determines your bleeding is caused by a hormone imbalance but medications just don't seem to help, there are also some surgical procedures that might do the job. While they won't alleviate any of the *other* symptoms related to hormone instability—like hot flashes or mood swings—the following procedures can help control or stop the bleeding, which for many women can go a long way in relieving many of the quality-of-life issues that can make perimenopause a difficult time.

D&C (Dilation and Curettage)

Although no longer considered the "gold standard" in treatment for heavy bleeding, this procedure can still be very helpful for many women. Usually done in an outpatient clinic or hospital, and often requiring general anesthesia, this procedure involves having a large portion of your uterine lining manually "scraped" away. This is accomplished by first dilating your cervix, and then inserting a thin scalpel or scraping tool, which your doctor then gently passes around the inside of your uterus, literally pulling the excess lining away from the endometrial wall and removing it. Although there can be some significant bleeding directly following the procedure, overall, recovery is quick. Usually in a few days you can go back to work, with all activities resumed in about a week. You can, however, continue to have a bloody discharge or light bleeding for about ten days. While your dysfunctional bleeding will generally stop after that, the respite can be temporary, with relief lasting only a few months. As soon as the lining begins to build again, the bleeding problems can resume. Often, repeat procedures are needed for effective control. Another option is to follow a D&C with birth control pills or progesterone to help prevent further excessive buildup of the uterine lining. In the event that your doctor seriously suspects your bleeding may be the result of uterine cancer (if you are past menopause or have a strong family history of this disease), it's important to note that a D&C is also a very effective way to test a large area of endometrial cells and ensure that no cancer is present.

Endometrial Ablation

In this procedure, your doctor will use one of several different methods to permanently destroy at least one layer of uterine cells. If you can imagine this, it's almost like rendering a piece of your garden "sterile"—meaning nothing you plant there will ever grow. Thus, no uterine cells will build up, so there is essentially no risk of future bleeding. While there are several ways of accomplishing this, the two most common methods are:

- *Laser Ablation:* In this instance, your uterus is flooded with a harmless saline-type solution and a computer-guided laser is used to literally vaporize or "burn off" the uterine lining.

- *Balloon Ablation:* Here, doctors insert a hollow "balloon" into the uterus, then fill it with heated fluid. The contact between the sides of the balloon and the surface of the uterus causes the cells to "shrink and burn" in much the way they would under laser power. The advantage over lasers is that the balloon conforms to the exact shape of the uterus, thus ensuring an even "burn" of all surface areas. There may be mild to moderate cramping up to twenty-four hours after this procedure, and vaginal spotting or discharge for up to thirty days.

Both procedures take between fifteen and thirty minutes and are usually done on an outpatient basis. Recovery time is generally short—you are usually free to leave the center or clinic within two to three hours. Afterward you need to avoid heavy lifting, exercise, and intercourse, all for about a week. As your uterus heals, however—which can take up to six weeks—you may experience a blood-tinged or yellowish discharge, particularly with balloon ablation. This is normal and not considered a sign of problems.

The downside with either procedure is, of course, that since your uterine lining is rendered permanently destroyed you will be unable to sustain a pregnancy—one reason these procedures are recommended only to women who can no longer conceive, or don't want to get pregnant. Both procedures also carry small risks of problems including infection and hemorrhage, and, with laser therapy, perforations of the uterus or other organs.

Important Warning: While this procedure can be helpful in many instances, there are at least some significant concerns that an endometrial ablation, using any technique, might, in some way, mask future cell changes in the uterus that could be an early warning sign of endometrial cancer. According to Dr. Allan DeCherney of the UCLA School of Medicine in Los Angeles, because not every bit of endometrial tissue is ablated, there could be remaining "nests" of cells that are left behind. And this, he says, can "provide a site of origin" for a malignancy to develop. DeCherney also says that in most of these procedures the lower portion of the uterus is ablated, so, in the event a cancer does deveop, there is often no chance for bleeding to occur. And that means you may miss an other-wise important signal that something is wrong. The end result: By the time a cancer is diagnosed, it would be in an advanced stage, making treatment far more difficult and complicated.

To avoid these risks, you may want to avoid any stimulating hor-mone therapy following ablation (particularly estrogen). In addition, Dr. DeCherny suggests that this procedure never be used as a treatment for endometrial hyperplasia with atypia (see "From the 'M' File: Will This Be Cancer?" later in this chapter) or any precancerous endometrial condi-tion.

Hysteroscopy

This procedure uses somewhat the same technique as an endoscopy exam: the same lighted probe, with camera attached, is inserted through your vagina and cervix into your uterus. In addition to the viewing equipment, surgical instruments are attached and can be used to remove any small abnormalities that could be causing or exacerbating bleeding, such as tiny endometrial or cervical polyps (see "If You Have Uterine Polyps," later in this chapter). In addition, this procedure allows your doctor the opportunity to sample a much larger area of tissue than what would be available via biopsy. This can also allow tissue sampling directly from any area that appears abnormal, due either to inflammation or exceptionally thick cell growth. Compared to a biopsy, which is said to be a "blind" removal of tissue (your doctor doesn't know where the probe will hit), samples taken during a hysteroscopy are thought to be much more accurate in ruling out conditions such as polyps, hyperplasia, or even cancer. The procedure takes about fifteen minutes, can be done under local anesthesia, and is frequently performed right in the doctor's office.

A second type of hysteroscopy, known as a rectoscopy, uses a hysteroscope with a built-in wire loop. The loop is attached to an electrical source so that very high-frequency electric currents can be used to cut or coagulate tissue. This procedure takes between fifteen and thirty minutes and almost always requires either general anesthesia, or sedation and a local anesthetic. It is considered to be more effective at removing large areas of tissue, particularly large polyps or small fibroids. Recovery takes several hours, but you can usually return home from the hospital the same day and return to normal activities within a few days.

Important to note: While a hysteroscopy itself won't stop heavy bleeding (unless the source of the bleeding, such as a polyp, is removed), this procedure is often recommended as a diagnostic tool when heavy bleeding persists.

An even more permanent solution than all these procedures is to have a hysterectomy—the complete removal of your uterus. You'll find out more about this option later in this chapter (see "Should You Say No?"

From the "M" File

WILL THIS BE CANCER?

Q: I'm only forty-five years old and my doctor diagnosed me with endometrial hyperplasia—and said it is a precursor to cancer. He is recommending a hysterectomy. I live in a very small town in the Midwest and I don't have a lot of access to medical care, but from what I've read his suggestion seems too drastic, especially for a condition that is only precancerous. What are the risks that cancer will develop? And how soon does it happen?

A: The problem you describe—endometrial hyperplasia—is an "overgrowth" or thickening of the uterine lining that occurs when you stop ovulating and estrogen becomes the dominant hormone. This, in turn, causes the cells of your uterine lining to split and divide, creating the overgrowth of tissue. This can occur in either isolated sections of your uterus or globally throughout the lining. Hyperplasia itself is quite common, occurring in about one in every one thousand women, oftentimes in those in your age group who are experiencing perimenopause. If you are overweight—usually indicative of an estrogen overload—hyperplasia is more likely to occur. In perimenopausal women symptoms of hyperplasia usually include bleeding between periods and an exceptionally heavy menstrual flow (soaking a pad or tampon every hour for up to twenty-four hours). In older gals who are past menopause, symptoms include any vaginal bleeding or unusual or heavy discharge. When these hyperplastic cells begin growing, the condition is always benign—meaning it is not cancerous. The key to whether or not your condition will *progress* to cancer lies in a more precise diagnosis of the cells themselves. The hyperplasia that is characterized as simple, cystic, or adenomous has a very small chance of becoming malignant. In this instance, the hyperplasia frequently regresses on its own and no treatment is needed. Or, the process can be hurried along via a D&C, followed by hormone therapy—usually progesterone (see Chapter

11)—or hormone therapy alone followed by a biopsy every three to six months for at least one year.

However, a fourth type of uterine cell growth known as hyperplasia with atypia is another story. This diagnosis means that cells have already begun to change and they have taken on some characteristics of a malignancy. If not treated, this condition has a much higher chance of progressing to cancer—according to some statistics as least 15 percent of women with hyperplasia with atypia do develop uterine cancer.

More than likely your hyperplasia was initially diagnosed via a biopsy, which studies show can be highly accurate. However, to be more certain of the exact type of hyperplasia you have and the extent to which it is occurring, a D&C or a hysteroscopy (see the previous section) can provide much more information. These procedures involve removing larger areas of the thickened lining so that cells can be examined for any specific cancer-related characteristics.

Because there is a significant risk that hyperplasia with atypia will progress to cancer, at least some doctors continue to believe a hysterectomy is necessary. However, an equal number believe that it's worth trying at least one D&C followed by about three months of progesterone therapy first. While hyperplasia with atypia does return in about 75 percent of women who have a D&C, if you are among the 25 percent in whom the procedure is successful, you can avoid a hysterectomy. If, however, even after progesterone therapy and a repeat D&C to check for resolution, you are still found to have hyperplasia with atypia, then yes, a hysterectomy would be the recommended procedure.

The bottom line: You should have a second opinion. And request a second biopsy to confirm a diagnosis of hyperplasia with atypia before considering a hysterectomy. If your diagnosis is confirmed, the one procedure you should probably avoid is endometrial ablation, discussed in this chapter.

If You Have Fibroid Tumors:
What You Need to Know

Although the word *tumor* has a frightening connotation, when it refers to fibroids it's not quite so alarming. That's because these growths—found in and around the uterus—are routinely benign and are not a cancer risk. Comprised of renegade muscle cells that come together to form a fibrous lump or "knot," they can grow singly or in clumps, all within the uterine wall. By some estimates up to 77 percent of all American women have at least one fibroid tumor—ranging in size from just under one inch to as large as a grapefruit—but most don't even know it.

While no one is certain what causes a fibroid, they most commonly develop in women between ages thirty and forty, and African-American women are at greatest risk. Being overweight may slightly increase the risks for all women. To date, at least one genetic link has also been identified, indicating that fibroids may run in families.

Doctors also know that fibroids are estrogen dependent—they thrive on this hormone, which can initiate wild growth spurts. That's one reason that tiny, almost insignificant fibroids can grow very large during pregnancy, when estrogen levels are high. It's also one reason why perimenopausal women must remain vigilant about fibroids, since sometimes the temporary estrogen dominance that can occur once ovulation stops can spark the growth of these tumors, causing symptoms that otherwise might never have occurred. In fact, one of the underlying causes of dysfunctional uterine bleeding in perimenopausal women can be fibroid tumors, even if these growths did not cause problems in the past.

Although all fibroid tumors have the same cellular makeup, they are categorized into three separate types based on their specific location within the uterus. They are:

- Submucosal fibroids, which lie just under the uterine lining and push into the empty space inside the uterus. These fibroids can cause heavy menstrual bleeding, pain, and infertility.

- Intramural fibroids, which reside between the muscles of the uterine wall. They are the most common type and when they grow large can cause a feeling of "heaviness" or pressure in the uterus, as well as some heavy menstrual bleeding.

- Subserosal fibroids, which extend from the uterine wall outward, to the outside of the uterus. If left to grow large enough they can push on other organs, causing bloating, pressure, and pain.

Fibroids can also develop a "stalk" or stem that allows them to dangle down into the uterus or grow outward into the pelvic cavity. If the stalks twist, they can cause significant pain. The twisting can also "strangle" the fibroid, which may start to degenerate, increasing the risk of infection.

While in many instances fibroid tumors cause no symptoms, this is not always the case. Depending on the size, number, and location of your fibroids you may experience longer, heavier periods, pelvic discomfort, or even pain as they press on other organs. If any of these symptoms do occur your doctor can check for fibroids during an ordinary pelvic exam—most can be felt during a manual examination. A transvaginal ultrasound can also help confirm the diagnosis.

One word of caution: According to fibroid expert Dr. Paul Indman, chairman of the editorial board of Laparoscopy & Hysteroscopy for OBGYN.net, in some instances fibroid tumors can be confused with adenomyosis, or enlarged uterus (see "The Uterus That Ate Cleveland," earlier in this chapter). This is because both can be felt or even visualized on an ultrasound as a pelvic "mass." However, it's vital that the difference be discovered, since they require very different treatments. When there is any possibility of confusion, Indman says, an MRI scan can provide detailed imaging of the entire uterus, making it easy to distinguish between the two conditions.

TREATING YOUR FIBROID TUMORS AT MIDLIFE

Discovering you have fibroid tumors at midlife can be both a blessing and a curse. It can be a blessing because fibroids are estrogen dependent. So, as you age, and estrogen levels decrease, fibroids are far more likely to shrink and even disappear without treatment. On the other hand, because of your age, your doctor may be more inclined to push you toward a hysterectomy, particularly if your fibroids are causing considerable dysfunctional bleeding. In fact, some 200,000 hysterectomies a year are performed for fibroid tumors.

Regardless of your age, even if your fibroids are a source of trouble, you don't have to have your uterus removed. There are a number of other options to try. And, in some instances, your age may be on your side. Indeed, since your estrogen levels are declining, your fibroids are less likely to *keep* growing—so some treatment options that offer only temporary relief for younger women may offer you a permanent solution.

Other than hysterectomy, the three main surgical treatments for fibroid tumors include:

- *Myomectomy:* This operation removes only the fibroids, keeping the uterus intact. This can be done either through an abdominal incision or via a hysteroscopy (see "Treating DUB," earlier in this chapter) or a laparoscopy, a form of minimally invasive surgery. Although the operation successfully removes the fibroids, they can grow back, but that is usually the case only in younger women, in whom estrogen levels remain high.

- *Uterine artery embolization:* This procedure is based on the principle that without a blood supply, a fibroid will shrink and die. So in this operation, doctors seek to block the blood flow to the fibroid by creating a type of medically induced blood clot in a vessel leading to the tumor. There is a small risk of infection and/or hemorrhage following this procedure, but it can be very effective for certain types of fibroids.

- *Myolis:* In this procedure doctors use either lasers or some form of electrical current or energy to destroy the fibroid. It is most often performed via a laparoscopy.

In addition to surgery, there are also several medications that can help shrink large fibroid tumors. They can sometimes be used prior to surgery, to make the operation less extensive, or even on their own as an independent treatment. If you are approaching menopause and your estrogen levels are already declining, some of these drugs may work especially well. Medications currently being used for this purpose include:

- *GnRH (gonadotropin-releasing hormone) agonists:* These drugs, which include Lupron, Synarel, and Zoladex, block fibroid growth by working against hormones that normally stimulate estrogen production. With less estrogen to stimulate growth, fibroids tend to shrink and sometimes disappear. The downside here is that these drugs generally exacerbate menopause symptoms such as hot flashes and night sweats. Also important to note: If estrogen levels remain high, fibroids can begin growing rapidly once these medications are stopped. In addition, because they can have a negative impact on your bones— mostly because they are dramatically halting estrogen production—it is not advisable to use these drugs for longer than three months.

- *GnRH plus hormone therapy:* This regimen begins with GnRH medications, followed within one to three months with the addition of low-dose hormone therapy. This is thought to help replace some of the estrogen suppressed by the GnRH agonist drugs, but in amounts still lower than what is produced by your body. Thus this therapy won't cause your fibroids to grow.

- *Ru486:* The controversial "abortion" drug mifepristine has shown promise as a fibroid treatment. It works by encouraging the tumor to shrink on its own.

- *GnRH plus Tibolone:* This drug combination is popular in Europe and other parts of the world where Tibolone, a type of "designer estrogen," has been in use for many years, particularly for the prevention of osteoporosis (see Chapter 12). In this instance the Tibolone acts like an estrogen in the bones and heart, but like an anti-estrogen in the breasts and uterus. So, it will discourage fibroid growth but won't interfere with GnRH. Still in clinical trials, Tibolone is not yet approved for use in the United States.

- *Interferon:* This drug, normally used to treat illnesses such as hepatitis C, is also being investigated for its potential to shrink fibroid tumors. In one case study fibroids remained small for up to seventeen months after treatment stopped, raising the possibility that it may have permanent or certainly long-lasting results. To date, this treatment is still considered highly experimental.

If You Have Uterine Polyps: What You Need to Know

Among the most common uterine problems occurring during perimenopause are polyps—localized overgrowths of endometrial lining that come together to form a nodule that can project into the uterus. Polyps can be as small as a pencil eraser—or as large as a lemon, as layers of tissue "roll" together to form the growth. Polyps that lie close against the surface of the uterus are called "sessile" and are usually broad based and more flat in appearance. More often, however, polyps develop tiny "stalks" or stems that cause them to dangle down into the open space within the uterus itself.

Though only 25 percent of women develop polyps, most do so during the perimenopausal years. In fact, they rarely occur before age twenty, and as we pass each decade of life, the chance of developing a polyp becomes greater. For most women, the incidence peaks in their fifties and then gradually declines after menopause occurs. Fortunately, polyps are rarely, if ever, malignant, with far fewer than 1 percent containing abnormal cells. They do, however, account for up to 25 percent of all dysfunctional uterine bleeding that occurs during perimenopause.

While many women don't even know they have a polyp, when symptoms do occur they usually include irregular and sometimes heavy bleeding—which is the case for up to 50 percent of women diagnosed with this problem. There can also be some spotting after each monthly period ends. Some women report several days of "brown blood" after each cycle. Many women also experience spotting between periods, or sometimes spotting or bleeding after intercourse. Using low-dose birth control pills when you have polyps may also cause some spotting. In fact, if you are bothered by breakthrough bleeding while on the Pill, before you stop or change formulations, talk to your doctor about the possibility of an undiagnosed polyp. Less frequently there may be extreme bleeding from polyps, sometimes resulting in a prolonged period or a very heavy flow.

DIAGNOSING AND TREATING POLYPS:
WHAT YOUR DOCTOR CAN DO

While your symptoms, particularly dysfunctional bleeding, can clue you and your doctor in to the possibility of a polyp, as you read earlier, in many instances the same symptoms can be caused by other problems. That's one important reason to make certain your condition is properly diagnosed. In some instances, a uterine biopsy will provide the answer when the tissue sample shows remnants of polyp cells. This, however, depends on your doctor hitting the polyp when doing the biopsy, something that does not occur very easily. This is particularly true when a biopsy is done "blind," with no visual point of reference guiding selection of the tissue sample.

A transvaginal sonogram can sometimes help, but according to Dr. Steve Goldstein, professor of Obstetrics and Gynecology at NYU School of Medicine, this tool frequently misses polyps that may be lying close to the surface of the uterus—or sometimes even those on a stalk. This is because the "wand" pushes against the lining, flattening the polyp and making it difficult to visualize. What can help, says Goldstein, is a saline sonogram, or sonohysterogram. "With this procedure fluid can be introduced into the uterus, which slightly separates the front and back walls from each other," says Goldstein. In this way, your doctor can more clearly see a difference between a thickened area of the lining representing a polyp and generalized thickening resulting from an abnormal buildup of tissue.

Another option is a hysteroscopy (see "Diagnosing Your DUB," earlier in this chapter). This allows your doctor to directly view the inside of your uterus and not only visualize any polyps firsthand, but also remove them during the same procedure. This is considered a fairly minor surgery that is usually followed by several days of light spotting and a return to normal activities within a day or two. While a small percentage of polyps do grow back again, for most women this treatment is considered permanent.

In rare instances a polyp might "self-abort," meaning it pulls away from the wall of your uterus on its own and is passed through the vagina much like a blood clot. And while it may resemble a clot, frequently a polyp will be more structured in appearance, often resembling a tightly wound cigarette butt, and may also bear a longer, thinner "tail." Polyps also fail to dissolve in water. A blood clot, on the other hand, is a shapeless mass and will usually break up quite readily in water. If you suspect you may have passed a polyp and not a blood clot, call your doctor as soon as possible. In some instances you may be able to save the polyp and send it to a laboratory for testing. In addition, sometimes heavy bleeding or "flooding" can follow a self-aborting polyp, so it's important that your doctor check you afterward. In the event that heavy bleeding does occur, you may need a D&C or other procedure to stop it.

Should You Say No?
Making the Hysterectomy Decision

Once upon a time the operation known as a hysterectomy was considered a woman's saving grace. Medically defined as removal of part or all of the reproductive system, this surgery included not just the uterus but oftentimes the ovaries, fallopian tubes, and cervix as well. And it was routinely performed for just about everything that went wrong—or could possibly go wrong—between a woman's belly button and her thighs. Fibroid tumors, dysfunctional bleeding, even menstrual pain were all, at one point, reasons enough for a hysterectomy.

Then in the 1980s and '90s the pendulum swung decidedly away from this surgery. Women were cautioned continuously to "just say no" anytime a hysterectomy was even suggested. In fact, in many states around the nation, health departments were mandated to produce patient information documents that clearly spelled out all major treatment alternatives for any condition for which a hysterectomy was recommended. Doctors were then cautioned to make certain patients received adequate counseling on all available treatment options—and not telling your patient that another procedure could be helpful was tantamount to malpractice in many parts of the country.

While this dramatically reduced the number of unnecessary hysterectomies being performed, the number of procedures still remained high. Today, some 700,000 hysterectomies are performed in the United States each year, many of which some experts say could still be avoided.

According to Dr. Ernst Bartsich, associate professor of obstetrics and gynecology at New York Hospital-Cornell Medical Center in New York City, only about 15 percent of hysterectomies performed today are medically necessary—a figure on which many doctors agree.

Complicating matters a bit further, over the past decade a number of different approaches to this operation have also come to light. Some experts sought to lessen the drama of this surgery by developing various operating techniques that ostensibly would reduce the severity of this procedure and in many instances make recovery faster and easier. Doing away with the large abdominal incision and instead removing organs either through the vagina or via a tiny incision made in the "bikini line" were two ways doctors sought to make this operation more palatable. Similarly, some advocated removing only the uterus while leaving the ovaries intact.

For those who continued to oppose this surgery—including Bartsich—offering these options to a woman is like playing a shell game with her decision-making process.

"Placing so much emphasis on how you do the operation only serves to take attention away from the real issue—which is that this surgery is still being needlessly performed over and over, every day, in hospitals throughout the United States," says Bartsich. Telling women there is a better or safer way to do this operation does not justify doing it, he says, and only makes the decision more difficult. "Too often women are swayed by the technique instead of influenced by the facts," he says.

WHY IS A HYSTERECTOMY SO BAD?

Clearly, if and when a woman is diagnosed with uterine cancer, then a hysterectomy is unequivocally the best way to save her life. On this point there is little to argue about. The same can be said of ovarian cancer, in which case an oophorectomy (removal of the ovaries) becomes necessary, and a hysterectomy—the removal of the uterus—likely a good idea as well.

But what about other problems for which this surgery is still routinely performed—such as fibroid tumors, polyps, dysfunctional bleeding, adenomyosis, endometriosis, or sometimes even menstrual pain? Clearly this operation will help all these problems—so, why is that bad?

UNDERSTANDING HYSTERECTOMY

In the event that you need a hysterectomy, there are a number of options to consider. These involve not only the scope of the surgery itself, but also how it's performed—all of which can vary greatly, depending on many factors. To help you decide, here's what you should know:

- **Total hysterectomy:** This operation removes the uterus and cervix. The ovaries and fallopian tubes may or may not be removed.

- **Hysterectomy with bilateral salpingoophorectomy:** Here the uterus, cervix, fallopian tubes, and ovaries are all removed.

- **Subtotal or partial hysterectomy:** This surgery removes all of the uterus but leaves the cervix intact. The ovaries and the fallopian tubes may or may not be removed.

- **Radical hysterectomy:** Here, the uterus, cervix, and all surrounding tissue, as well as the upper vagina and some pelvic lymph nodes are removed. This operation is reserved for treating only the most invasive and severe cancers.

Additional surgical options for hysterectomy:

- **Total abdominal or "open" hysterectomy:** This involves a large incision in the abdomen that allows full open access to the uterus. Usually reserved for large pelvic tumors or suspected cancer. The incision is four to six inches in length; your

One reason, argue critics, is that very often the side effects of this operation can prove worse than the problem for which it was performed. According to the HERS Foundation, an independent research organization dedicated to disseminating information about hysterectomy, the effects can be devastating for many women. According to HERS, in

hospital stay is three to six days, and recovery time a full six weeks.

- **Vaginal hysterectomy:** In this procedure the uterus and, if need be, the cervix are removed through an incision in the vagina. This method is frequently used when the uterus is not enlarged, or when it has dropped down into the bladder area. The incision is small, and made into the vagina where a scar cannot be seen. Hospital stay is one to three days, with about four weeks of at-home recovery.

- **Laparascopically assisted vaginal hysterectomy (LAVH):** In this variation on the vaginal hysterectomy, your doctor will also make a tiny incision into your abdomen, into which is inserted a laparoscope—a telescope-like device that provides a look inside the entire pelvic cavity. This procedure is often used when the ovaries also have to be removed. Your hospital stay is between one and three days. And at-home recovery takes about four weeks.

- **Laparoscopic supracervical hysterectomy (LSH):** The newest type of hysterectomy, this procedure removes the uterus through a laparoscope but leaves the cervix intact. Some studies indicate this technique may reduce the risk of postoperative incontinence or pelvic floor prolapse. This requires several tiny incisions into the abdomen or navel, but they are less than a quarter-inch in length. Your hospital stay will be just twenty-four hours and recovery is six days or less.

addition to whatever operative injuries may occur, other common consequences include an increased risk of:

- Bone, joint, and muscle pain and immobility
- Loss of sexual desire, arousal, sensation

- Painful intercourse, vaginal damage

- Displacement of bladder, bowel, and other pelvic organs

- Urinary tract infections, urinary frequency, incontinence

- Chronic constipation and digestive disorders

- Profound fatigue

- Chronic exhaustion

- Altered body odor

- Loss of short-term memory, blunting of emotions, personality changes, despondency, irritability, anger, reclusiveness, and suicidal thinking

While many doctors continue to believe the uterus functions only in regard to reproductive activities, according to HERS reports—including a study of more than six hundred women who have had this surgery—the impact can be felt bodywide. In one jaw-dropping study out of the University of California at San Francisco, hysterectomy increased the risk of incontinence by a whopping 60 percent. For some, the problems may not even show up for ten or twenty years after the operation. Since the average age for a hysterectomy in the United States is forty-four, that leaves an awful lot of time to spend with your legs crossed trying not to pee!

Of equal concern has always been the effect of hysterectomy on sexual function, which according to the HERS Foundation, and many physicians, can be significant. Indeed, some experts contend that the uterus plays a much bigger role in sexual pleasure than previously believed and that losing this organ can blunt a woman's pleasure center in far more ways than once thought. Certainly, the number of women who contend that this *is* the case for them is staggering. However, in one study, published recently in the *British Medical Journal*, a group of doctors from the Netherlands found this *wasn't* the case at all. In their research involving over four hundred women who underwent hysterectomy for benign disease, those who did not have sexual problems prior to the surgery did not have them after the surgery. This was true regardless of the type of hysterectomy performed.

So what accounts for the vast difference in opinion and medical findings? Dr. Irwin Goldstein, a specialist in women's sexual function at Boston University, may have the answer. He believes the way in a which a woman experiences orgasm may be the telling factor regarding whether or not her sex life will be affected by a hysterectomy. According to Goldstein, if a woman reaches orgasm through deep vaginal stimulation, then a hysterectomy is likely to cause major problems. The reason, he says, has to do with the fact that the uterus is deeply intertwined with sensation-sending nerves that go right to the vagina. When you cut those nerves, says Goldstein, you sever connections to the vagina as well, so nearly all sense of sensation or pleasure vanishes—and you can't get it back. If, however, a woman experiences sexual pleasure and climax via clitoral stimulation, then a hysterectomy is less likely to affect the way she feels afterward. And while there are few, if any, statistics on the number of women who reach orgasm via vaginal stimulation compared to clitoral stimulation, something tells me that this is one time you don't need a bunch of numbers to help you make a decision—since clearly you know where the juiciest fruit in your basket lies!

MAKING THE HYSTERECTOMY DECISION

The more time I spend doing medical research, and the more studies I read, the more I am convinced that there is no one right medical answer for all women—and that includes hysterectomy. Certainly, when possible, always avoid any kind of dramatic surgery in favor of less drastic measures—whether it involves your uterus or your big toe! And to this end, I hope this chapter has provided you with some less drastic treatments for many of the problems that were previously treated via hysterectomy. At the same time, every medical decision, no matter how big or small, must take many factors into consideration, including not only the specific medical problem for which you are seeking relief, but also your personal health history, your lifestyle, and your expectations.

Certainly, in the event that you are diagnosed with uterine or ovarian cancer, a hysterectomy can be a life-saving operation. In other instances, when you are in pain or bleeding profusely—particularly if other treatments have failed to help you—then yes, a hysterectomy can be a powerful medical solution as well. If it turns out that a hysterectomy is your life-saving alternative, you will be glad to know that this operation has been vastly improved, even over the last several years.

At the same time, if there are other options for you to consider—be they in the form of medications or procedures—I urge you to find out all you can about what is available to help you. In addition to the information in this chapter, and in the chapters that follow, you will also find some important sources in the resource section at the end of this book. Hopefully, this information will guide you to a more meaningful discussion with your own doctor or, if need be, help you find a new physician—one who is willing to take your personal opinions and desires as well as your medical needs into consideration when deciding on a course of treatment. And on this count, I want to offer you still another word of caution. While many women count on their doctors to be truthful concerning all their treatment options, at least one study shows this may not be true. In a survey of more than eight hundred gynecologists published in the journal *Obstetrics and Gynecology* in August 2003, nearly 50 percent acknowledged that they routinely perform a more dramatic form of hysterectomy than may be medically necessary. More than 60 percent admitted they never gave their patients the option of choosing a less dramatic operation, even though that option was clearly available. No real reason was given for their decision to withhold the information from their patients.

So, while it's important to remember that you always have the right to say no to a hysterectomy (or any medical treatment), before you do you owe it yourself to investigate not only this surgery, but all your options. Then make your decision based on wise counsel and education, and not "gut reaction." Knowledge is power, and nowhere is this truer than when making decisions about your health and your health care.

4

Standing at a Pay Toilet with No Spare Change

Why Your Midlife Bladder Has a Mind of Its Own

Y ou should only hear how my friend Samantha makes fun of all those incontinence commercials on TV. You know the ones . . . where the woman is about to take a walk on the beach until she realizes that she won't be anywhere near a bathroom, so she declines.

"Didn't she ever just think she could pee in the ocean?" Sam says, giggling, as she continues to describe her vision of a conga line of fifty-something female celebrities dropping their drawers all along the shoreline of Malibu.

"Really, I think women spend way too much time worrying about whether or not they're near a bathroom," she's been known to announce anytime our little group was out to lunch and one of us was forced to cut a high-speed chase to the ladies' room. My other friend, Kathy—a few years older and a few wet sanitary napkins closer to reality—always rolls her eyes and shakes her head knowingly, fully aware that Sam, now aged forty-four, is not all that far from getting "up close and personal" with dribbles and leaks herself.

While many of us are like Sam, believing that incontinence is something strictly associated with "old age"—like orthopedic stockings and pillbox hats—the truth is that by the time we reach our mid-thirties, one in six women is experiencing this problem. By age fifty, that number jumps to one in two, so if it's not you, then you can rest assured it's your best girlfriend. According to Dr. Cynthia Hall, a specialist in women's pelvic health at the Cedars-Sinai Health System in Los Angeles, urinary incontinence—or loss of bladder control—is twice as common in women as in men. And while it's not a sure thing that every woman who passes through menopause will have to face this problem, don't be the least bit surprised—or embarrassed—if you find yourself among those who do.

The good news is that even if you do, there are a plethora of things that can help, from natural and behavioral treatments you can do on your own, to medicines your doctor can prescribe—there are even medical procedures that can help. Hall reports that more than 80 percent of women who pursue treatment for incontinence find the help they need.

Of course getting that help also means admitting you have a problem, and then not feeling so embarrassed or intimated that you fail to seek a doctor's advice. I know, I know . . . talking about this topic doesn't come easy. But you have to remember, we're the generation that changed the world in a multitude of ways. If you're old enough to need the information in this book, you probably remember when the only way they could advertise the Playtex "Cross Your Heart" bra on TV was if the model put it on over a turtleneck sweater! Now if you think about the recently televised Victoria's Secret fashion shows . . . well, you get my drift. The world has changed. We are the generation that took pretty much everything "out of the closet"—and then went ahead and redesigned the closet! Why not keep the ball rolling now? By recognizing and accepting reduced bladder control as a fact of life, we can not only feel better about our problem but also do something about it. And, as is the case with most things in life, success often begins with knowledge. Knowing just a bit about what's happening to your body—and what's changing in this area of your physiology—you can not only better cope with what's going on but also figure out which treatments might be right for you.

Understanding Your Midlife Bladder

Regardless of your age, your urinary system is designed to do just one job—filter your blood and remove any waste products that might upset the delicate balance between various tissue salts and water. While it sounds complicated, the whole system is surprisingly simple. As your kidneys filter your blood, the waste products—which are now in the form of urine—travel through two thin tubes called the ureter to your bladder. There, the urine is stored waiting for you to release it by urinating. When you do, it travels through another tube called the urethra, which transports it from your body.

To help the whole process function swiftly and efficiently, there are a number of muscles and nerves involved. In the wall of your bladder, for example, lies what is called the detrusor muscle. It allows your bladder to expand according to how much liquid you consume and then helps you hold the fluids until you are ready to urinate. So, when you gulp down that twenty-two-ounce Starbucks Mochaccino while driving on the freeway, you can thank your detrusor muscle for helping you stay dry until you get home.

Also helping you achieve this feat are two additional sets of muscles called sphincters. They are located at the juncture where your bladder meets your urethra—the tube through which urine leaves your body. The internal sphincters are involuntary muscles that keep a constant pressure on your urethra. The external sphincters are under your control, and are the very same muscles you taught your children to use when you were toilet training them.

In addition, a network of ligaments and muscles known as the pelvic floor supports your entire urinary system, along with part of your intestines and your reproductive system. It extends from your pubic bone in front all the way to your tailbone behind, with openings for the urethra, as well as your anus and your vagina. For the most part, these muscles remain firm and tight, helping to keep everything in place. You have the ability to tighten these muscles even further, which, along with controlling your external sphincter, controls urination.

Pulling the whole act together is a set of nerves designed to control reflex actions that ultimately control the timing of when you urinate. And if you've ever toilet-trained a child, then you know exactly how this works. Indeed, when we are babies, a group of sensory nerves located in the detrusor muscle send a signal to our spinal cord that the bladder is beginning to fill. In turn, a set of motor nerves located in the spine send a message back to the bladder telling it to contract, while signaling the urethra and pelvic floor muscles to relax. Together, these actions force urine from the body. Because in the beginning of life all this is automatic, babies urinate at will—whenever their bladder is full. Gradually, however, as the brain matures, we are able to learn how to override this automatic system and literally stop the signal that tells the bladder to empty. That is essentially what toilet training is all about.

As time passes and the bladder becomes more accustomed to control, it also becomes better at holding larger amounts of fluid. Eventually, when full control is assumed, we can command when and how often we urinate—at least up to a point. On the other hand, if anywhere along the line a snafu occurs in the system—either in the muscles that control the bladder function or the nerves that control response—urinary incontinence can occur. While there are a number of factors that influence these functions—including childbirth, a hysterectomy, diseases like diabetes, or nerve damage due to disease or injury—right now we'll concentrate on how the hormonal ups and downs of menopause, along with the natural aging process, can interfere and sometimes cause incontinence.

YOUR HORMONES AND BLADDER CONTROL

When my friend Natalie was in the throes of her perimenopause, she became withdrawn and quite sullen—more so than what might be expected, even with menopause mood swings. She stopped coming to lunches, constantly turned down invitations to dinner parties, and even begged off our famous shopping expeditions on Red Hot Sale days. It was, in fact, right after Natalie—a self-confessed shoe-a-holic—turned down my invite to attend the now famous "Shoes On Sale" breast cancer fund-raiser at the Pierre Hotel that I knew *something* had to be wrong. The following Saturday afternoon I paid her a visit, determined to pry that reason out of her!

"So, you *finally* have enough shoes, is that it?" I joked as we sat at her kitchen table sipping some herbal tea. Natalie was no dummy—she knew what I was getting at.

"Okay, so I've been begging off a few invites these last few months—what's the big deal?" she said, pushing her chocolate pastry around on the plate with far less enthusiasm than anything made of chocolate deserves!

"Natalie . . . it's not just that we miss having you around . . . it's that we're worried about you." I could see she was becoming uncomfortable with the conversation, so I tried to lighten things up. "I mean, if you're having this glorious affair with a Brad Pitt look-alike and he's simply taking up all of your time—hey, you go, girl!"

My friend smiled, grateful for my attempts, but it seemed as if she was still looking for a way to broach what was on her mind. "But if it's something else . . . you can tell me—honest—maybe I can help," I said, trying to sound as encouraging as I could.

Natalie took a deep breath and closed her eyes. She thought for a minute, and then spoke. "I'm wetting everything," she finally said, blurting it out like a shot from a cannon. "I mean, it's the bed one night, my jeans the next day, the couch one afternoon when I took a nap—they tell you about hot flashes, they prepare you for night sweats and mood swings—but nobody, *nobody* tells you you're going to wet the couch," she said, heaving a giant sigh of both relief and exasperation.

As lonely and isolated as incontinence made Natalie feel, I explained that she was far from alone in her distress. And while there was always a possibility that her condition was caused by an infection or even disease—such as undiagnosed diabetes—I was pretty sure her hormones were to blame. Remember when I told you that estrogen receptors are found throughout your reproductive tract? Well, they're also found in your entire urogenital system as well. For example, estrogen-sensitive cells line the urethra, helping to produce secretions that create a tighter seal between your bladder and the tube through which your urine flows. Estrogen also affects muscle tone, particularly in the sphincter muscles that surround the urethra and control the bladder. And it is also the estrogen receptors found throughout the urinary tract that increase blood flow to this entire area. This keeps cells healthy and prevents inflammation from developing. So, it's probably not hard to see how, when estrogen levels start to really take a drop—as they do when you are very close to reaching menopause—the opportunity is wide open for urogenital problems to occur. This includes not only urinary incontinence but also an increased risk of urinary tract infections.

And while it seems intuitive that so long as estrogen is behind the problem, HRT would help, doctors are somewhat mystified that this appears not to be the case. In fact, a study reported in *Ob. Gyn. News* in June 2003 showed that HRT might actually increase the risk of certain types of incontinence by more than 50 percent. In some instances, women who use hormones may be *four times* more likely to experience these problems than women who don't. What's more, the study also showed that the longer you use hormones, the greater your risk for urinary problems. But why does this occur?

One plausible explanation rests in the type or preparation of the commercial estrogen products used for HRT. In essence, they may simply not have the same effect on the urogenital system as the natural estrogens we produce in our bodies. Another possibility is that the synthetic progestin used in conjunction with estrogens may also yield a negative effect. Whatever the case is, what's clear is that while a lack of estrogen may be behind your problems, tossing back an estrogen prescription is not likely to help you. So what will? The answer depends a great deal on the specific type of incontinence you are experiencing. And to this end, it's important that you pay close attention to the explanations that follow. Not only will they help you to identify your specific problem, but they can also point you in the direction of the treatments that might help you the most.

PEEING IN YOUR PANTS: WHAT HAPPENS AND WHY

While all incontinence problems may have the same ultimate result—you lose bladder control—they can fall into two very distinct categories. The first is called *stress incontinence*—and no, you don't get it from the crazy demands of your boss, your teenage son's irritating girlfriend, or your husband who is trying to turn the family room into a hockey museum every chance he gets. Instead, this term refers to the *physiological* stress on your bladder whenever certain physical motions are made. Bladder muscles may be inherently weak already, particularly if you have given birth to one or more children, so once estrogen deficiency is added into the equation, problems can quickly ensue.

If your urinary problems are not so much "leakage" as a continuing urge to pee—even when your bladder isn't full—then you may have what doctors call "detrusor instability" or *urge incontinence.* You may know it as "overactive bladder"—at least that's what they call it on all those TV commercials! But whatever you call the problem, it involves overwhelming feelings of having to urinate, followed shortly by a total loss of urine, usually before you can make it to the bathroom. This was what Natalie experienced, causing her to wet her clothes and even her couch.

Essentially, urge incontinence develops when your body can no longer control involuntary bladder muscle contractions that dictate when urine leaves your body. While this can be caused by a number of factors, including nerve damage or disease, often there is no identifiable cause beyond the natural aging process itself. In women, however, declining estrogen also plays a role, altering the cells lining the bladder and impacting muscle control. In addition, many women can experience "bouts" of urge incontinence, often precipitated by urinary tract infections, which also increase during perimenopause.

If, like my friend Natalie, you appear to have urge incontinence, don't be surprised if you *also* experience some symptoms of stress incontinence—such as "leaks" when you engage in physical activity, including sex. A good percentage of perimenopausal women experience both types—a condition doctors call "mixed incontinence."

Finally, for a small percentage of women who experience still another midlife problem known as prolapse, a type of incontinence known as "overflow" can occur. Because prolapse causes either the bladder or uterus to drop from its normal position to a lower spot inside your pelvic cavity (see "When More Is Drooping Than Just Your Drawers," later in this chapter), when either happens a kink can develop in your urethra—much the way it does if you run over your garden hose in the driveway. That bend in your "internal hose" then interferes with the ability of urine to leave the bladder. The end result: Since your bladder never completely empties, it can become so full that it pushes hard on the urethra, causing urine to leak out, or overflow, at various intervals.

From the "M" File

KEY IN THE LOCK SYNDROME

Q: I've heard several women in my office use the phrase "Key in the Lock" Syndrome to describe incontinence problems. What does this mean?

A: You pull into your driveway after a long ride, lug the groceries out of your car trunk, and drag yourself up the walkway to your front door—all without feeling the urge to pee. But the minute you put your key in the front door and hear the lock click open, suddenly the "urge" becomes so overwhelming you barely make it to the bathroom in time. If this sounds familiar, then you too have experienced "key in the lock" syndrome—also known as "latchkey incontinence." It occurs when we regularly hold back the urge to urinate—like on the drive home from work, for example—only to "let loose" the minute we know a bathroom is nearby. If you do this often enough, you create a bladder-to-brain signal that automatically associates urinating with certain activities—like putting the key in the door. So, every time you do this, your brain registers that a bathroom is near, and sends a message to your bladder that it's okay to let it go! Eventually the association can become so strong that your bladder gets the signal to empty every time you put the key in the lock, even when it's not full. Of course the "I've got to pee this instant" association can involve any destination or activity—like when you arrive at work, or when you get into bed. The point is, whatever you train your bladder and brain to link with urination can trigger an automatic reflex action. The good news is, even old bladders can learn new tricks! You can retrain your bladder and your brain to respond in a different fashion and cut the association and the urge incontinence. The best way to do that is via bladder-retraining rituals, which you'll learn more about in the next section.

Getting Back Control:
What You Can Try on Your Own

If your incontinence is mild to moderate, there are a number of *simple* solutions that you can easily try on your own. In many instances, you may find it's all the help you need to permanently overcome your problem. And even if it turns out that you do need additional care, most of these self-help techniques can still be beneficial, sometimes helping you avoid more dramatic forms of treatment.

Based on guidelines recommended by the American College of Obstetricians and Gynecologists, as well as experts from the Harvard Medical School, what follow are some suggestions for ways you can begin taking back bladder control.

SOLUTION #1: BLADDER RETRAINING

If your problems involve a frequent need to urinate, along with urge incontinence, then it's possible you may have unknowingly conditioned your bladder to respond with a "gotta go now" signal, even if you really don't. This can occur, say experts, when you routinely urinate before your bladder is really full, which is often the case for those women who are afraid they *might* lose control. The only problem is, the more often you urinate, the more often you need to. Thus, this therapy involves retraining your bladder to hold increasing amounts of urine without causing you discomfort. The simplest way to accomplish this involves the following steps: First, keep track of how much you urinate during a twenty-four- or forty-eight-hour period. This includes the number of times you go to the bathroom and the number of "accidents" you have. Calculate the amount of time you generally wait between urinations. Then, start your retraining by adding ten to fifteen minutes to the shortest time between bathroom visits. If you typically wait two hours between urinations, try waiting two hours and fifteen minutes. Gradually increase your intervals over several weeks or months. To increase your ability to do this, you can also try both fluid management and pelvic floor exercises (see Solutions #2 and #3).

SOLUTION #2: FLUID MANAGEMENT

While it may seem as if you drink an "average" amount of fluid every day, you may be surprised to discover just how much you are actually consuming—and how easily you can control incontinence problems by simply controlling how much you drink. And even if you feel you aren't drinking a lot, remember, soups and cereals with milk also count as a liquid, as do fruits, which can be high in water content and contribute to urination.

If you're not certain just how much to cut down, doctors say that if your urine output is more than forty ounces a day, you may be consuming too much fluid. While this isn't harmful, it can certainly make your bladder work overtime, and exacerbate almost any incontinence problem, regardless of the cause. At the same time, remember that if your urine output drops much lower than thirty ounces daily, you increase your risk of a urinary tract infection—so strive for a balanced intake between thirty and forty ounces daily. In addition, the Harvard Medical School Special Report on Incontinence suggests the following tips:

- Don't drink more than eight ounces of fluid at one time.

- Limit fluids to between six and eight cups a day.

- Drink slowly—the faster your bladder fills, the greater your urge to urinate.

- Minimize consumption of caffeinated beverages and carbonated drinks—both help move fluids through your body more quickly.

- Decrease or eliminate alcohol consumption—this too can increase urination.

- If you are thirsty—from exercise or heat—drink water rather than other beverages. It's more likely to replenish the fluids your body needs rather than going straight to your bladder.

SOLUTION 3: EXERCISE

If you have had a baby, then you are probably already aware of one of the most effective exercises for incontinence. It's called the Kegel—and it was developed specifically to strengthen pelvic floor muscles that can weaken after childbirth. But even if you've never given birth, the hormone losses of perimenopause can also affect muscle strength, leaving your entire urogenital system with less support than what is necessary to control urine output. To this end, the Kegel exercise can help. To correctly perform a Kegel try the following techniques:

- While urinating, contract your pelvic muscles and try to stop your flow in midstream—then remember how it feels. Then at other times of the day (when you are not urinating) try to constrict these same muscles, holding each contraction for several seconds and then releasing. If you repeat ten contractions several times a day, you will strengthen the muscles involved in bladder control.

- Another technique involves tightening your vagina around a tampon—and remembering the muscles involved. Remove the tampon and try to re-create the feeling—then tighten and hold those muscles for several minutes at a time, up to ten times. Repeat three times a day for up to thirty contractions daily.

- To keep from contracting abdominal muscles, hold your hand over your stomach and press gently while doing the Kegels. Also be certain not to contract your thigh or buttock muscles or lift your pelvis while holding the contraction.

In addition to doing these exercises every day, you can also use this same muscle-tightening technique if you have any "warning" before you cough, sneeze, laugh, or do any activity that causes urine to leak. By quickly contracting these muscles and holding for up to one minute, you may quickly and easily offset the leak.

EXERCISE PLUS

In addition to Kegel exercises, you can also try using a weighted vaginal cone to help increase pressure and build muscles faster. This technique utilizes a series of specially designed, ultrasmooth tampon-shaped cones of varying weights, which are inserted, one at a time, into your vagina to help increase muscle tone. You begin with the lightest cone—about one ounce—and, while standing, contract your pelvic muscles to hold it inside. If the cone comes out with pressure, try inserting it deeper, or put your hand on your tummy and bear down to ensure you are not pushing it out with your abdominal muscles. If you can keep the cone in your body for three to five minutes while standing, then you are doing the exercise correctly. It should be done twice a day, gradually increasing the amount of time. Once you can hold the cone in your vagina while walking, coughing, laughing, or walking up or down stairs, you are ready to move on to the next-heaviest cone. Ultimately you should aim to hold in the heaviest cone for fifteen minutes, twice a day. Your doctor or pharmacist should be able to tell you where you can purchase the weighted cones. You can also talk to your doctor about renting or purchasing a home biofeedback machine. This tiny, handheld electronic device uses a vaginal sensor (either covered with a condom-like protector, or purchased for individual use), which helps relay the strength of your muscle contractions. When used in conjunction with Kegel exercises, the biofeedback can measure the strength of your contractions so you know when you're doing it right.

In still another high-tech technique I like to call the "lazy girls" (of which I am definitely one!) exercise, a similar vaginal sensor is used to deliver low levels of electrical current directly to your pelvic muscles. These short spurts of harmless electricity contract your muscles for you, accomplishing results similar to a Kegel. The strength of the currents can be customized, along with varying the time intervals of the contractions. According to experts at the Harvard Medical School, electronic stimulation helps stress incontinence by strengthening the muscles involved in controlling urination. For urge incontinence the electrical current may help "reset" the triggers that allow your nervous system to control urination. Portable devices are available for use at home, while larger, more powerful units are frequently used in doctors' offices.

Bladder Control:
How Your Doctor Can Help

While it's important to give your self-help solutions at least a few months to begin working, sometimes, no matter how long you Kegel, the leaks and floods just don't improve all that much. When this is the case, it may be time for you to see your doctor. While oftentimes your gynecologist can help you, if your symptoms are significant and your incontinence is interfering with your social or work life, then you may want to schedule an appointment with a urogynecologist—a doctor who specializes in female incontinence problems.

To give either doctor a better understanding of the nature of your specific incontinence experiences, it may be helpful to keep a "bladder diary" for at least a few days prior to your appointment. This should document the amount of fluid you drink, when you drink it, and when you have your "voiding accidents." In addition, you may also want to prepare ahead for your visit by jotting down answers to the following questions—information that your doctor is likely to need, including:

- When your problem started.

- Whether you have a problem with "leakage" or more significant urine loss.

- If your problem is worse at night or during the day.

- Any foods, activities, or specific liquids that make your problem worse.

- If you have an incontinence problem during or after intimate relations.

- The amount of your urine loss: A little means your underwear is damp; a moderate amount means your underwear is soaked; a lot means your clothing is soaked and your bladder completely empties during each episode.

- The amount of fluid you consume daily including not only drinks but also soups and fruit, including what and how much of each.

- The number of times you visit a bathroom to urinate during the day, and evening; if you get up during the night to urinate and if so, how often.

- If your continence problems are interfering with your social or work life.

- Any medications you are taking for any reason, including both hormones and herbal preparations.

- Your menstrual history—including the last time you had a regular period, if you are experiencing any menopause-related symptoms, if you have had any gynecological surgeries, if you have given birth, and if so, how many times.

YOUR INCONTINENCE EXAM: WHAT TO EXPECT

Once your doctor has had a chance to assess your health history and your incontinence information, he or she can choose from a number of different diagnostic tests or procedures—each designed to help discover the specific source of your problem.

In general, however, your exam will likely include the following:

- A test of your reflexes, as well as an observation of your muscle strength and your nerve health—all of which can often be determined by a series of pinpricks in your foot or leg. To test the nerves in your genital area your doctor may stroke the skin near your lower back or anus to check for muscle contraction.

- A thorough pelvic exam to assess the strength of your pelvic floor muscles, and to check for the position of your bladder and uterus. Your doctor may also gently tap on your clitoris looking for a contraction—a sign of good muscle tone in this area—and check your vaginal lining for signs of atrophy or other indications of significant estrogen loss.

- A test of your muscle control that involves standing with one leg raised on a stool or box and coughing as you hold a paper towel over your genital area. If urine appears on the towel, then it is likely you have a stress incontinence problem.

- If stress incontinence is suspected—but the "paper towel" test is negative—your doctor may send you home with a supply of sanitary pads that have been carefully weighed. You will be asked to wear the pads over a twenty-four-hour period, changing every few hours and saving the removed pads in a sealed container. The pads will be returned to your doctor and weighed again to determine how much urine you lost over the course of one day.

If your exam does not reveal enough specific information, your doctor may suggest a number of other more detailed tests designed to further zero in on the source of your problems. These can include:

- *Uroflowmetry:* In this test you will urinate into a funnel that helps measure amount and flow, which can in turn help determine if your bladder muscles are weak.

- *Postvoid Residual Volume:* This test involves catheters or tubes that are inserted into your bladder to test how much fluid is left after you urinate.

- *Cystometry:* This also involves the insertion of a catheter designed to check the pressure in your bladder, the amount of urine it can hold, and the point of fullness at which you get the urge to urinate.

- *Electromyography (EMG):* Here, painless electrode patches applied to your genital area help measure the activity and coordination of the muscles involved in bladder control.

- *Cystography:* In this test an X-ray is used to help determine if blockages exist in your urinary passage.

- *Ultrasound:* Harmless sound waves are used to measure the placement and size of your urogenital organs and to detect any abnormalities, such as tumors or kidney stones.

- *Cystoscopy:* This test uses a lighted telescope similar to the instrument used during hysteroscopy to diagnose uterine abnormalities (see Chapter 3). It is inserted through your urethra and into your bladder.

INCONTINENCE TREATMENTS:
THE MEDICATIONS THAT CAN HELP

Depending on what your test results show, your doctor may "prescribe" nothing more than the self-help techniques described earlier in this chapter. In other instances, however, some additional medical help may be warranted. If so, the first line of defense is often medication—one of the various types of new drugs designed to aid bladder control. If, like my friend Samantha, you too have noticed those beachy, dreamy, shampoo-type commercials about incontinence, then you are probably already aware of what some of these medications are. If not, what follows is a short guide to what's available. While you'll need to rely on your doctor's advice as to which ones are right for you, having this information on hand should help you to open the discussion and find the right medication to suit your needs.

- *Anticholinergics:* This group of medications includes drugs such as oxybutynin (Ditropan), hyoscyamine (Levbid, Cytospaz), and tolterodine (Detrol), as well as the newer, once-daily extended-relief drugs Ditropan XL and Detrol LA. They are most commonly prescribed for urge incontinence and are thought to work by inhibiting bladder contractions while increasing your ability to hold more fluids. They can also be used to delay the initial urge to urinate, thus reducing the discomfort of trying to "hold it in." Although approximately 80 percent of patients who try these medications are satisfied, up to 20 percent have to quit, mostly due to side effects. These include dry eyes, dry mouth, headache, constipation, rapid heartbeat, and confusion. However, clinical trial data shows that at least some of these problems occur to a much lesser degree when using the new extended time-release once-daily formulations.

- *Antispasmodics:* While this is a broad category that includes many different medications, the two most commonly prescribed for incontinence are flavoxate (Urispas) and dicyclomine (Bentyl). They are frequently recommended for urge incontinence and work to relax the bladder muscle. This controls contractions, which in turn controls urination. Both medications also have some anticholinergic properties as well, which can also increase their effectiveness. Side effects for these drugs include weakness, dizziness, drowsiness, hallucinations, insomnia, dry mouth, and restlessness. Although both medications are commonly prescribed and have been for years, recent studies have suggested that Urispas may have much less value as an incontinence treatment than previously thought.

• *Alpha-adrenergic agonists:* The drugs in this category include ephedrine and pseudoephedrine, two ingredients commonly found in over-the-counter decongestants and some diet pills. While they are not approved specifically for urinary problems, women who take them for other reasons often report they help stress incontinence. They are thought to work by stimulating the muscles around the neck of the bladder and urethra, causing them to contract and form a tighter "seal." This in turn keeps urine from leaking during times of physiological stress, such as laughter or exercise. Side effects include agitation, insomnia, anxiety, dry mouth, and headache. You should not take these medications if you have heart disease, glaucoma, diabetes, an overactive thyroid, or high blood pressure. In addition, you should not use these medications for stress incontinence without your doctor's okay.

• *Antidepressants:* While experiencing incontinence can easily leave you feeling depressed and even withdrawn, antidepressant medications are not prescribed for this reason. Instead, in low doses they can act much like the newer incontinence drugs to quiet bladder spasms and contractions and help control urge incontinence. The specific drugs in this category include older medications known as tricyclic antidepressants, including imipramine (Tofranil) and amitriptyline (Elavil). Because they can cause drowsiness, these medications may also help you sleep through the night without being woken by frequent urges to urinate. Side effects include drowsiness, blurred vision, constipation, and dry mouth. The newer class of antidepressants known as SSRIs (like Prozac, Zoloft, and Paxil) is not effective against incontinence.

• *Antidiuretic hormone:* If your main problem is holding urine overnight, then this type of medication can help. The body naturally produces a hormone known as vasopressin. It originates in the pituitary gland but quickly sends a signal to the kidneys to control the amount of urine produced. A synthetic version of that hormone—a drug known as desmopressin (DDAVP)—can tell the kidneys to do the same thing while you sleep. Much the way a diuretic helps drain water from your tissues, an antidiuretic helps you retain fluid. Side effects include fluid retention at a level that can be dangerous if you have high blood pressure or any degree of congestive heart failure.

• *Cholinergics:* If your doctor diagnoses a weak bladder muscle and urinary overflow, medications in this group (drugs like Urecholine or Duvoid) can help. Essentially they work by strengthening bladder contractions, which in turn prevents the overflow from occurring. Side effects include shortness of breath, blurred vision, sweating, and dizziness. If you take these drugs before meals you may avoid an upset stomach. You should, however, totally avoid these medications if you have asthma, hyperthyroidism, or Parkinson's disease or if you have recently undergone any urogenital or gastrointestinal surgery.

• *Estrogen:* While oral HRT can make incontinence worse, ironically, when topically applied, estrogen alone may help, mostly by strengthening the tissues in the urinary tract. Creams, suppositories, gels, tablets, and devices that secrete estrogen have all been found useful— and most do not need progesterone to balance their effects. While there is little in the way of *scientific* proof that topically applied estrogen works, many women report anecdotally that it does. As with all hormone therapy, risks are often dictated by your personal and family health history—including whether or not you are at risk for breast or endometrial cancer. For a complete report on natural estrogen creams see Chapters 8 and 10.

GOING WITH THE FLOW:
DEVICES FOR INCONTINENCE

While many women find that medications alone provide all the help they need, my friend Natalie ultimately found her saving grace when her doctor introduced her to one of several vaginal devices available to "catch" urine overflows and leaks. Working somewhat like a menstrual cup that is inserted near the cervix, a urine collection device is placed near or sometimes into the urethra and serves as a kind of "well," preventing urine from leaving your body. Although some are available only by prescription, others are found in pharmacies, and you can buy them on your own. Still, it's important that you don't purchase these items until you have at least one incontinence consultation with your doctor. It's important that you know the nature of your problem before you attempt to use this solution. That said, here's a rundown of the vaginal devices that are available, and how they can help.

VAGINAL FOAM PADS

Sold under brand names such as Miniguard, Softpatch, or UroMed, these soft foam pads with an adhesive coating are placed over the opening of the urethra, where they create a seal that prevents urine from leaving the body. Obviously they must be removed prior to urination, and replaced with a new one afterward to prevent further leakage. If you don't have urge incontinence, the pads can be safely worn for up to five hours without removal, so they are excellent if you have a social event, business meeting, or other circumstance where it would be difficult to get to a bathroom. They can also be worn during exercise, but some women report a certain degree of slippage when activity is brisk. They cannot, however, be worn during sexual intercourse. In studies of women with mild to moderate incontinence, the foam pads were shown to cut the number of "accidents" nearly in half. In women with severe incontinence—about thirty-four "leaks" or more per week—the incidence was reduced by nearly two-thirds, down to ten leaks or less per week. When leakage did occur, it was said to be very slight.

As effective as these pads are, there are a few cautions to consider. They should not be used if you have any urinary or vaginal tract infections, or if you have had surgery for incontinence. Also, they must be used

From the "M" File

UTIs AND HOT FLASHES

Q: Am I the only woman in America whose major menopause symptom is urinary tract infections? I am forty-eight and haven't had much in the way of hot flashes, night sweats, or even mood swings, but ever since my periods started becoming irregular (sometimes every two weeks, other times not for two months), I've been getting all these urinary tract infections. It seems I just get rid of one and another pops up. Is there a reason for this? And is it hormone related?

A: First—you can relax. No, you're not the only one this is happening to—although I must say about a zillion women right now are wondering how come they got all the hot flashes and you don't have any. Lucky girl. That said, UTIs (urinary tract infections) round the clock are not much fun either—and yes, they are apt to occur more easily during this time of life. Here are the reasons: Whether or not you are experiencing hot flashes or other common signs of estrogen deprivation, if your periods are irregular and you are forty-eight years old, it's highly likely your hormone levels have already started to plummet. As they do, estrogen receptors within your urogenital tract don't receive the normal amounts of stimulation. This results not only in a thinning of the vaginal wall and symptoms such as urge or stress incontinence, but also in an increased risk of UTIs. According to experts from the North American Menopause Society (NAMS) a lack of estrogen also results in shrinkage of your urethra—the already short tube (short compared to

for stress incontinence only and are not considered a treatment for any other type of urinary tract problem.

URETHRAL SHIELDS

These are small, round silicone "caps" that attach by suction and support the inner muscles that control urine flow. An ointment is applied first to

a man's) that carries urine out of your body. The shorter the urethra, the more vulnerable you are to infection, since bacteria have a relatively short walk from the outside of your body to the inside. In addition, NAMS experts say that as estrogen levels drop, the acid level inside your vagina changes to a more alkaline environment—an atmosphere that helps bacteria thrive. So, any little bugs that make their way to your vagina (which can happen simply from careless bathroom hygiene, as well as during sex) can multiply quickly and then hop right up into your urinary tract.

Most important, are you certain you are having urinary tract infections—and not just a case of stress or urge incontinence? Commonly, their symptoms can overlap. And while most UTIs cause pain and burning on urination and incontinence problems generally don't, if you are continually using sanitary napkins or even incontinence pads for protection, you could be experiencing a burning irritation similar to what is experienced during an infection—even if none is present. The bottom line: If you haven't already done so, make certain your doctor diagnoses at least one UTI with a urine culture for bacteria. Next, if it is a UTI, take whatever antibiotic he or she prescribes for the full amount of time—don't stop just because symptoms let up. Lastly, talk to your doctor about whether or not local estrogen therapy can help you—specifically, vaginal estrogen creams that, by some reports, can increase the thickness of the vaginal wall beginning as soon as ten days after use (see Chapters 8 and 11). You can also talk to your doctor about prophylactic antibiotic treatment, which involves taking a very low dose of antibiotics whether you have an infection or not, to "cover" you for a period of time.

help create a vacuum seal that holds the cap in place. When you urinate, you must remove the cap, wash it with soap and water, and then reapply it after you are done. Sold under brand names such as CapSure or FemAssist, they have been clinically shown to work for many women. In one study of patients with stress incontinence, CapSure successfully reduced urine leaks by 96 percent within seven days. Of those patients 82 percent reported they were completely dry. In a study on FemAssist, 47 percent of women experienced complete cessation of incontinence, while 33 percent reported their urine loss was cut by some 50 percent. In addition, FemAssist was equally effective for stress, urge, or mixed incontinence. Side effects of these devices include a slight risk of irritation and urinary tract infections. In addition they can be inconvenient to use, since you may frequently have to remove and wash them in a public restroom.

URETHRAL TUBES OR SLEEVES

These devices work in a similar fashion to the cap shields, catching urine before it leaks out of your body. In one product known as the Reliance Urinary Control Device, a tiny balloon attached to a thin tube is inserted into the urethra via a reusable syringe. Once it is inside the body, the syringe helps inflate the balloon, which presses against the urethra. This helps seal the opening and block the urine leaks. Although the device works well, it must be removed each time you urinate (you pull a string that deflates the balloon) and replaced with a new one. This device also carries a high risk for urinary tract infection and some degree of discomfort. If you want to try it, however, you'll need a doctor's prescription, since your urethra must be measured in order to get the correct size balloon.

A slightly different version is a product called FemSoft. Made of silicone, this tubelike device sits inside a liquid-filled sleeve. You insert the tube into your urethra, and the sleeve conforms to the exact shape of your body. This creates a seal at the neck of your bladder that prevents leakage. FemSoft must be replaced after urination. So far there have been no adverse reports of increased risk of irritation or infection.

VAGINAL DEVICES

These are a series of devices that, although inserted into the vagina and not the urethra, can still offer some support to the urogenital system and in this way reduce leakage and flow. Among the most popular is a vaginal pessary, a doughnut-shaped device that, once inserted into the vagina, helps support the internal walls. Usually made of silicone, they are reasonably comfortable but must be measured and fitted by a doctor first.

Once the proper fit is attained, most can be left in place for a number of days, or sometimes even weeks, before being removed, cleaned, and reinserted. While some women can do this easily on their own, don't be surprised if you need your doctor's help, at least the first time you try this. Your doctor should also advise you as to how often your pessary should be removed. Although a small number of women report it does interfere with intercourse, most often it can be worn comfortably during sex and cannot be detected by your partner. In addition to helping with incontinence these devices are also effective for vaginal prolapse (see "When More Is Drooping Than Just Your Drawers," later in this chapter).

Along these same lines you can also try the Introl Bladder Neck Support device—a kind of flexible ring that is also inserted into the vagina. The design is such that it presses against the vaginal wall, which in turn presses on the urethra, offering support there as well. Using this device will require a doctor visit, since you must be measured internally in order to get the correct fit. Once you do, this device is up to 83 percent effective against stress incontinence. While it can be left in during urination, it has to be removed and cleaned at some point afterward. Some women report a degree of discomfort, and studies show it might increase the risk of vaginal or urethral infections.

When Surgery Is the Answer: What You Should Know

Although many women find relief through products, devices, or sometimes simply exercise, there are those, like my friend Stephanie, who found that surgery was the best approach for her.

"I just want the problem to be over—I don't want to mess with devices and I tried the exercises and they just don't help enough," she said one day as we discussed the pros and cons of urogenital surgery. And the more we talked, the more it seemed that surgery would be her best option. As a fashion photographer she frequently traveled all over the world and often found herself not only on long flights but also in exotic locations, which, as she is fond of reminding me, is "not so glamorous as you would imagine." Indeed, she one time found herself having to take a

From the "M" File

TAMPONS FOR INCONTINENCE?

Q: My best friend says that using tampons can help incontinence—I say she's nuts and doesn't know her own anatomy! Maybe what she read is that sanitary napkins work, which makes sense. But tampons? She has got to be wrong!

A: Best friends sometimes do know best! Although I see your point about the anatomy lesson, the truth is tampons can be helpful, but not in the way you are thinking. When used to control stress incontinence, the tampon serves to push on the vaginal wall, which in turn compresses the urethra. This gives the muscles some added support and may help you control urine flow when you laugh or sneeze. Many report it's also an excellent method for controlling leaks during exercise. In one study 86 percent of women who had mild stress incontinence found the tampons kept them completely dry while working out. In addition, nearly 30 percent of those with severe incontinence also found the tampons helped. If you try this method, be certain to apply a good amount of KY Jelly on the tampon to make insertion easier, and to keep the fibers from sticking to your vagina. Remember, however, that when used for this purpose a tampon should only be kept in for a short period of time—to cover you during an exercise session, for example. Without the normal fluids and secretions present during a menstrual period, irritations and even infections can ensue if a tampon is left in too long. And of course, as you pointed out, sanitary pads, or even incontinence pads, can help as well. While they won't stop the leaks, they can prevent them from reaching your clothes and causing you an embarrassing stain.

cargo flight through the jungles of South America to reach a fashion shoot for a top magazine—on a plane, she said, that didn't even have seats, let alone a toilet. So for her, surgery was beginning to sound as if it was the right option.

If you, too, want the problem to "just be over" with minimal maintenance in the future, then you should definitely speak to your doctor about the advantages of having a surgical procedure to correct your incontinence. Remember, you will have to consult with a urogynecologist or urological surgeon in order to get the best advice. Most gynecologists have only basic knowledge about these procedures. In addition, because stress and urge incontinence are treated somewhat differently, particularly in the surgery arena, it's imperative that you be correctly diagnosed before planning any type of operation. Having the wrong procedure will not only fail to correct your problem, it could make things worse.

To find out the latest surgical options for incontinence, visit www.yourmenopause.com.

When More Is Drooping Than Just Your Drawers: What to Do About Bladder Prolapse

My friend Leigh called me one day on the verge of hysteria. "My vagina is falling out—I swear to you—I can see it and I know the menopause gods are punishing me for dumping that younger guy I was dating at work." Despite her sense of humor, she was clearly upset.

"You want to give me that again? I didn't know you were dating a younger guy," I said, hoping she would relax just a few decibels.

"I'm not kidding you—something looks as if it's coming out of my vagina—like I'm giving birth to some alien."

"Are you in pain—or bleeding?" I asked.

"No—no pain, no bleeding—just my insides looking as if they are going to land on the kitchen floor any minute—I am *so* scared I don't know what to do."

I told my friend to sit tight—I would hail a cab and with any luck be there in ten minutes. Predictably, by the time I arrived she had worked herself up to near hysteria, standing in the doorway of her apartment with her hand pressed firmly against her crotch—looking a lot like Madonna, only without the leather breast cups.

Although I was pretty sure I knew what was wrong with Leigh, I hauled her downstairs, into the taxi, and off to the doctor's office to be sure. Within an hour, we both knew what I had suspected from the start: She was diagnosed with a "Grade 3 cystocele," otherwise known as a severely fallen bladder. It happens when the wall that lies between the bladder and the vagina becomes so weak it can no longer hold things in place. As a result, the bladder pushes down so far it begins to bulge out through the opening of the vagina. That's the "alien birth" Leigh described on the phone. And while it's certainly a frightening experience, it's not nearly as dangerous as you might think—considering that a part of your body that belongs on the inside is now clearly on the outside!

And, in all fairness, this didn't just happen "out of the blue" the way Leigh made it sound. She admitted having had some incontinence problems for a while, *and* her doctor said she had suspected it might come to this. In fact, cystocele occurs in three stages, or "grades." In its mildest form (known as Grade 1) the bladder drops only a short way down into the vagina—so you don't really see anything on the outside. Most often incontinence is the only sign that something is wrong. Occasionally your gynecologist may notice the drop during a pelvic exam—or more likely with the help of a vaginal sonogram, but this is not always the case.

More severe effects can be seen with a Grade 2 cystocele—which means that your bladder has dropped low enough to approach the opening of your vagina. While you are not likely to see anything different, you can sometimes feel it if you place your finger inside your body—and your doctor is likely to see and feel the problem during a pelvic exam. In a Grade 3 cystocele—the type Leigh experienced—the bladder drops so far down into the vagina that it actually begins to bulge out through the opening, and it can be easily felt and even seen. Frequently, doctors can diagnose a Grade 2 or Grade 3 cystocele on sight because it's easy to see what's going on, particularly on an OB/GYN exam table. To help diagnose a Grade 1, or sometimes a Grade 2, cystocele, your doctor may ask you to take a cystourethrogram—essentially, an X ray of the bladder during urination. Other tests (see "Your Incontinence Exam," earlier in this chapter) may be required as well.

Although many women develop cystocele after giving birth—particularly if they have a hard labor and do lots of pushing—it can also come about as a result of other significant straining. If you lift something very

heavy, for example, or if you repeatedly strain when having a bowel movement. From the perimenopause standpoint a cystocele can develop from
a simple lack of estrogen. As you read earlier, it is estrogen that helps keep
the muscles around the vagina strong, which in turn helps keep the bladder in its proper place. As estrogen levels plummet, muscles can get
weaker, and when they do sometimes even a small strain can cause the
bladder to shift and fall, sometimes dramatically.

TREATING BLADDER PROLAPSE: WHAT YOU CAN DO

If your cystocele is a Grade 1, frequently no treatment will be required—
particularly if it is not causing you any significant problems. You should
avoid lifting anything heavy or straining, particularly when having a
bowel movement. If you are suffering from constipation (another common perimenopause symptom) you should talk to your doctor about prescribing a stool softener. Unlike a laxative, which moves your bowels for
you, a stool softener simply makes your stool softer so your natural bowel
movement becomes easier.

If your cystocele is a Grade 2 or if it bothers you, a pessary device
placed in your vagina (see the earlier section on vaginal devices) may help
keep your bladder in place. Sometimes local applications of estrogen
cream, with or without a pessary, can also be helpful, particularly if you
have already passed menopause. If, however, your problems are severe—
a Grade 3 cystocele—you may need surgery to reposition your bladder.

Bladder Control:
Out of the Closet and Back into Life

As if hot flashes and night sweats and mood swings and weight gain
weren't enough of a kick in the butt, yes, it's true, wetting your thong can
be part of the aging process. But as I said when this chapter began, what
sets our generation apart from most others is our relentless dedication not
only to finding answers to our problems, but to bringing many of these
problems to light.

I remember about fifteen years ago—right after I wrote my first book on pregnancy—I wanted desperately to write a book on menopause, much like the one you are reading now. I prepared a proposal and submitted it to my publisher at the time—a much older but very well educated and very savvy gal—who I was certain would just love the idea. Boy was I wrong. She called me up soon after reading my book outline and told me what she thought.

"Are you crazy," she almost whispered in hush tones into the phone. "Women don't talk about these things, much less read about them—who would buy this book?"

Of course I was nowhere near perimenopause at the time, but I did know many women who were—and I remembered how much my own mother suffered with symptoms. I tried to convince her she was wrong, but it was "no soap." She didn't want the book and neither did a half dozen other publishers, all of whom had pretty much the same reaction she did. Frustrated, I simply gave up on the idea—but I'm glad someone else didn't. That "someone" is the now critically acclaimed author Gail Sheehy. The book was *The Silent Passage,* and it was the first of the new ilk of menopause books—and the knife that cut the emotional duct tape that had kept this subject bound and gagged for way too long. Finally, our "secret" was out of the closet! And much like PMS, menstrual pain, breast cancer, and other strictly female problems, menopause was *finally* being talked about as well. Our generation has done that—for us, and for all of our daughters and granddaughters who follow.

I'd like to see the same thing happen for all of you who may be suffering with incontinence problems. Although the discussion of this subject is much more open than in the past, I can still see that this topic is a source of great embarrassment and upset for many women—so much so that many of you reading this chapter, and suffering with these problems, may simply avoid getting medical help.

So, let's make a deal: Let's decide here and now that our generation *can* take women's health the whole way home. Just as we have brought menopause and so many other women's issues into the public arena, let's do the same for incontinence problems as well. No woman should ever have to be embarrassed or ashamed or frightened to seek medical help— particularly when there is so much help available. So if you have this problem, don't ignore it, and don't put off seeing your doctor. And if you're one of the lucky ones—someone who solves this problem with some of the self-help remedies in this chapter, or maybe even has no problem at all—then please, pass on this encouragement to your sister or your best friend, who may still be suffering. Lend her your support and understanding, and encourage her to seek help. It's the least we can do for ourselves and each other—and our generation.

5

Getting Back Your Groove and Your Glow

Droop, Drop, and Wrinkle Advice for Midlife Skin

Our names are different. Our faces are not the same. Even our ages can vary dramatically. But in many ways, our stories are remarkably similar. One unsuspecting night we kick off our slippers, pull on our PJs, snuggle under the covers, and drift off to sleep a relatively hot-looking midlife mamma. Next morning, we wake up, look in the mirror . . . and scream bloody murder! There, staring right back at us like some Palm Beach matron from a pink-neon bingo parlor, is this aging stranger—right there in the mirror, some incredibly older woman who looks remarkably like a great-aunt we barely knew! How the heck did it happen? And so fast?

Wrinkles. Lines. Creases. Sags, droops, and jowls, and a face that we swear was not there even eight hours ago. And while I can't quite figure out how it all happens so quickly (though my friend Robyn swears it has something to do with how often you wash your bathroom mirror), when it hits, it hits hard—worse than the first time a delivery boy calls you "ma'am." And more obvious than when you walk into the office cafeteria with your twenty-seven-year-old secretary and realize how amazingly well you are blending in with the wallpaper. And if it hasn't happened to you yet, trust me, my sweet, if you're over forty-five, you're just a few bottles of moisturizer away from that blood-curdling scream.

Fortunately, you only have to scream the one time. Because once the realization passes, it all gets *much* easier—or at least it can. Are you ever going to look twenty-five again? Sorry, no—not even with an Extreme Makeover. But you can get back your groove—and your glow—and become an amazingly sexy, vibrant, healthy, and, yes, gorgeous middle-aged siren with a whole lot less effort than you might think!

How Your Skin Ages—and What You Need to Know to Look Young

My friend Leigh tells me she hates the way her skin looks. But oddly enough, when I ask her what is it about her skin that she hates, she never really has a specific answer.

"I just look old," she always says, "like I'm somebody's mother."

"But you are somebody's mother," I gently remind her, as I tick off the names of her three teenage sons.

"Yes, but I never thought I would actually *look* like somebody's mother—like, like *my* mother—at least not this soon," she says, placing her fingertips on the corners of each cheekbone and pushing the extra flesh toward her ears in a kind of mock face-lift.

If you feel pretty much the same way—like you just look "old" and you don't really know why—then believe me, you're not alone. While it may seem as if this whole aging thing happened overnight, in truth, experts tell me that's because the whole sneaky process starts a lot sooner than most of us realize—sometime in our mid-thirties. If we look very carefully, that's when we begin to see some of the "subtle" changes in our epidermis—the first of the three layers of our skin. Those changes are centered around a process called "cell turnover." This is the natural life-and-death cycle of skin cells that allows your complexion to renew itself every fifteen to thirty days—at least when you are young. Indeed, as old cells die, new ones come forward from the deeper layers, pushing upward and casting the dead cells out of the way. The newer the skin cells, the more moisture they can hold and, ultimately, the younger and fresher your complexion looks. So, rapid cell turnover is a distinct advantage.

But beginning around age thirty-five, the cycle of skin cell renewal starts to slow down—and the process gets even slower as more birthdays pass. Eventually, new cell growth slows to such an extent that our "old" cells are forced to hang around on the surface of our skin for a truly extended period of time—which is what creates that dull, "lifeless" look that my friend Leigh and so many other women see in the mirror beginning around age forty. Since the "older" cells are on the surface of your skin, the drier and more "rough" your skin can look, and the texture of your complexion seems to change as well. Makeup doesn't look quite the way it did before, for example, and you may find that your foundation or even your blush seems to be exaggerating fine lines and creases.

As a little more time passes, even more changes can become apparent—thanks to activity that has been going on in the dermis, or second layer of your skin. This is where your collagen supply is manufactured—a kind of connective tissue that helps plump your skin and give your face that "bloom of youth." In fact, 70 percent of your skin's collagen is made in cells called fibroblasts, located in this second layer of skin. As you age those cells begin to work less efficiently, so less collagen is produced. As a result your skin begins to lose some support from underneath, allowing fine lines and wrinkles to become even more apparent. While no one is quite certain what causes collagen production to falter, researchers now believe it may actually be linked to a corresponding drop in estrogen. Reporting in the *Journal of Molecular Medicine* in 2002 a group of Polish dermatologists documented the existence of estrogen receptors in those collagen-making fibroblast cells. When these cells are flooded with estrogen—as they are when you are young, and especially during pregnancy—collagen production thrives. The end result—your skin looks plump and juicy and young. You have that "glow." But as you age, and estrogen levels fall, fibroblasts can be literally "starved" for hormone attention. When they are, collagen production slows significantly—and your skin suffers the blow.

Down one more floor is the subcutaneous layer of your skin, where quite a bit of aging activity is also silently taking place. Deep in this third layer lie some key fat reserves that, along with collagen, help to give your skin support and add shape and definition to your face. As you age, some of those fat reserves begin to break down—and that can dramatically impact the way your face looks. Cheekbones may not seem as high, while eyelids, brows, and even your forehead seem to droop. Since the least amount of fat is found just under the eyes, even a tiny loss in this area can result in deep indentations, almost creating a hollow in the area between your lower eyelid and your cheekbone.

Interwoven between all three layers of your skin are elastin fibers— bands of connective tissue that give your skin support from underneath. Think of it as scaffolding for your face! As a result of simply growing older—as well as the effects of years of environmental abuse, like sun exposure and pollution—those fibers begin to break down, losing some of their elasticity. Remember how the scrunchie you used to tie your hair back last summer needed to be wrapped around your ponytail a few more times by the fall? Well, that's what losing elasticity is all about—and as you pass from the summer to the autumn of your years, that's somewhat the same thing that is happening to the elastin "bands" that crisscross underneath the skin on your face. The end result: Gradually your skin begins to droop and drop. The nasal labial lines (running from your nose to the corners of your mouth) become more pronounced, as your cheeks begin to "slide south." Eventually your jowls begin to drop as well, and you may start to notice the skin that covers your jawbone, as well as your neck, beginning to look less taut and firm.

Speeding this whole aging process along are environmental factors, as well as genetic influences. Sun exposure, for example, can facilitate the breakdown of collagen and elastin as well as impact cell turnover. Exposure to pollution and particularly cigarette smoke can do the same. Stress, diet, and nutrition can also play a role in how quickly your skin ages, as can the use of certain medications. Ultimately, your genetics may matter the most, since the rate at which your skin ages, as well as the amount of collagen and elastin you start out with in life, is influenced by what you inherit from both Mom and Dad.

Now if all this is beginning to sound pretty discouraging, hold on! While you may not be able to stop the hands of time from moving altogether, there is lots you *can* do to tie them down and impact the way your skin looks, right now and in the future. Of course I can't promise that you'll look like you do on your senior prom picture—and truthfully, I'm not sure any of us would even want to (bad gowns, bad shoes, and reaaaaally bad hair!). But if you give me a chance, I *can* offer you the ways and means to take control of the way you look right now, change the way you feel about "getting older"—and maybe even make a difference in where you see yourself going in the future. And it can all be easier, and take less time and money than you realize.

Turning Back the Hands of Time: What to Do First

When your mom—or even more so, your grandmother—was going through menopause, pretty much all she had to counter the effects of aging was a jar of Ponds Cold Cream and a prayer. Not so today. Over the past decade, and particularly since 2000, the field of anti-aging skin care has literally exploded, as the lines between medicine and cosmetology have been significantly blurred. In the last five years alone many esteemed researchers have joined forces with top cosmetic companies to produce products that definitely straddle the fence between treatment and cosmetic—and in the process allow us to achieve some nearly miraculous results, all from a bottle or a jar. Renowned dermatologist Dr. Albert Klingman of the University of Pennsylvania even coined a brand-new phrase just to describe this exciting new treatment trend—and that word is *cosmeceutical.* If you're not already familiar with the products that come under this new definition, chances are you soon will be.

On the other hand, if you're anything like me, spending just fifteen minutes browsing the now vast selection of skin-care treatments in your local pharmacy—or, heaven forbid, department store—causes your eyes to glaze over in some kind of catatonic *Vogue*-induced stupor. In short, there are now so *many* choices I have *no idea* what to try—or certainly what to buy. And here is where a little research really pays off. After talking to dozens of dermatologists and plastic surgeons, and even some skin-care companies, I discovered that, in most instances, the most successful product lines—those that are clinically proven to work—are based on less than a dozen key ingredients! How well they work—and what they accomplish—is usually determined by the concentration of those ingredients and how often they are applied.

Does this mean that any products that don't contain these key ingredients won't work? Certainly not. Since cosmetic companies are not required by law to do clinical trials it's entirely possible there are far more compounds that can do the job—we just don't know what they are yet, at least not from a scientific point of view. Which is to say, if you have already found a product that you just love, but it doesn't contain any of the newest anti-aging "buzz words," by all means keep using it.

At the same time, if you find yourself getting so confused about what to buy that you buy nothing at all, then I invite you to make use of my research, and use the list of key ingredients that follows as your guide. Remember, however, that while many products may boast one, two, or even more of these factors, how much they contain is key to how well they will work. In a perfect world, all skin-care companies would clearly label the percentage of ingredients in their products. But sorry, that's not happening. What they must do by federal law, however, is print ingredients in descending order—so what is first on the list is most plentiful, and so on down the line. So, if a treatment boasts a certain key ingredient—but you can see by the label it's got thirty-five others ahead of it—then chances are there's not going to be enough of it to do you much good. If you use a little common sense—and read the labels—when selecting products, you should get the most out of your skin-care dollar. If you're not sure about a product, you can also contact the manufacturer via e-mail or letter and inquire about the ingredients, particularly how much of any one key substance is being used. The ones that choose to answer you are usually the ones who have nothing to hide!

Also remember that now, and especially in the future, it's likely you may need more than one type of product and more than one key ingredient to achieve satisfying results. This is certainly true as we age and various different types of problems begin to surface. In addition, many women report better results when they use a variety of products anyway, alternating them on different nights, or between morning and evening. Doing so can help keep your skin from becoming so "used" to a product that it stops working as efficiently.

So . . . if you think you're ready to begin, take a good hard look in that magnifying mirror (and wouldn't you just like to smack whoever invented magnifying mirrors), figure out what your skin needs most, and go shopping!

The Top Ten Anti-Aging Ingredients: What Really Works

Most of the time, most of the ingredients on the following list can be found in a wide assortment of products—including day creams, night creams, cleansers, moisturizers, serums, and sometimes even masks. In fact, most companies now package entire "lines" around certain key ingredients, so that you get a little help with each product you use.

That said, you frequently don't *have* to use the whole line to get the result. So, if you can afford to buy only one product, choose the one where the key ingredient is listed highest on the label. Usually this will the "cornerstone" product of the line. Sometimes it is also the first one introduced with a particular ingredient. In addition, look out for key words such as "serum" or "night cream." Very often these formulations contain higher concentrations of the key ingredient, and choosing them may help you do away with the other items in the line. That said, here's a rundown of the hottest anti-aging ingredients, and what they promise to do.

1. RETINOL/VITAMIN A

Arguably the most clinically researched skin-care ingredient, retinol is the purest and most active form of vitamin A. The synthetic version is called tretinoin, better known as the prescription drug Retin-A. In recent years, however, an over-the-counter version has become available and is found in many products under the simple name "retinol." Once applied, it is converted in the skin to tretinoin, the active ingredient that makes the product work. The most outstanding quality of retinol is its tiny molecular size, which gives it the ability to penetrate deep into all three layers of skin. When it does, it helps to stimulate your natural production of collagen—which, as you just read, can help keep your skin plump and youthful, prevent fine lines and creases from forming, and help to reduce the appearance of those that are already in plain view. It also increases cell turnover and exfoliation, giving your skin a more "youthful" glow (see "The Anti-Aging Prescriptions," later in this chapter).

Best Suited For: Early treatment of fine lines and wrinkles; improving skin's texture and clarity; correcting a sallow complexion and hyperpigmentation; improving the look of enlarged pores; increasing moisture content; reversing photo-aging damage caused by the sun.

What You Should Know: In the prescription dosage, these products can cause redness and flaking of the skin early on during treatment, and even with the "buffer" ingredients found in over-the-counter versions, Retin-A–based products can still be irritating to sensitive skin. You should also remain out of the sun and always use sun block, even with the over-the-counter retinol products. You can expect to see some kind of result in several weeks, but it usually takes three months of daily use to see the full results. In addition, correct manufacturing standards and packaging are key to this product working, as light and heat diminish its potency. Concentrations of retinol must fall between 0.04 and 0.07 in order to work, and it should be packaged in a container that keeps out light and air. Check with the manufacturer if the product *doesn't* state concentrations on the label.

2. ALPHA HYDROXY ACID (AHA)

Formulated from natural acids derived from fruit or dairy sources, all AHA products work to dissolve the "glue" that holds the top layer of dead cells together on the surface of your skin. This, in turn, speeds cell turnover and encourages newer cells to come forward faster—much the way they did when you were young. The end result: Your skin looks smoother and more even in terms of tone, with seemingly fewer fine lines. The most powerful AHA is glycolic acid. It is made from sugarcane and its molecules are the smallest, so it easily penetrates the skin. However, it's also the harshest and most potentially irritating. Other forms of AHA include lactic acid from sour milk, citric acid from citrus fruits, malic acid from apples, and phytic acid from rice. In addition, tartaric acid, made from grapes, is also extremely powerful but is usually only found in products that blend several AHAs together.

Best Suited For: The exfoliation of dead skin cells, improving skin's clarity, and brightening a "dull" complexion. Through the exfoliation process, it may also help reduce the appearance of some fine lines and small wrinkles. Some studies also show that in high concentrations, glycolic acid can increase collagen production, plumping the skin and also adding to a more youthful appearance. Results are usually visible in three to four weeks, or sooner.

What You Should Know: These products can be irritating to sensitive skin. If you have a finicky complexion, start with a milder acid (such as citric or malic), and if your reaction is good, work up to the lactic or glycolic acid. In addition, concentrations higher than 10 percent can cause hyperpigmentation and uneven skin tone, which are more likely to occur in darker complexions. Women of Asian, Latin, Eastern European, or Middle Eastern backgrounds are especially prone to this. In addition, never use an AHA product on the same day or night you are applying a retinol or bleaching product, and always use a sunscreen. Also important: The concentration of ingredients makes all the difference in how effective an AHA product will be. Most cosmetic counter formulations contain between 4 and 8 percent, which will give you some effects but clearly not extremely dramatic results. For that you will need higher concentrations of 10 or 12 percent—usually found only in professional beauty supply stores. If you do decide to use a product that is at 10 percent acid concentration or more, check with a dermatologist first to make certain your skin can "take it." In addition to the high amount of fruit acid, many of these products can also have a low pH—often below 3—which means they can be extremely irritating to the skin.

3. BETA HYDROXY ACID (BHA)

The primary ingredient in these products is salicylic acid—an anti-inflammatory compound made from the bark of willow and sweet birch trees. While BHA works in much the same way as AHA—to speed skin cell turnover—because it's oil soluble, it can penetrate the cell buildup in pores more easily, and that may make the exfoliation process easier. It's also reportedly milder than AHA, so those with sensitive skin may have an easier time tolerating these treatments. In addition, a BHA in a 2 percent concentration is less irritating than the standard 4 to 8 percent glycolic acid but can accomplish nearly as much.

Best Suited For: Restoring skin clarity and smoothing the complexion, with some ability to smooth fine lines. It also has an anti-inflammatory effect, so it can be used even if you have acne, or the skin inflammation rosacea. Results can usually be seen in a few weeks.

What You Should Know: Although it's less irritating than AHA, it may not have the same effect on deep lines and wrinkles. Plus, it can still cause some problems for those sensitive to BHA. However, for "early" lines, or surface wrinkles that are not deep furrows, this can be an excellent way to hold off Mother Nature well into your fifties.

4. POLYHYDROXY ACIDS

Of the newest "generation" of acid products, many experts believe the front-runner is the ingredient gluconolactone, a type of sugar acid that occurs naturally in the skin. It is often paired with a second ingredient known as lactobionic acid, as well as vitamins A, C, and E. The "skin-friendly" structure of this formulation—including larger molecules that make penetration a bit slower—means these products are generally gentler and easier on sensitive complexions than AHAs, and cause little or no burning, itching, or stinging. Still, when used over a period of time, they manage to yield good results. Depending on the formulation, they can also provide excellent moisturization and some antioxidant protection.

Best Suited For: Rapid cell turnover; exfoliation; smoothing skin; reducing roughness and redness; smoothing fine wrinkles and lines; increasing moisturization.

What You Should Know: Definitely not as effective as AHA or BHA in the short run, so you may need to use it for a longer period of time to see results—between four to six months, or longer.

5. PEPTIDES

A common buzz phrase bouncing from page to page of the most popular beauty magazines, peptides are a compound of two or more amino acids. As the building blocks of protein the peptides frequently function as chemical messengers, transporting signals that direct the body in a number of metabolic functions. In the case of skin, that function is the production of collagen. So, it's no wonder that peptides were of great interest to those in the skin-cream game. One of the newer anti-aging skin therapies is built on copper peptides, which are believed to play a vital role in the production of collagen, elastin, and a substance known as glycosaminoglycans (GAGs). This is the "glue" that bonds tissue cells together and keeps skin looking firm and young. In addition, copper can help fuel enzymes that increase the body's natural ability to rebuild and repair tissue, which can also impact how your skin looks and feels. According to the American Academy of Dermatology, double-blind, placebo-controlled medical studies have shown that skin creams containing copper peptides yielded improvement in fine wrinkles, facial pigmentation, and overall photo damage. Skin also increased in thickness by nearly 18 percent. These compounds are said to be non-irritating and relatively inexpensive. Using a slightly different approach are creams containing compounds known as pentapeptides—many of which are making headlines as an important new anti-aging technology. Groups of long-chain amino acids, pentapeptides are reportedly directly involved in instructing the body to make collagen (see "Stretch Mark Cream in Perimenopause," later in this chapter). The whole peptide theory stems from a concept seen in wound healing. Here, naturally occurring peptides stimulate collagen production so that skin which has been severely damaged can be renewed. Whether or not this same physiological response can be triggered by a peptide applied topically to skin that is not damaged is a subject of great debate. Those who manufacture peptide-based products, however, claim that studies confirm it's not only possible, but perhaps the quickest route to younger-looking skin.

Best Suited For: Wrinkled skin that is losing its elasticity. These creams can help your skin look plumper and smoother and revive a dull complexion while increasing moisture levels deep in the cells. What they can't do: Combat "sagging" or bagging under the eyes, or lift a sagging jowl. The other results, however, are usually evident in about a month or less.

What You Should Know: If there is a problem with a peptide product it's usually due to whatever secondary ingredients are part of the formula. The peptide itself is not likely to have any ill effects on the skin.

6. VITAMIN C

Vitamin C is necessary to the production of collagen. In fact, some research shows that, when applied topically, at least one form of vitamin C, known as L-ascorbic acid, appears to send a signal to collagen-producing genes to work more efficiently, while at the same time activating two skin enzymes that help your skin use the collagen that is produced. So, products containing sufficient levels of L-ascorbic acid may help your skin naturally produce more collagen, resulting in a younger, firmer, more youthful complexion. In addition, vitamin C can also protect against damage from the sun and prevent UV immunosuppression—the effect of the sun on the immune system that occurs in up to 90 percent of all skin cancer patients. The key, however, is the form of vitamin C that is used. While there are a ton of C-rich products on the market, unless they contain L-ascorbic acid, you might not get the results you are seeking. That's because at least some studies show this may be the only form the body can fully utilize in a topical preparation. Derivatives of vitamin C, such as ascorbyl palmitate and magnesium ascorbyl phosphate, may have some benefits on the skin but have not been shown in studies to work the same way, or accomplish the same things, as L-ascorbic acid.

Best Suited For: Skin that is sun damaged or photo aged—damage that occurs due to the UVA or UVB rays of the sun. It can smooth the appearance of fine lines and wrinkles and firm the skin by promoting the synthesis of collagen.

What You Should Know: Some topical vitamin C preparations can cause irritation to sensitive skin, particularly when used in conjunction with AHA or BHA products. Once L-ascorbic acid gets into the skin, it cannot be washed off, rubbed off, or perspired off for up to seventy-two hours—so to avoid overtreatment leave at least that much time between applications. In addition, you should also know that vitamin C can be a very unstable ingredient—meaning it loses its power and potency rapidly. If possible, purchase preparations in single-capsule form, in concentrations of 10 percent or greater. A low pH (under 4) will help speed absorption. Results can usually be seen in about four weeks.

7. GREEN TEA

The real value in green tea is its antioxidant properties—specifically, a polyphenol compound known as epigallocatechin (EGCG), which has been shown to be one hundred times more powerful than vitamin C and twenty-five times more powerful than vitamin E in finding and destroying free radicals when taken internally. These are the natural compounds that develop from sun exposure and pollution and can literally gobble up collagen and elastin. On the skin's surface, some researchers claim that green tea protects against aging by holding a reserve of protective antioxidants in skin cells—however, there have been no published studies to back up this research. There is, however, some evidence that it may help protect against UV damage from the sun.

Best Suited For: Sun-damaged skin and photo aging; fine lines and wrinkles; loose skin due to wrinkling.

What You Should Know: The higher the concentration of EGCG the more effective the product. Ideally, it should be listed in the first few ingredients to be effective on the skin. Generally there is no downside to using a product containing green tea, unless you have a sensitivity or allergy to other ingredients frequently used in these compounds, such as

herbs or flowers. Protection is ongoing and the longer you use it, the better it gets. However, some results are evident within a few weeks' time.
And if you're wondering whether or not drinking green tea can have similarly good results on the skin, it can—simply because it is a powerful antioxidant that can help your body in myriad ways, including providing
protection and nourishment for the skin (see "Anti-Aging from the Inside
Out," later in this chapter). However, for optimal concentration in the
skin cells, it's a good idea to use it topically as well.

8. TOPICAL ESTROGEN

Yes, the same hormone that makes your hot flashes disappear and eases
your mood swings can also increase collagen production in your skin,
making your complexion more supple and giving your face a smoother,
more youthful appearance. The key lies in estrogen receptors deep within
the skin. Much like inserting the right key in the right lock, filling these
receptors can help encourage your body's natural production of collagen.
Both topical estradiol and the weaker estriol (see Chapter 11) have been
found to work. However, studies on estriol found that in addition to an
increase in collagen there is also a marked decrease in the depth of wrinkles already present on the skin. Topical estrogen also increases the ability
of skin to hold moisture by increasing levels of hyaluronic acid.

Best Suited For: Dry, wrinkled, aging skin, or, when used preventively, to
stop fine lines from developing. It also increases moisture and helps restore elasticity.

What You Should Know: Because the use of oral estrogen, alone or as part
of hormone replacement therapy, has been found to increase the risk of
certain cancers, most doctors do not advise taking oral estrogen to help
keep your skin young. Topical estrogens, however, have not had these
same negative effects. Although studies are somewhat limited, there is at
least some research showing that when creams containing 0.01 percent
estradiol or 0.3 percent estriol are used topically, blood levels are not elevated, suggesting the effects may be local to the skin. So, be certain that
any estrogen cream you purchase does not exceed these amounts, unless

approved by your doctor. In addition, some women report better results when using creams made from bio-identical estrogens—so-called "natural" hormones—identical to what is made in the body, as compared to synthetic estrogens (see Chapter 11). While they can require a prescription (depending on the type and strength of the estrogen you want to buy), generally they are available in pharmacies that compound their own custom formulations (see the resource section at the back of this book for compounding pharmacies).

WARNING: If you are at risk for a hormone-sensitive cancer, particularly breast or uterine cancer, you should avoid the use of all estrogens, even natural estrogen creams, unless recommended by your doctor.

9. NATURAL BOTANICALS

The most popular natural ingredients include coneflower (echinacea), lotus blossom, grape seed extract, shea butter, and soy—each of which can be found alone, or in combination, in a wide variety of moisturizers and other anti-aging products. While each has its own specific properties (coneflower, for example, has been practically elevated to cult status for its ability to smooth and tone a wrinkled neck), essentially, they all work to lubricate the skin and in some instances fight free radical damage (see "Diet and Your Skin," later in this chapter).

Best Suited For: Moisturizing dry skin, softening fine lines and wrinkles, increasing suppleness. What they won't do: Increase collagen, impact deep lines, or lift extremely saggy skin.

What You Should Know: While many products contain botanicals, a great many don't have enough to yield any significant results. Your best source of information is the product label—the botanical should be listed within the first several ingredients. And the closer it is to the number one position, the more likely you are to reap the benefits. Depending on the condition of your skin results can be evident in about four to twelve weeks.

10. ARGIRELINE

You may not know the chemical name, but there's no doubt you've heard the buzz about argireline (pronounced ar-ju-LEAN), now touted as the Anti-Botox and a way to get similar muscle-relaxing results without injections. The treatment is built on the premise that at least one cause of wrinkles is an involuntary tensing of micromuscles deep within the skin. When the muscles continually tense, the skin on the surface contracts, and a wrinkle is formed (kind of like the "laugh lines" that form around your eyes). In any event, natural chemicals known as catecholamines mediate the muscle contractions linked to wrinkles. According to experts, when argireline is applied topically, it works to inhibit the production of catecholamins by the muscles in that area—thus reducing or stopping the minute contractions. Eventually, they say, the muscle relaxes, and so does the wrinkle. In clinical studies, wrinkle reduction occurred by up to 30 percent in thirty days—and the longer you use this ingredient the more powerful the result.

Best Suited For: Skin that is beginning to wrinkle; easing the look of fine lines and creases. May have some impact on very deep wrinkles if used for an extended period of time, usually six months or more.

What You Should Know: This ingredient caught on fast and is now widely used in many products—but at least in this instance, there is no guarantee of safety in numbers. Because it's a "cosmeceutical" and not a drug, it didn't require any FDA testing or approval, so there are no long-term studies on the effects of blocking production of catecholamines, even on a local level. In addition, many dermatologists say that if argireline could actually impact catecholamine production it would have to be classified as a drug—so the effects, if any, have to be minimal.

Still, so far, anecdotal reports are that the ingredient has some effect on wrinkles—with no reports of adverse reactions. It is, however, important to note that for argireline to be effective, it must be present in at least a 10 percent concentration. If your product doesn't state the amount on the package, don't buy it until you can confirm what it contains. It's an expensive ingredient, and there's a good chance that many companies will use the power of the name without giving you enough to make a difference.

The Buzz Before the Buzz: Four Cutting-Edge Anti-Aging Ingredients

In addition to the anti-aging ingredients just mentioned, there are also a number of "super cutting-edge" developments—ingredients so new that testing of any kind, even by manufacturers, is sorely limited. At the same time, preliminary results are so exciting they have even dermatologists buzzing about their potential. Although you might find some of these ingredients in a few select products right now, over the next year or so, the buzz will either grow deafening or fade out—depending on what researchers find.

But to get in on what's generating the "buzz before the buzz," here's what to look for:

- *Growth Factors:* Taken from cultured skin cells, placental cells, human foreskin, and sometimes plants, growth factors act as chemical messengers, telling cells what to do. One cell-derived growth factor known as kinetin has been shown in studies to reduce fine lines and wrinkles and lighten sun-damaged pigmented skin.

- *Alpha Lipoic Acid:* This powerful antioxidant is generating a lot of interest, though much of what is known is garnered only from laboratory tests. What makes this naturally occurring antioxidant so special is that it is soluble in both water and oil, so it can easily penetrate skin cells (which are oil heavy) yet still do its job once inside (where the water content is high). It can also protect against the destruction of vitamins C and E, which can also protect skin cells. While results thus far are impressive, many doctors believe more studies must be done before all of its benefits can be verified. Still, it might be the one to watch!

- *Dimethylaminoethanol (DMAE):* This ingredient claims to boost skin's firmness, lifting those droopy jowels and creating a tighter, more taut, more youthful complexion—and this is the first time these kinds of claims come even close to being proven. According to the American Academy of Dermatology, some studies show appreciable lifting of the eyebrows, jowls, and cheeks after using products containing DMAE, though doctors can't fully explain why. In the past, DMAE has been used as a dietary supplement to improve both mental and physical performance. Currently industry-sponsored studies are under way to ascertain how DMAE works topically, if results are cumulative and/or permanent, and what, if any, problems may come to light.

· *Spin Traps:* They may sound like something connected to your twelve-speed bike or maybe your golf game, but spin traps are really a cutting-edge compound known for their ability to bind free radicals—those collagen-gobbling molecules generated by aging influences like the sun. Said to be more powerful than an antioxidant, spin traps work to "trap" the damaging free-radical molecules and "disarm" them before they can damage skin cells. So far, they've only been used in laboratory settings, but spin traps have been shown to have powerful anti-inflammatory and anti–free-radical properties. Currently, products containing spin traps have been useful in treating rosacea and sunburn. Several companies are now in the development and testing stages of spin-trap compounds for anti-aging.

Making Up the Difference—Your Midlife Makeup Bag

You can laser-peel away the wrinkles. You can slough off the dead skin cells. You can even pick it all up and tuck it all in with a surgical needle and thread. But if you don't polish off the look with a contemporary cosmetic image, you're still going to look old! Indeed, experts say that one of *the* biggest makeup mistakes women over forty make is that they wear the same products—or colors, or styles of makeup—they wore twenty years or more before.

"You can always tell the happiest time in a woman's life—just look at her makeup and you'll know where she's stuck in time," says legendary

From the "M" File

HOME ON THE RANGE WITH
WEATHER-BEATEN COWBOY SKIN!

Q: The older I'm getting, the more my face is taking on that sort of "weather-beaten" look—my husband says it's like a cowboy who's spent one too many nights on the range (thank you, darling, and look for divorce papers shortly!). I'm from southern California, so I have spent a lot of time outdoors—but I have friends who have done the same and don't have this look. Why did it happen to me, and is there anything I can do about it?

A: The problem you describe (the one with your skin, not with your man!) is what doctors call elastosis. This refers to changes in the connective tissue underneath your skin that ultimately cause a change in its elasticity, or ability to remain taut over the muscles and bones of your face. Essentially, it occurs as a result of free-radical damage caused by the sun. In short, both UVA and UVB rays gobble up both collagen and elastin, and when this occurs skin cells begin turning over in a more irregular fashion. This, in turn, can result in either scaly patches of rough skin or an overall "weather-beaten" complexion. In addition, as we age—including photo aging from the environment—skin cells become slightly misshapen, almost lying on top of, instead of alongside, each other. The end result is more of that rough, weather-beaten look. As to your hubby's analogy—well I don't love it that he associates you with cowboys on the range, but it is true that those who spend a lot of time outdoors, like the proverbial cowboy, are more likely to take on this appearance. While you can't turn back the hands of time, there are treatments that can help—including dermabrasion and face peels, two dermatological procedures that can smooth rough skin and "resurface" your face (see "The Top Ten Medical Anti-Aging Procedures," later in this chapter). Also, topically applied retinol products and AHAs can help (see the earlier section on anti-aging ingredients).

celebrity makeup artist Adrien Arpel. Too often, Arpel says, women are knee deep in a "cosmetic time warp," inexplicably bound to a look and a style that is clearly from another decade of their lives.

"No woman would be caught wearing a thirty-year-old dress or a twenty-five-year-old pair of shoes—but yet so many are still wearing the same makeup they wore when they were in high school or college—and many more are duplicating the look they had on their wedding picture," says Arpel. Even when products are updated—to a pricier brand, for example—most women still stick to the same color palette and, she says, seldom take chances or think outside the box to find a new look.

So where do you begin putting on the new face of glam for the second half of your life? Experts say updating can be easy if you begin with products geared to compensate for the changes that occur in midlife— like thinning lips, or a change in skin coloring or texture. To help point you in the right direction, Arpel, along with makeup artists Laura Geller, Bobbi Brown, and Valerie Sarnelle, offers the following suggestions for a midlife makeup bag that can help you look as young as you feel.

THE EIGHT COSMETICS EVERY WOMAN OVER FORTY HAS TO HAVE

1. FACE PRIMER

The number one product all our experts agree is essential for midlife skin is a "face primer"—a relatively new kind of product developed to smooth the skin and give you the equivalent of a freshly spackled canvas upon which to paint. A good primer not only evens out skin tone, it can even fill in some tiny lines and wrinkles, make enlarged pores less visible, make foundation and blush slide on easier, and stay on longer, *and* put a layer of protection between your skin and the makeup. This means less gets in your pores, so more color *and* product stays on your face longer.

- **APPLICATION TIPS:** Apply after cleansing and moisturizing, using fingertips or a sponge. *Don't* "rub" it in, like you would a moisturizer— instead pat into your face, applying sparingly much the way you would a liquid foundation.

2. SKIN ILLUMINATOR

Also known as "skin brighteners," these must-have creams, liquids, and powders contain microscopic particles that work like tiny mirrors to reflect light onto your skin. The end result is a radiant complexion that looks younger than springtime!

"Illuminators are important and a great breakthrough in makeup technology because they reflect light and make the skin look smoother—which also makes you automatically look younger," says celebrity makeup artist Laura Geller. "But," she cautions, "there are illuminators and there are frosted illuminators—you want the low-level products with a soft pearlized glow that can be blended into foundation or used on the entire face." To emphasize that glow, look for products tinted a light peach or warm beige tone.

- **APPLICATION TIPS:** Since, on their own, illuminators *won't* cover like a foundation, you need to add them to your makeup, or put them on *over* foundation. So, the primer goes first, then foundation, then an illuminator or brightener. If your skin is dry, definitely choose a liquid illumination product. If your skin is oily, and you don't have a lot of fine lines or wrinkles, then a face-brightening powder works best.

3. CONCEALER

Designed to cover and conceal discolorations around the eyes, these ultra-creamy "super-foundations" can be a midlife woman's best friend. The reason? As we age, the already thin skin under our eyes thins out even more, letting tiny blue and red veins underneath suddenly appear. Add to this a few sleepless nights, and you have the makings of dark, discolored *aging circles* around the eyes. In addition, as estrogen levels plummet and the collagen reserves in our skin begin to decline, we lose definition in our cheekbones—which in turn can cause a "dip" under the eye that creates still another shadow. The end result can add up to ten years to your appearance. A really good concealer can solve all these problems, plus make your eyes look brighter and your face look more rested and youthful. The trick to finding a good concealer is to skip the heavy products and go for a thin application you can "layer."

"If you have low points on your face, pat on concealer, let it dry a few seconds, and pat on another layer—slowly building up the areas where you want or need to add brightness or lightness to your skin," says Beverly Hills makeup guru Valerie Sarnelle.

She also says you don't need a heavy product to cover shadows—just one in the right color, which, she says, should have pink-orange undertones. "It lightens the whole area, and the orange tones neutralize the bluish veins underneath," says Sarnelle.

The biggest concealer mistake women make: Using under-eye cover in white or very light beige. This, says Sarnelle, draws attention to puffiness and dark discolorations.

• **APPLICATION TIPS:** Make certain your product is creamy and not drying—and be sure to moisturize around your eyes before applying concealer. Also, make certain to pat concealer in place using your ring finger (for minimal pressure on the eye area) and always put it on last—after foundation. If you put concealer on first, followed by foundation, you're likely to dilute the product and end up with less coverage.

4. LIGHT-DIFFUSING FOUNDATION

If you haven't changed your foundation in the last five years, it's time to do so now! The reason: the brand-new light-diffusing foundations, products that can work miracles on midlife skin. Among the newest formulations are those that replace most of the water with microscopic silicone "beads," which keep pigment uniform and give your face a soft, even glow. And because the tiny silicone spheres don't evaporate or get absorbed (like water) your skin stays fresh and naturally pretty all day. In addition, because the silicone lies on the very top layer of your skin, it won't get deep into fine lines and wrinkles. In fact, it can provide a surface "fill" while also covering large pores and even some acne scars.

"If you can't or don't want to use a primer, then choosing a cream foundation containing lots of natural 'butters'—like shea and cocoa—is the best way to have a youthful-looking complexion," says Arpel. Once you find a formula that you like, Arpel says, buy it in two shades: one that matches your skin tone, one two shades lighter. You can use the lighter shade under your eyes in place of concealer, as well as around the mouth, which tends to look darker and shadowy as we age.

• **APPLICATION TIPS:** If you use one of the new synthetic "techno" brushes to apply your foundation, you'll get more coverage with less product and ultimately a more natural look. In case you haven't seen these brushes, they are anywhere from one-half to one inch in width and have white or beige nylon-like bristles and a "slick" feel, all of which helps the foundation glide over your skin rather than into the pores and fine lines. If your skin is very oily, feel free to add a layer of translucent powder, but look for one that is "micro-milled"—usually an Italian-made product with such a fine consistency it can keep from settling into fine lines and wrinkles. Or, try the new moisture-rich powders that are "shot" through an air compressor and mixed with aloe vera, giving them a moist look and feel on the face. If, however, your skin is very dry, beauty editors at *Harper's Bazaar* magazine say, skip traditional powder. Even the ones that are finely milled are likely to age you, emphasizing wrinkles and lines and reducing your "glow."

5. BRONZER

Different from a permanent tanning product, a bronzer is a cosmetic that can add a glorious temporary glow to your skin and a shimmer of summer color all year long. Experts say it's perfect for midlife skin, since as we age we tend to lose color from our faces—one reason behind that "pasty" look that adds years to your appearance. While bronzers used to be available only in powder form, the newer products also come in crème and gel formulations, which can add even more glow to a dry midlife complexion. If your skin is very oily, however, you can still use a powder bronzer—or even a "loose" mineral powder in a bronze color.

• **APPLICATION TIPS:** According to Victoria's Secret makeup artist Charlie Green, for the most natural look select a bronzer no more than two shades darker than your natural complexion. Fair-skinned gals should look for products with a yellow/peach undertone, while dark-skinned ladies need reddish-brown tones. If your skin is very pale, use a cream blusher in a pink shade applied to the "apples" of your cheeks first, *before* applying bronzer, says Green. And regardless of your skin color *never* put a bronzer *all over your face.* Instead, hit only the "high" points where the sun normally kisses your skin: Tops of cheekbones, down the center of your nose, and on the chin. Blend in upward toward the temples, and if there's any left on the brush, sweep it across the top of your forehead and into your hairline.

6. CREAM OR GEL BLUSH

If you use nothing else on your face, a cream blush can be your single most important anti-aging cosmetic. Not only can it add a sheer wash of much-needed color to your face—*very anti-aging*—it can also leave you looking healthier, and what could be more youthful than that? The key is to keep it looking as natural as possible—as if the glow is coming from within and you're keeping some wonderful *sexy* secret! And for all but the oiliest of complexions, a cream or gel blush achieves that healthy glow without the "cakey," aging look of some powder blushes. To select the right color, according to editors at *Allure* magazine, "pinch" your cheeks, and then look to duplicate that shade. Generally speaking, however, they advise women with pale, pallid skin to seek out plum or blue-based pinks; medium-toned skin needs the warmth of apricot or coral colors; olive tones need bolder colors, like bright coral or soft red. African-American skin tones look best with golden shades that highlight face structure.

• **APPLICATION TIPS:** To get the most wear out of your cream blush, say *Allure* magazine editors, pat it onto your cheeks—don't rub it in like a moisturizer or cream. Since oil in a foundation can break down color and cause it to rub off quickly, try a silicone-based primer or foundation first for great staying power. To get the natural glow of cream blush and the staying power of powder, use the powder blush first, then add a cream blush in a lighter shade on the tops of the cheekbones. To make all blush look better on your skin, experts at *Allure* suggest exfoliating your skin weekly with a facial scrub, and always applying under bright daylight for the most natural glow.

7. ANTI-FEATHERING LIP PENCIL/LIP GLOSS

If you've always used lipstick as your primary lip color, it's time to cap the tube—at least for a little while. As we age, our lips get thinner and smaller and often lose their defining shape. In addition, tiny lines around the mouth can cause whatever lipstick you do use to "travel" upward and leave lips looking messy and undefined. The solution: an anti-feathering lip pencil. Designed with a "harder" colored lead and less oil and wax, they won't smear into lines and will give lipstick and gloss an "anchor" to hang on to.

Additionally, nothing says "young, juicy lips" like a gloss—it's the ultimate supermodel anti-aging trick that works for women of any age. While it's true that glosses do have a tendency to "walk" their way from your lips to your nose, if you look for a slightly "tacky" consistency *and* always outline and fill in your lips with anti-feathering pencil first (see the application tips that follow), that final coat of gloss can take five to ten years off your appearance, as compared to a matte or even a satin-textured lipstick.

- **APPLICATION TIPS:** Look for a color that is close to that of your natural lips, and then draw a "soft" line, putting only as much pressure on the pencil as necessary to see the color, says makeup artist Valerie Sarnelle. This, she says, will give you a softer, more natural lip line. To make an aging thin mouth look fuller, Sarnelle says, cover your entire lip area with foundation or primer first, then use the pencil, guiding it just along the outside edge of your lip line. This will add fullness without changing the basic shape of your mouth. Once the outline is in place, fill in the remainder using the same pencil *lightly* on the rest of your top and bottom lip. Then apply gloss in a clear, neutral, rosy, or brown tone. If you feel you must use lipstick, avoid dark red or wine colors in matte finishes, because they can make lips look thinner and smaller. And always top your lipstick with a clear gloss. If you're careful not to take the gloss all the way to the edge of your lip line, you'll get more anti-feathering control, says Sarnelle. In addition, don't match your lip liner to your lipstick. Instead choose a neutral shade closest to the color of your natural lips. This will allow you to build fullness without the heavy "outline" look that is definitely aging.

8. LASH EXTENDER

Whether or not you wear eye makeup—particularly shadow or liner—is entirely a matter of personal choice. However, what you should never go without is mascara, and especially a lash extender. Why? As we age, our lashes thin out—and if you want to call out your age, nothing does it louder than skimpy, sparse fuzz framing your eyes. In fact, if you do nothing else, experts say a good mascara and a lash extender can automatically put you in a different demographic—unconsciously sending a message to those looking at you that you are younger than your years. Some say the right lashes can take ten years off your appearance!

"Lashes are a dead giveaway of a woman's age—when they are sparse she just looks older," says Geller. While there are always false lashes to turn to, there is also a whole cache of brand-new lash-lengthening technologies that can give you a far more natural and youthful look. Now if you're thinking of the clunky, gooey, stiff lash thickeners of the past, think again. Today's products blend technology with science *and* beauty, relying on ingredients like down-soft polyester fibers or even real silk for a whole new approach to lash lengthening.

- **APPLICATION TIPS:** Don't overdo! While it's great to go from lashless to sultry, sweeping, flirty eyes, says Geller, use too much of these products and you end up looking like a cartoon of Bessie the Cow. Instead, she says, use them sparingly and apply one coat at a time—and always, always start with a good-quality, non-sticky mascara.

Finally, regardless of what makeup tips you choose to try, remember to put your cosmetics on in direct sunlight—get away from the bathroom vanity and instead take a hand mirror to the nearest window and put your cosmetics on in this light. Doing so will help ensure that you don't over-paint your face, which can be the best anti-aging secret of all. Remember, as you age, less is best—so the lighter and more natural your makeup looks, the younger and more vibrant you will look.

Getting the Biggest Bang from Your Beauty Bucks

In case you're wondering how you're going to find all these wonderful new products, I'm happy to tell you that you don't have to spend a lot of money in order to get in on the latest buzz. While frequently it's the

From the "M" File

SAY GOOD-BYE TO PROM HAIR!

Q: I've always had long, shoulder-length hair, ever since I can remember. But now that I've turned forty-five my sister insists that my long hair has to go. Are there any "rules" about when it's time to cut your hair—and why is it that so many older women do get cropped do's as they age?

A: Uh-oh—your phrase "ever since I can remember" frightens me just a little bit. Are we talking your wedding day, your college graduation, or (yikes!) your senior prom? Well, we'll get to *that* part of your question in a minute. But first, the good news: There are no rules—at least not when it comes to style and age. Short, long, natural gray, bleached, dyed, or highlighted—it's *all* a matter of personal choice. That said, it is also true that lots of women do seem to cut their hair short—or shorter—beginning in middle age. For some it's a practical decision: As our lives grow more complex and hectic, we have less time to fuss with personal grooming, and sometimes—though not always—short hair can be easier to handle. Another consideration—hot flashes. Many women suffer terribly with both hot flashes and night sweats, so a short do is simply a way of coping. It can be cooler, plus it's easier and faster to wash and dry if you do perspire a lot. Finally, many women cut their hair short when it begins to thin because it's true, a shorter, layered style generally does hide hair loss better than a long straight look (see Chapter 6 for more information on midlife hair loss).

If, however, none of these situations apply, then wearing your hair long is perfectly acceptable—just ask some fabulously long-locked forty-plus gals like Suzanne Somers, Cher, Star Jones, Goldie Hawn,

higher-priced, department-store brands that do the most advertising of the flashy new ingredients and products, more often than not most drugstores or cosmetic retail shops will also carry lines that feature some of these same advances—and often in formulations that are amazingly close

Susan Lucci, and Meredith Vieira—they look fabulous, and I wouldn't snip even their bangs! However, getting back to your "ever since I can remember" hairstyle—now that can be a problem, long or short. In fact, regardless of the length of your hair, if you are stuck in a style rut that has left you with the *same* hairdo since your thirties or even your twenties, then sweetie, it's time for a change! Nothing, I mean *nothing* dates a woman more than a hairdo from another decade! At the same time remember that "change" doesn't have to mean a haircut—it can mean a new color or highlights. Sharon Dorram-Krause, star colorist at New York's John Freida salon, recently told *Harper's Bazaar*, "Always go lighter as you age," she says, because the darker your hair the more prominent wrinkles and lines can seem. If you're less than 50 percent gray, Krause says, try a semipermanent color, in one or two shades up from your natural color, and you'll have automatic highlights without the work! If you're more than 50 percent gray, your hair may be color-resistant, so talk to your hairdresser about what to do beforehand to increase color absorption. You should also speak to your hairdresser about a new "do"—one that suits your personality and your personal sense of style, with or without a cut. One more point—if you are thinking of joining the league of soccer moms and shearing your locks but are fearful of making the commitment, visit a local wig shop and try on styles in various lengths (and colors!). This will give you a great opportunity to check yourself out in a new look and see how you feel. You might even consider purchasing a wig in a new short style and "living with it" for a month or more to see how you like it. If you do, then head to the hairdresser *in the wig* and tell him or her to duplicate the look with your natural hair. While it doesn't always look exactly the same, you will at least have an idea of how you'll look before the scissoring begins.

to the very high-priced brands. For example, Cellex C offers an incredible vitamin C line of products—but the price of just one jar can set you back a mortgage payment. At the same time, Adrienne Arpel's Signature Club A line, sold on the Home Shopping Network, will net you a whole bag full of vitamin C products—and the tote bag to boot—for less than the cost of one Cellex C item. More importantly, the key ingredient—the L-ascorbic acid form of vitamin C—is present in both. The same is true for Avon's vitamin C serum. For anywhere between $10 (when it's on sale) and $20 (full price), you can get a 10 percent L-ascorbic acid serum that is as potent as anything you'd pay $100 or more for in a department-store brand. While the higher-priced items sometimes do contain larger amounts of the key ingredient, this is not *always* the case, so this is one time where shopping around—and reading labels—always pays off. (And when doesn't it?!)

In fact, no matter what ingredient or product type you are seeking, there are clearly some mid-priced and even discount lines that can offer you terrific bargains. When searching out any of the ingredients featured in this chapter—or *any* that may catch your eye in a beauty magazine— check out the following companies for some of the best cosmetic and skin-care buys.

You can also visit www.yourmenopause.com for a continually updated list of the top products for women over forty.

THE BEST BEAUTY BARGAINS

- *Avon*
  (www.Avon.com)

- *L'Oréal*

- *Oil of Olay*

- *Neutrogena*

- *Le Club des Créateurs de Beauté, Paris*
  (www.ccbparis.com)

- *Signature Club A*
  (www.hsn.com)

- *Dr. Jeannette Graf Skin Care*
  (www.hsn.com)

FROM ITALY, WITH LOVE, FOR YOUR FACE

When it comes to glamming up our forty-plus faces, there is perhaps no better partnership than that which has formed between the United States and Italy, where a combination of U.S. smarts and Italian style have come together in a remarkable way! The end result is a development of an assortment of finely milled powders and foundations so creamy they are like a dream come true for midlife skin. In fact, if you think that getting older means giving up foundations and powders—mostly because they *all* seem to settle in fine lines and creases and make us look *decades older* than we are—you owe it to yourself to try the new Italian-made generation of these products, which can actually do the opposite.

Although a number of U.S. companies are now importing these technologically advanced cosmetics, among the best you can try hail from two surprisingly moderately priced lines. The first was developed by legendary makeup artist Jerome Alexander. Of particular note is his Studio Stick foundation, a creamy, high-pigmented product that covers *everything*, without a cakey look or feel. It *never* settles in fine lines, yet it covers flaws, including enlarged pores, leaving you with a flawless complexion that lasts all day.

To polish off the look, seek out his Bronzi blushing powder. It starts out as a creamy liquid that is then poured into terra-cotta pots and baked for hours until it forms into a solid powderlike consistency. The end result is a finely milled bronzer that will not go into fine lines, moisturizes your skin like a cream blush, but lasts on your face like a powder. It's a combination that can't be beat.

Using still another Italian technology is Adrien Arpel's line of Buttery Cream foundations—a combination of eight moisturizing butters, including mango and shea, which come together to produce a foundation that not only covers but gives your skin a rich, natural glow. Complemented by face powders and a golden patina bronzer that are infused with hydrating aloe vera and niacin, and then milled to an ultrafine consistency, they are like a kiss of heaven for over-forty skin.

Both product lines are reasonably priced and available from the Home Shopping Network at 800–284–3100 or online at www.hsn.com.

- *Serious Skin Care*
  (www.hsn.com)

- *Revlon*

THE BEAUTY BOUTIQUE AND SPA BUYS

Whether online or in the mall, the gap between pricy department-store brands and the drugstore shelf is often filled by boutique and spa lines—products that, while they don't have quite the cachet of Estée Lauder, Prescriptives, Dior, or Chanel, can still offer you some of the best midlife skin care and makeup at a fairly reasonable price.

Lines to die for include:

- *Laura Geller Cosmetics*
  (www.qvc.com and www.laurageller.com)

- *Diane Young*
  (www.dianeyoung.com)

- *Bare Escentuals*
  (www.qvc.com)

- *Victoria Principal's Principal Secret*
  (www.principalsecret.com or www.qvc.com)

- *Illuminare*
  (www.illuminarecosmetics.com or www.hsn.com)

DERMATOLOGIST IN A JAR

Among the latest trends in "boutique" skin care are what I like to call "dermatologist in a jar" products—skin care that is developed specifically by noted dermatologists to meet their exacting standards. While many doctors routinely offer products under their own label to their patients, oftentimes these are what is known in the industry as "generics"—private-label skin care and cosmetics that can be pretty much the same from doc-

FROM PARIS, WITH LOVE

There's three things the French seem to know more about than any-one else: Romance, champagne . . . and skin care! And when it comes to anti-aging skin care, in my book French scientists and der-matologists are right up there with Nobel Peace Prize winners in terms of coming up with some truly great advances.

Among the crème of "la crop" is the private skin-care line known simply and quietly as G. M. Collin, Paris. Developed by a group of French researchers in 1957, and now headquartered in Montreal, you won't find them in major department stores or even fancy upscale cosmetic boutiques. But if you're willing to venture off the beaten path and into one of the 1,300 dermo-corrective salons around the United States and Canada, I think you'll be amazed at what you discover—unique blends of extremely high-quality botanicals and marine ingre-dients paired with the latest technology to form a system of skin care that really works.

While the line boasts over forty face- and body-care products, for me the cornerstone is their Visible Lifting Cream and Visible Lifting Serum. Chock-full of the pentapeptides generating the loudest anti-aging buzz, it also contains a "cocktail" of other important ingredi-ents, including sweet almond proteins that quite remarkably act like a "net" to produce a visible lifting effect on the skin, while moisturizing and polishing. There's also a complex of botanicals and other ingre-dients that work to drain idle lipid cells of fluids to redefine the facial contours and reduce that saggy, jowly look around the chin line. So you not only end up with fewer wrinkles and tighter skin, but also a better contour—and they have the results of clinical trials to show it works.

To learn more about the line, visit their website at www. GMCollin.com—or call 800–341–1531 (U.S.) or 800–361–1263 (Canada) for the dermo-corrective clinic near you. While you don't need to have a treatment there, professional aestheticians can advise you on the best products for your skin type.

FROM ITALY, WITH LOVE, FOR YOUR BODY

If your over-forty skin is just crying out for some tender loving care, then you don't want to miss a line of Italian bath and body products that is positively *legendary* when it comes to kissing your all-over body complexion with hydrating love. That line is Perlier, and their American sister company Elariia, both of which rely on some of the finest European botanicals—and some formulations that go back generations—to bring you body care on a par with some of the most expensive European spas, at a price you can really afford.

Most notable for those with forty-plus skin is their complete olive oil–based line—totally nongreasy formulations that are literally infused with nourishing botanicals, including olive oil, that can give even the toughest, driest "alligator" skin a smoother, younger-looking *and* -feeling body complexion. The line includes crème bath liquids, moisturizers, body butters (my favorite and just *divine*), and an olive-oil hair masque that is not to be believed!

Also worth trying are their honey line, including a royal bee jelly face-and-body cream that is extraordinary when it comes to ultimate moisturization; their shea butter line of products; and their Banana Nourishing Body Treatment cream.

You can find Perlier in most major department stores, but you'll get the best buys on these products, as well as the Elariia line, on the Home Shopping Network. You can order by phone at 800–284–3100 or online at www.hsn.com.

tor to doctor, only the label is different. But the new breed of "doctor creams" is something quite different—products that frequently contain ultrapremium ingredients, and in many cases tout the latest cutting-edge skin technologies. Whether they can or can't accomplish more than a mass-market or even boutique product is a subject of great debate—particularly among dermatologists. That said, most of the top products have a legion of followers that often include some of Hollywood's most cele-

Soy Sense for your Skin

Among the most popular natural approaches to menopause symptoms is the use of soy-based foods. As you will read later in this book (see Chapter 11), properties in soy may mimic those of estrogen—and in doing so help ameliorate some of the symptoms that develop when hormone levels begin to fall.

This same concept of replacing estrogen with soy is now being explored for midlife skin care. The idea here is that because estrogen helps keep collagen production high and wrinkle formation low, when applied topically soy may do the same thing.

Among those pioneering this research is skin care and cosmetic guru Adrien Arpel. She recently developed "Richer Than Rich"—a line of soy-based skin care that promises to deliver at least some of the topical benefits of estrogen, without the associated health risks. I'm happy to report the theory seems to hold up, with skin appearing moist and younger looking almost immediately. Other natural ingredients include echinacea, black cohosh, and flax seed oil.

Products start at about $30. However, you can find some amazing deals—including kits that include five products for less than what you'd pay for just one—if you shop her line on TV at the Home Shopping Network, or online at www.hsn.com.

You can also find soy-based skin-care products at some health food stores—but be certain to check the ingredients label to ensure you're getting enough of this potent ingredient to make a difference.

brated beauties—so clearly, they are doing something right. Although these products can be pricey, often costing upward of $75 for a single cream, and sometimes running into the hundreds of dollars per treatment, for those adventurous souls with a little cash to burn, here's the latest buzz on what to try.

You can also find the latest products from these and other dermatology lines at www.yourmenopause.com.

- *Doctor's Dermatologic Formula:* Clearly, Park Avenue meets Hollywood in this line, developed by New York City dermatologist Dr. Howard Sobel.

- *Murad:* This line was created by noted Los Angeles dermatologist Dr. Howard Murad, an assistant clinical professor of dermatology at UCLA.

- *N.V. Perricone:* Products developed by Yale dermatologist Dr. Nicholas Perricone.

- *Re Vive:* This product line is created by University of Louisville dermatologist Dr. Gregory Bays Brown.

- *Erno Lazlo:* The Hungarian dermatologist Dr. Erno Lazlo passed away in 1973 at the age of eighty-two. His line of legendary products lives on, however.

- *Dr. Brandt:* The label bears the name "Dr. Brandt" on all products, but there are actually six different lines in all—and all created by noted Miami/Manhattan dermatologist Dr. Fredric Brandt.

Diet and Your Skin: The Latest News

In addition to what you put on your face, what you put in your body—in terms of the foods you eat—can also have an impact on the aging process of your skin. In the not so distant past most doctors pooh-poohed the idea that foods could influence skin health, but this is not so anymore. Today, the most forward-thinking experts know there are important links between diet and dermatology, particularly in the area of anti-aging skin care. In fact, there are some who go so far as to say that if you don't eat the right foods, your skin may age faster no matter how many expensive creams and lotions you lather on.

Again, the reason has to do with the effects of free radicals—molecules that are generated in large amounts by sun exposure, chemicals, and pollution. As you read earlier, the link to aging occurs when these molecules attack skin on a cellular level and prematurely break down collagen and elastin—which increases wrinkle formation and even pigmentation problems. So where does diet fit in? First, some foods—like those high in animal fat—contribute to the creation of free radicals when they are metabolized. In other instances, foods that contain antioxidants—like fresh fruits and vegetables—disarm the free radicals so less damage is done to your skin.

According to a meta-analysis of over fifty studies conducted by assistant professor Harvey Arbesman at the University of Buffalo, a diet rich in antioxidants—like fruits and vegetables—can actually ward off premature aging of the skin, and may even reduce the risk of some skin cancers and precancerous lesions. How many fruits and veggies do you need a day? Some experts say five servings are enough—but if your skin is already aging, boost your intake to ten per day and you may have even better results.

A third nutritional factor—omega-3 fatty acids, found in great abundance in fish—can also play a role in your skin's appearance, mostly by inhibiting the formation of inflammatory factors that can dull your complexion. According to Dr. Nicholas Perricone, famed anti-aging expert and professor of dermatology at Yale University, if you eat a dinner of fresh salmon with a salad drenched in olive oil and lemon, plus a wedge of cantaloupe for dessert, for just three nights in a row, your skin will look smoother, younger, and more radiant, almost immediately.

And do you get your eight glasses of water a day? Although the overall health benefits of this philosophy have been challenged, when it comes to your skin most dermatologists agree it's still an important tenent. If you don't drink enough water you could end up with dry, flaky, even wrinkled skin. But increase your intake and, like a rose garden in a spring rain, your skin will blossom with a dewy and more youthful appearance. Drink more than eight glasses and you may see even more dramatic results. Remember, soups, juices, and decaf beverages count—but there is still some evidence to show that anything that contains a lot of caffeine negates some of the effects by pulling water from your skin.

Finally, if your complexion is very dry and wrinkles are forming on your face faster than on a white linen suit on a hot summer's day, cut

From the "M" File

LIVER SPOTS AND SKIN BLEACHING

Q: I remember my grandmother always having these flat, brown spots on her hands—she used to call them "liver spots." My mother had them as well—and now, at age fifty-one, it looks as if I'm getting them too. Is this a hereditary condition—and is there anything I can do to stop it or prevent more from coming out?

A: The problem you describe is medically known as lentigines—but you're right, most of us know them as "liver spots," or sometimes "age spots." No matter what you call them they are small, flat, brown or tan markings that appear on the backs of the hands, arms, shoulders, forehead, and sometimes the face—and yes, they do seem to occur more frequently as we age. The important thing to remember is that they are not dangerous and not indicative of any problems with your liver! These markings are also not hereditary. Essentially, they come from sun exposure, which causes permanent changes in the pigment of groups of skin cells, which, in turn, form the flat, brown spots. The process takes a while, though, which is one reason why they don't normally show up until the middle years, or later.

Although the American Academy of Dermatology reports that over-the-counter skin bleaching creams won't fade liver spots, they do say that some prescription creams, as well as laser therapy, can make them all but disappear. That said, there is also much anecdotal evidence—mostly from women themselves—attesting to the power of certain over-the-counter fade and freckle creams to at least lighten, if not completely fade, brown spots, so they can certainly be worth a try.

down on your daily cocktails or glasses of sangria and see your glow return. Studies show that as little as one or two glasses of wine a day can dehydrate tissues, making wrinkles appear more prominent, plus adding a puffy, bloated look to your face. Stronger alcoholic drinks can have an even greater aging effect.

When it comes to bleaching ingredients—both prescription and over-the-counter—among the most well known are hydroquinone (the only FDA-approved product for skin bleaching), kojic acid, and Mandelic acid. All work by killing off the melanin-producing cells in the skin—the ones responsible for pigmentation. Hydroquinone in concentrations of 4 percent works best, but will require a doctor's prescription. Among the most well-known brand names is Lustra. Over-the-counter preparations are available in strengths of 2 percent or under—less effective, but they still offer *some* help. Either version should not be used more than three months, or you can develop a permanent discoloration that is difficult to fix. You also need to stay completely out of the sun while using these products. Kojic acid works in a similar fashion, but has been shown to be less irritating. Mandelic acid is not technically a bleach, but instead an alpha hydroxy acid made from bittersweet almonds that has been shown to have some skin-lightening properties. It is the only bleaching agent safe for use on dark complexions and is generally non-irritating even on sensitive skin.

In addition to age spots, skin bleaching is also an effective way to lighten any area of face or body that takes on a gray or "muddy" look—something that can occur as a natural result of the aging process. However, be careful not to overuse these products—either in terms of length of time, or how much you apply. In this instance, less is definitely more.

One other word of caution: Before you bleach anything, be certain to have your doctor give any irregularly shaped skin growths the once-over. Many skin cancers can be quite benign looking at the start—and if there is any question that your growth could be an early cancer, you need a professional opinion before you treat it yourself.

Anti-Aging from the Inside Out: The New Beauty Vitamins

My friend Renee has this incredible knack for simplifying *everything*. From her laundry routines to her work schedule, even to her shopping

From the "M" File

STRETCH MARK CREAM IN PERIMENOPAUSE?

Q: I fell down laughing when my fifty-two-year-old sister said she had to purchase some stretch mark cream—it's been more than thirty years since she was pregnant! But she tells me this is the latest trend in anti-aging skin care for the face. Is this true? And if so, how does it work, and are there any downsides to trying it?

A: No doubt your sister was referring to a stretch mark cream called StriVectin-SD, a topical product that was indeed developed to help fade the stretch marks that form during pregnancy. Not long after it was marketed, however, it developed a cult following as a wrinkle cream, mostly because of a key ingredient called oglio-peptide—one of the new peptide, amino-acid formulations found naturally in the skin. Although it was not intended as a wrinkle remedy, in July 2002 a totally independent study was presented at the twentieth World Congress of Dermatology in Paris. There, doctors compared the wrinkle-fighting power of oglio-peptide to creams containing retinol, vitamin C, or placebo. According to the study result, the oglio-peptide was miles ahead of the other ingredients in terms of improving wrinkle depth, length, and volume and skin texture. Women in the study also reported less irritation, fewer wrinkles, and faster results with the peptide concentration than with either the retinol or the vitamin C. Once the word got out that StriVectin-SD included this peptide ingredient . . . well, the rest is Hollywood history. One caveat—StriVectin-SD is costly, about $135 a tube. However, the manufacturer says that when used on the face, one tube should last about six months. It's important to note that the new product line by L'Oréal known as Regenerist also contains a similar peptide complex and claims similar results—at about $20 a jar.

trips, Renee always seems to find the fastest, easiest ways to accomplish *anything*—one reason I really paid attention when, one Sunday afternoon, I found her tossing all her skin-care products in the trash.

"I'm free," she said with a kind of reckless abandon I'd not heard since she gave up wearing pantyhose.

"Free—like from the ravages of political torture? Free from the confines of your low-carb diet? Free from your addiction to QVC?" With Renee there could be a lot of "frees."

"No, silly, look at my garbage can," she said, rattling the glass jars that were sitting at the bottom of the metal container. "I'm free of skin care!" she said with an almost hysterical joy in her voice.

"And that's because you're dating a plastic surgeon now?" I said, wondering if it actually could be true. She sighed and rolled her eyes, clearly disappointed that I didn't know *what in the world* she was talking about.

"I would have thought that *you,* more than anyone, would be up on the latest buzz on skin care," she said, sounding just a little smug, I thought.

"And that would be . . . "

"Vitamins, you silly girl—good old-fashioned C and E and A and D—and, oh, a few other nutrients I can't quite remember, but I read this book and I'm convinced it not only works, it's so much simpler than trying to figure out what to buy to put *on* your face," she said. There's that word again—simple.

After a bit more prodding I found out my friend was referring to the books written by Dr. Nicholas Perricone, the new anti-aging skin-care "guru" who, as you just read, has written an awful lot about the power of our diet to impact the way we look. But he's also a great proponent of vitamin and nutrient supplements for the skin as well. And, in fact, in the time since Dr. Perricone first made his theories known, a whole gaggle of traditional beauty companies (like Avon and Olay and L'Oréal) have come forward with their own line of *skin vitamins*—"neutraceuticals," as they are now called in the medical community. The premise here: that feeding your skin from the inside out may be at least as beneficial as topical care—and in some instances, maybe more so. And many experts tend to agree.

"In many ways, you can accomplish a lot more with vitamin supplements than you can with creams," says Zoe Diana Draelos, M.D., an associate professor of dermatology at Wake Forest University and a member of the American Academy of Dermatology. While topical creams and lotions can help, Draelos believes that what you put *on* your face could never fully replace what is needed *internally by your body* to keep your skin healthy and looking great. And that's where she says supplements can play an important role.

"A cream is never going to replace a faulty diet—if you're not getting enough of a certain nutrient, you aren't going to replace it with a cream or serum," says Draelos.

Nicknamed "vanity vitamins"—because you're more likely to see bottles of these nutrients on your dressing table than next to the kitchen sink—these skin nutrients are beginning to make their way into the beauty culture, manufactured not just by traditional skin-care companies, but also a number of large vitamin manufacturers as well. Among the most popular formulations are powerful blends of antioxidants—vitamins like A, C, and E, and plant-based ingredients such as lycopene (found in tomatoes). Perhaps it's no coincidence that these are also many of the same ingredients that have grown in popularity in topical products as well.

And while the medical research supporting their use in skin care is sketchy at best, theories do abound attesting to their usefulness. One of the most popular involves the ability of antioxidants to destroy free radicals. As you learned earlier, these are dangerous molecules that are formed by exposure to the sun or pollution or sometimes even a result of the foods we eat. In the skin, free radicals destroy collagen—and as you also learned earlier, this can contribute to aging in a big way. In fact, it's one reason why spending a lot of time in the sun can leave you looking older than your years. Putting antioxidants *on* the skin is thought to help block some of the damage of free radicals. Now experts say taking it internally may boost the effects even further.

"These vitamin and nutrient formulas were specifically developed for the skin—and the effects go much deeper than just antioxidant protection," says Amy Newburger, M.D., a New York dermatologist and spokesperson for the new Olay line of beauty nutrients. At least some of the new skin nutrients, she says, play a distinct and important role in collagen production. So, by taking steps to protect against a deficiency, you are helping ensure your body has what it needs to keep collagen production perking—and your skin looking younger—for as long as possible.

While that seems like an awfully good idea, the question remains whether or not the products will work if a nutrient deficiency *doesn't* exist—which is probably the case for most of you reading this book. This is particularly true since vitamins like C and beta-carotene (the form of vitamin A most of these vitamins contain) are automatically excreted when we reach our saturation point. Or, as my friend Leigh the scientist says, "You just end up with *really* expensive pee."

Be that as it may, there is clearly some anecdotal evidence to validate the effects of skin vitamins, and even a study or two leaning in that direction. New York University nutritionist Samantha Heller says it may be that some of us even have "subclinical" vitamin deficiencies—*slightly* lower-than-normal nutrient levels—that are too small to be measured in a test but might, over time, affect our skin.

"Let's face it, there are so many things in our world stressing our skin, and so many of us have a really poor diet, it wouldn't surprise me that subclinical deficiencies are out there, maybe more than we realize," she says.

But do we have to take a "beauty nutrient" to do something about it? Most experts say no. If your diet is fairly healthy—lots of fresh fruits and vegetables as well as whole grains, and a good supply of omega-3 fatty acids found in foods like salmon (see "Diet and Your Skin," earlier in this chapter)—you probably already get most of what your skin needs. Further, if you take a multivitamin, chances are you are in even better shape and ensuring that your skin is getting all it needs.

However, some research into the "skin vitamins" on the market right now also showed me that there are specific nutrients you probably aren't getting in your diet or your regular multivitamin—like evening primrose oil, green tea, alpha lipoic acid, and pycnogenols. And while there may not be any solid research to back up claims that they can affect your skin, they can certainly impact your overall health, and that can only be good for your complexion. Or, as my grandmother was fond of saying, "I can tell where you've been, how long you stayed, and some of what you did—just by the color of your cheeks." And while I'm certain that at least part of that was a guess, it's clear that our faces do give away a few secrets, not the least of which is our age.

The bottom line: If you're not happy with the skin-care regimen you're using, you might want to give these skin nutrients a try. But I wouldn't toss the jars of creams and lotions just yet. Even the beauty companies making these vitamins agree that treating skin from both the inside *and* the out-side is the best approach. After all, it does seem to cover all the bases!

If you do want to try skin vitamins, look for those by reputable beauty companies, such as Olay, Avon, and L'Oréal—all three have new products on the market. Also, don't overlook what you might find in a health food store, or even on the shelves of your local grocery. Many vita-min companies now have their own versions of "beauty vitamins," in-cluding Hair, Skin and Nails by Andrew Lessman, sold on the Home Shopping Network, Natrol's Skin, Hair and Nails and Dermavites, sold in most drugstores; and Ultra Mega Beauty and Vitality and Hair Skin and Nails, sold at General Nutrition Centers nationwide.

For more on skin vitamins, visit www.yourmenopause.com.

Medical De-Aging:
How Your Doctor Can Help

Once upon a time, anti-aging medical treatments were a luxury reserved for the rich, the famous, and (mostly) the Hollywood elite. While golden screen goddesses got to zap their wrinkles before they ever even appeared, the rest of us were pretty much relegated to our proverbial gene pool—and what we could buy in a drugstore—to maintain our good looks.

Not so anymore. Today there are a host of medical procedures and treatments that both dermatologists and plastic surgeons alike offer, at prices much less than what you might expect to pay. While it's clear that the cost is going to go far beyond that jar of moisturizer or even an ex-pensive bottle of anti-aging serum, because results are often longer last-ing, in the end you might wind up paying about the same, or even less, for the medical procedure.

So, if you happen to find yourself in the middle of what my friend Jeannie likes to call "an all-out aging extravaganza"—and creams and serums just don't seem to help—then yes, there are ways that your der-matologist or plastic surgeon can, at least temporarily, stop the hands of time and, if you're lucky, even reset your glamour clock back a few years.

To help you know a little more about what is available, what it can do, and how much it will set you back, I've put together a guide to the most popular procedures and treatments being performed today. Based on information provided by the American Society of Dermatologic Surgeons and the American Academy of Plastic Surgeons, it can help open the door to discussion with your own doctor, who can best advise you on which of these procedures might be right for you.

Note: Costs are approximate, based on national averages. They may not include the cost of anesthesia, medications, or other charges by the surgical facility or doctor's office.

THE TOP TEN MEDICAL ANTI-AGING PROCEDURES

I. CHEMICAL PEELS

This in-office procedure utilizes a customized chemical solution to gently "burn" away the outside layers of aging skin. It can help with the appearance of surface lines and wrinkles (great for around the eyes and mouth), skin discolorations, age spots, and acne scars, as well as improving skin texture. The peels are available in light, medium, and deep strengths, depending on the degree of damage to your skin.

- *Approximate cost:* Between $1,000 and $2,000.

- *Approximate downtime:* Redness and scaling last three to five days for a light peel; up to fourteen days for a deep peel, with blistering and peeling.

- *Frequency:* Light peels—every four weeks for up to several months, followed by a peel every two to three months for maintenance; medium peels—once yearly; deep peels—once per lifetime.

FYI: At-home peels using vitamin C or chemicals are available from a number of companies. They are not as strong as what you can get in a doctor's office but will offer some results at a fraction of the cost.

2. DERMABRASION

A form of cosmetic "sanding," this procedure utilizes special instruments, or sometimes "micro crystals," to mechanically remove the top layer of skin. It reportedly smoothes out irregularities and can correct scarring, combat some aging effects of sun damage, and reduce pigmentation problems. It can also improve the appearance of fine lines and wrinkles.

- *Approximate cost:* $1,700 and up.

- *Downtime:* About ten days, but you should avoid sun for three to six months afterward. Makeup is often required for up to twelve weeks to cover the temporary "pink" discoloration caused by the procedure.

- *Frequency:* Once or twice per lifetime.

3. LASER RESURFACING

The heat created by certain types of lasers helps vaporize damaged skin tissue, layer by layer. This uncovers fresh new skin that has fewer wrinkles and lines and less sun damage. The highly focused beam of either a carbon dioxide or erbium YAG laser allows a dermatologist to precisely remove skin cells in a specific location.

- *Approximate cost:* $1,300 and up.

- *Downtime:* Aftereffects and recovery time vary greatly depending on the procedure, and on how deep the treatment goes.

- *Frequency:* Once or twice a lifetime

4. NON-ABLATIVE RESURFACING

Similar to laser resurfacing, but with a faster healing time, this rejuvenating procedure smoothes aging and sun-damaged skin to remove surface wrinkles and creases. Special light-pulsed lasers and "cold" electrical energy gently resurface the face without wounding the top layer of skin—so postoperative healing is fast. Good for highly pigmented skin and great for removing scars.

- *Approximate cost:* $1,300 and up.

- *Downtime:* Mild to moderate swelling for up to one month.

- *Frequency:* Once or twice a lifetime.

5. MICRODERMABRASION

Described as a "blast of liquid sandpaper" across your skin, this surprisingly painless technique uses tiny particles that are sprayed onto the surface of your face and then "vacuumed" off, taking with them layers of dead skin cells. This forces a rapid cell turnover that encourages fresh new skin cell growth. Because this procedure touches only the very top surface of the skin, it's best for those with mild to moderate skin damage and moderate wrinkles. Usually more than one treatment is needed to achieve results, but downtime is limited.

- *Approximate cost:* $150 per treatment.

- *Downtime:* Minor pinkness lasting up to a few days.

- *Frequency:* No more than twenty times a year; twelve times yearly average. Once the treatments stop, the aging process will eventually continue as before.

6. THE "FILLERS"

These procedures involve injecting various substances known as "soft tissue fillers" underneath the wrinkle, to plump and fill out the skin with a variety of filler materials (see "The New Wrinkle in Skin Care," in the next section). Fillers are best used for plumping deep wrinkles above the lips, augmenting the size of the lips, relaxing nasal labial lines (from nose to mouth), and plumping wrinkles on cheeks. They are not suitable for around the eyes.

- *Approximate cost:* $75 to $150 per injection.

- *Downtime:* Several hours.

- *Frequency:* Effects last from three to twelve months depending on the substance used, and the procedure can be repeated as often as needed.

7. BOTOX

This is an injection of a tiny amount of the same poison that causes botulism, a severe form of food poisoning. As scary as that sounds, the theory behind this treatment is that in very tiny amounts, this same organism can cause a temporary paralysis of tiny muscle fibers that lie just under an area of wrinkled skin. When the muscle relaxes, so does the wrinkle—and the skin appears smooth and furrow-free. It can improve the appearance of lines, wrinkles, and that "grouch frown" between your brows and can sometimes be used on areas of the neck for smoother-looking skin. Although it's widely popular, it is not FDA approved for cosmetic purposes so testing and evaluation remain somewhat limited. However, some patients have anecdotally reported a loss of some facial expression after Botox injections. Because muscle paralysis is involved, depending on the location of the wrinkle you want to relax, and the skill of the doctor administering the injection, it's possible you may lose some ability to form certain facial expressions during the time the Botox is active in your system. Most of the time, expressions return when the Botox wears out.

- *Approximate cost:* $400 per injection.

- *Downtime:* About thirty minutes.

- *Frequency:* Lasts about three to four months. It can be repeated when needed.

8. FACE-LIFT—TRADITIONAL

The oldest and most well-known cosmetic procedure, a face-lift is the only sure way to pull up a sagging, drooping face—including lifting the jowls and putting those cheeks that have gone south up where they belong! To perform this surgery an incision is made—usually in the hairline or behind the ear—and the excess skin is pulled up and cut, while the remaining skin is stitched into place. An "eye lift" is similar, with excess skin pulled away and, often, stitched into the lower lash line. New surgical techniques make this operation faster and easier than ever, with little or no scarring. Still, it's major surgery, requires anesthesia, and should be done in a hospital setting.

- *Approximate cost:* $5,500.

- *Downtime:* Surgery lasts several hours; bandages removed

within five days; stitches removed after five to eight days; several weeks before all puffiness and swelling subside; minimal sun exposure for at least several months.

- *Frequency:* Results generally last around ten years

9. THE PERIMENOPAUSE LIFT—RADIO FREQUENCY THERAPY/LASER LIFT

For those between forty and sixty who simply want a rejuvenated look, these procedures—and there are several—use various types of lasers to send heat deep into the inner layers of the skin. This, in turn, causes a wounding of the skin cells (you can't see it), which the body responds to by producing large amounts of collagen. It is this collagen which then produces the final result in about three months—including a plumper complexion and a "tightened," more taut look to the skin, as well as a lifted brow or eyelid, or even a tighter, less "jiggly" jowl line. It's being called the "perimenopause lift" because it works best for those women in their late forties to mid-fifties—before any "major" lifting is required.

- *Approximate cost:* $500 to $700 per treatment, with three to four treatments usually necessary.

- *Downtime:* Ten minutes for procedure; no recovery time.

- *Frequency:* Approximately once a month for four months. With good skin care the overall effects should last for several years.

10. LIPOSUCTION

In this procedure, tiny tubes attached to a vacuum are used to suck fat cells out of specific areas of the face and body to sculpt a new shape. Once associated with chubby thighs and hanging bellies, today liposuction is commonly used to sculpt the face, creating the look of higher cheekbones and removing a "double chin."

- *Approximate cost:* $2,100 and up.

- *Downtime:* Three to seven days.

From the "M" File

THE MIDLIFE ITCHES

Q: I'm forty-nine and smack in the middle of peri-menopause. I don't have a lot of problems with either hot flashes or mood swings, but I am going nuts with dry skin, and particularly an all-over body itch that is *relentless*. Is this common—and is it hormone related, or something else entirely?

A: In much the same way that estrogen depletion affects your facial complexion, it can also affect the skin anywhere on your body. For most women, skin does seem drier, rougher, and more difficult to moisturize. Because when skin becomes dry it can begin to itch, many women in perimenopause complain of the "overall" body itching you describe. The key is, of course, to use what I like to call "industrial strength" moisturizers—like Lubriderm or Neutrogena Swedish Formula, or any body cream containing alpha hydroxy acids, such as Adrien Arpel's Lemon Verbena Revitalizing Body Treatment. What can also help: avoiding hot showers and baths, and when you can, skipping bathing altogether. In addition, many women report that switching from a moisturizing gel body wash to a moisturizing soap such as Dove, Oil of Olay, or Caress,

---

- *Frequency:* This procedure offers permanent results. Even if you gain weight, you will not gain in the same place, simply because the fat cells were removed from the area.

The New Wrinkle in Skin Care:
Youth in a Hypodermic!

Move over, Botox—collagen injections step to the side. The road to the fountain of youth is about to be repaved with a slew of new injectables—"volume-filling" chemicals placed just under the top layer of skin to change angry wrinkles into happy smiles.

Unlike Botox injections, which, as you just read, stop wrinkles by

can help as well. As pleasant as body washes can be to use, if you compare their ingredient label to that found on a bar of moisturizing soap you may be quite surprised by the difference. In short, the soap accomplishes moisturization with only minimal chemicals, while the body washes are generally *loaded* with ingredients that have the potential to irritate any skin condition, and even cause itching.

That said, there is also a problem known as "formication"—a neurologically based itching that can make some midlife women feel as if their skin is literally crawling with bugs. Some describe it as pins and needles, while others simply say it's an intense "all-over itching and tingling." There is little known about this condition except that it sometimes occurs in conjunction with diabetes. However, it has also been found in women with no blood sugar problems—and perimenopause seems to be the link. Unfortunately, this condition has even most doctors stumped, and there is little information available on treatment options. However, some women report relief via the use of hydrocortisone cream, alone or in combination with some form of hormone therapy, including natural progesterone. Finally, all-over skin itching can sometimes be a symptom of kidney or liver disease. So, you should bring your condition to the attention of your doctor and find out if further testing is warranted to rule out problems in either of these two organs.

paralyzing tiny muscles underneath the line, the new injectables work by plumping up the underlying tissue and in this way help to "erase" lines, wrinkles, and crow's-feet. In some instances they can also be used to actually build up areas of the face where natural collagen reserves have diminished, such as cheekbones and chin. Costing between $750 and $1,500 per injection, most offer promising and immediate—though mostly temporary—results from a single treatment. Recovery is quick as well: within several hours there will be nary a trace that you had anything done—except, of course, your terrific new look!

So, what's available for you to try? The injectables generating the loudest beauty buzz right now include the following:

1. RESTYLANE, RESTYLANE FINE LINES, AND PERLANE

All three of these preparations are essentially a form of hyaluronic acid, a fluid that is found naturally in human joints like wrists, elbows, and knees. If you've ever purchased a pricey skin cream it's likely you've seen topical forms of hyaluronic acid on the ingredient label, since it has long been considered a super moisturizer. Dermatologist Dr. Robin Ashinoff, who did some of the clinical testing on Restylane at NYU Medical Center in New York City, reports it's a nontoxic sugar that when injected under the skin offers much longer-lasting results—lasting some seven to twelve months—than traditional collagen shots, which usually last just three to six months. Because it's so safe, Ashinoff says, no allergy testing is needed. All three of these products contain essentially the same ingredient but are used for different purposes. Restylane is primarily for wrinkle correction and lip augmentation; Restylane Fine Lines is for thin superficial lines around the mouth and forehead; Perlane is for larger areas, and is often used to reshape facial contours like cheeks or chin, and for plumping very deep wrinkles.

2. HYLAFORM

A slightly different twist on hyaluronic acid, this product is made from hyaluronan, a natural substance that, in a different form, is found in your skin. This form, however, is derived from rooster combs, and because of that the American Society of Plastic Surgeons warns that there may be a small risk of allergic reaction—not to mention some unpleasantness for the rooster! It does, however, have an excellent safety profile, with results that last from three to six months.

3. RADIANCE

This volume filler is composed of tiny particles derived from calcium—not unlike what is found in teeth and bones. Currently it is FDA approved for treating vocal cord paralysis and some types of incontinence, but many dermatologists and plastic surgeons are using it as an anti-aging volume filler as well. The pluses include long-lasting results, anywhere from two to five years, with a very small risk of allergic reaction. Minuses include a small but significant risk of "granuloma," a localized skin reaction that can result in tiny, hard bumps at the site where the injection was given—and they can last months or years. The American Society of Plastic Surgeons warns that the lumps can also migrate to other parts of the body, and long-term consequences are not known.

4. ARTECOLL

This formulation combines 75 percent collagen with 25 percent synthetic micro beads in a material similar to Plexiglas, and it works slightly differently from other injectables. While the collagen content helps to immediately fill the wrinkle, the micro beads cause an irritation just under the surface of the line or crease. This, in turn, causes your body to respond by manufacturing a kind of scar tissue to grow around the bead. When it does, it becomes a "permanent" wrinkle filler. And, in fact, Artecoll's results are said to be permanent—one injection and the wrinkle is gone, for good! Although results are said to be astounding, there is a significant risk of granuloma, which can be permanent. What's more, while the product's manufacturer says the body does not absorb the micro beads, experts at the American Society of Plastic Surgeons say that the beads can migrate to other parts of the body, with no information on what, if any, consequences may result. To date, Artecoll has not yet been approved by the FDA for use in the United States. However, it is under consideration, and that approval could come in the very near future.

5. COSMOPLAST AND COSMODERM

Helping to bring collagen injections into the twenty-first century are these two new compounds that are derived from human collagen grown under strict laboratory conditions. Unlike bovine collagen injections (extracted from cows), which can have a high allergic reaction rate, these new forms are considered so safe there is no need for skin testing prior to injection. Like the bovine collagen, they are used to fill tiny lines and creases, particularly around the mouth. Results, however, are still limited to around ninety days.

6. FAT INJECTIONS

Love the idea of looking young—but hate the thought that anything unnatural is crawling under your skin? Then you might be the right candidate for fat injections. In this procedure doctors harvest fat cells from other parts of *your* body—like your stomach or thighs—and inject them under the lines and creases of your face. The effect is similar to that of other injectables, and lasts between six and twelve months. However, it does require an extra surgery to harvest the small number of fat cells used in these injections. In case you're wondering, no, it won't make much of a difference in the area from which the fat cells are harvested—only a tiny amount is removed.

Waking Up Your Midlife Skin: What to Do Right Now

My good friend Tina called a few weeks ago to tell me that her face had fallen asleep.

"Excuse me . . . like in pins and needles—and do we need to call 911?"

"No, no, no," she said, heaving a sigh like she couldn't believe I didn't get it right off.

"I mean tired, as in lifeless, dull, boring-looking, no sparkle, plastic and not crystal, the 'I'm not J. Lo' lack of a glow. You know, tired."

I stifled my urge to say, "Well, that's because you're *not* J. Lo, who, by the way, is young enough to be your daughter." But actually, I knew exactly what my friend meant. And if you're even two hours past forty, you probably know it too. Because the truth is, while we all whine and worry about the threat of wrinkles, lines, creases, sagging, and, heaven help us, age spots, in reality, what frequently makes the most difference in the way we look is the *overall* appearance of our skin.

While much of what you've read in this chapter will help you get that glow going eventually, if you're anything like me, you want a change and you want it now! Perfectly understandable. That's why I've hunted down some of the world's best beauty experts and *hounded* them incessantly for some *immediate* solutions—things we can do *this very instant* to put a little "umph" back in our complexion and get our groove going, or at least take it out of "park" for the night!

So, with the help of makeup goddesses Adrien Arpel, Valerie Sarnelle, Laura Geller, Bobbi Brown, and Holly Mordini, I pass along these simple but effective ways to look a lot better by the time the sun rises tomorrow!

SIX SIMPLE WAYS TO LOOK BETTER IMMEDIATELY!

I. GET A FACIAL

From Adrien Arpel to Diane Young, from the spa at La Costa in San Diego to The Spa at the Plaza Hotel in New York City, there isn't a beauty expert that doesn't advocate facials for an instant pick-me-up—for not only your face, but your mind and spirit as well. Although there are a wide variety of products and ingredients, as well as types of facials for specific results, essentially the message here seems to be the same: They clean out your pores, enhance your circulation, help remove toxins from skin cells, and leave your face looking and feeling relaxed and refreshed. And you'd be amazed at how much a little relaxation can help ease worry wrinkles and lines and help you look younger! The only caveat here: Don't get your first facial the day of a big event or important moment in your life. In some rare instances a facial can leave your skin red and blotchy for about twenty-four hours—so until you know how you'll react, do it the day before any major event. In addition, says Genevieve Sparby, spa director at the famed New York City Plaza Hotel, never go out in the sun directly after a facial. Again, wait at least twenty-four hours.

2. STOP WASHING YOUR FACE WITH SOAP

Regardless of what your mother told you about washing your face, if her suggestions involved soap, give them up! According to L'Oréal consulting dermatologist Dr. Lydia M. Evans, most soaps are drying to the delicate skin on your face, stripping your epidermis of natural oils needed to moisturize and soften your complexion. They can also alter the delicate pH or acid balance of your facial skin, and this can result in a drier complexion that makes lines and creases far more noticeable. Indeed, dry skin looks like old skin, so to get the glow going, use a cream cleanser, rinse with lots of cool water, and follow with a toner to close pores. You won't believe the difference in how your face looks!

3. USE MOISTURIZER

Most women use it after cleansing in the morning, it's true. But I'm talking about putting it on several times a day! This is particularly important if you live or work in a dry climate, or spend a lot of time in heat or air-conditioning. As the day moves on, skin gets drier—and waiting until your evening cleansing routine to give your face a boost is waiting too long. If you choose a water-based moisturizer—and gel formulations are best—you can add a few drops to the palms of your hands, rub together, then gently pat your face, several times a day. It won't disturb your makeup, and the result is a dewy, moist, much younger-looking complexion.

4. REMOVE UNWANTED FACIAL HAIR

Nothing screams "menopause" more than those stray facial hairs or more-than-peach-fuzz sprouting on your upper lip or at the corners of your mouth. The culprit here is estrogen—as levels drop, hair grows in all the wrong places, including your face. Using a chemical or mechanical hair remover will go a long way in giving you a more youthful appearance.

5. GET ENOUGH SLEEP

When we sleep, the body secretes a series of biochemicals, including growth hormones. They in turn help restore cells, particularly in the skin. So, when those directions on your jar of night cream say to apply it at night—there's a reason! Additionally, not getting enough sleep can not only net you some nasty dark under-eye circles, it can also cause uneven skin tone, and a gray, almost "ashy" look to your complexion. Conversely, get those eight hours—even one night—and see a remarkable radiance return to your skin, almost instantly!

6. STOP SMOKING

Yeah, yeah, you've heard it all before—smoking dries out your complexion and helps form all those funny little lines around your mouth that let your lipstick creep up toward your nose. But I'll bet you didn't know that smoking can actually break down the *collagen reserves in your skin*. Researchers from King's and St. Thomas' School of Medicine in London found that smoking activates a gene that triggers an enzyme deep within the skin's structure—and that in turn sends a message for collagen to begin breaking down. The report, published in the journal *Lancet* in 2001, explained how all this action takes place not externally, but *internally*—the result of what you actually inhale when you smoke. And here's a real eye-opener: According to the researchers, if you do smoke, middle age actually begins in your mid-*thirties,* at least in terms of comparable damage to your skin. The good news: Stop smoking and see an almost instant halt to at least a part of the aging process of your skin!

Caveat Emptor Lipstick: Beauty Buyer Beware!

There is no question that with a little bit of effort and even a tiny self-care budget, you can clearly look better—and oftentimes younger—than your mother could at half your age. Undoubtedly, beauty technology has gone a long way, and if you hitch your wagon to even a few of the advances available right now, you just might see a significant difference in how your skin looks—and how you feel about the way you look.

That said, it's also important to remember that even when products claim to have clinical trials attesting to their benefits, it is rare to find one published in a medical journal. That's an important distinction because when a journal does publish the results of a study it means the research has been subjected to independent "peer review"—and that means a panel of doctors and researchers not involved in the study review not only the findings, but the methods used to gather the data. Without peer review status, many physicians consider studies of little value—one reason why doctors are frequently so reluctant to "buy in" to claims made by skin-care companies, even if the products have some legitimate benefits to offer. Another problem: Even when skin-care companies do conduct studies, often it is on a *very* small group—sometimes as few as six or eight participants. By comparison, drugs must be tested on thousands of people before gaining FDA approval.

So, should you believe everything you read? Of course not—you don't need me to remind you of *that*. Indeed, you should approach your choice of skin-care products and cosmetics with the same healthy dose of skepticism you use when looking over the chopped meat selection or picking through the vegetable bin in your local grocery store. Certainly, if you can afford to try the newest, greatest lotions and potions, regardless of price, go for it—because you're bound to find at least some that do terrific things for your skin. But on the other hand if you find you're missing car payments or stealing from your kids' college tuition fund just to hide a wrinkle or soothe a furrowed brow, it's time for a reality check: Aging is a natural process and nothing in a jar, no matter the price or the promise, is going to freeze your face in time forever. So use a little common sense and a lot of shopping savvy, and I promise you will soon be the best you can be.

And be sure to visit www.yourmenopause.com for continually updated information on all the hottest new ingredients and product lines.

6

Hair Today,
None Tomorrow

Solving the Riddle of Midlife Hair Loss

W hen the phone rang at seven A.M. I knew it could only mean
trouble. As I am a bona fide "night person," my friends all
know that phone calls before noon are reserved for winning
the lottery, getting nominated for an Academy Award, or being knee deep
in an overwhelming personal tragedy. I'm pretty sure now that my friend
Gail's seven A.M. call did not qualify for any of these categories, but I will
say that at the moment, she was definitely having a problem.

"It's happened, it's finally happened . . . what am I going to do?" she
sobbed pathetically into the phone that cold winter morning.

Being somewhat dramatic myself—particularly when waking up
from a sound sleep—I naturally assumed the worst.

"Oh, my goodness—how did it happen—how did he die?" I said in
my most sympathetic tone, assuming, of course, she was referring to the
untimely passing of her high-cholesterol, chili-dog-loving husband,
Roger.

"Huh . . . what are you talking about?" she said, temporarily snapping out of her grief.

"It . . . *it* finally happened, you said—I'm thinking Roger finally ate one too many chili-dogs—am I right?" I was just a little sarcastic as I began to realize this was probably not anywhere close to the tragedy I had imagined when I first picked up the phone.

"Oh . . . don't be silly, Roger is fine," she said very matter-of-factly.

"O . . . kay . . . Since I know the Academy already announced their awards for this year—and you weren't on the list, by the way—why the heck are you calling me at seven A.M.?" I asked, trying to wipe the remaining night cream from my eyes without poking one of them out. Gail heaved a big sigh—partly realizing that she was overreacting, but also letting me know she was still upset.

"It's . . . it's . . . my hair," she finally said in a much more quiet tone. "I'm sorry, I know I'm probably overreacting, but I just finished washing it and there were so *many* hairs in the sink this time, and this bald spot is really starting to show . . . I just freaked. Do you want to go back to sleep?" She was now talking in a *really* quiet voice, which I know means she's *really* upset.

"No, it's okay—I'm up now—but you know, we talked about this before, and you know that thinning hair is part of the midlife picture," I said, reminding her of a discussion we had about this topic five or six months ago when her problem first began.

"I know, I know . . . but when you said 'thinning hair' I thought you meant, like, a little less pouf in my . . . pouf. I didn't think you meant handfuls of hair down the sink and patches of white shiny scalp in my head! This is awful," she said, her voice starting to crack.

The truth is that, while thinning hair is a part of the menopause picture for many women (and you'll learn why in a few moments), some, like my friend Gail, do hit the extreme end of the spectrum. And while there is no way to tell who will score the highest on the Loss-O-Meter, what Gail didn't seem to recall from our earlier conversation was that there are important steps she could have taken to guard against the dramatic problem she was experiencing now.

As our conversation continued I refreshed her memory—and promised we would meet later that day to talk about it more, reminding her that there were still treatments she could try. But that phone call from Gail did more than just wake me from sleep—it was a wake-up call that made me realize how little we gals are willing to acknowledge the very real problem of midlife hair loss—until something dramatic like this occurs.

In fact, if you're like most women—and my friend Gail—you probably associate middle age with only one hair consequence: going gray. And Clairol and Revlon notwithstanding, that is something that, sooner or later, we all do have to face. But what very few of us are willing to confront is the equally common but somewhat more distressing problem— and that is, getting older also means having *less* hair, and sometimes it even means losing a whole lot of it. According to the American Academy of Dermatology, there are currently some 30 million women in the United States alone facing this very problem.

But what exactly is the cause—and why does midlife seem to set it all in motion? In order to make sense of the answer to that question, it's important to know a little something about how your hair grows during all the stages of your life.

Your Midlife Hair: What Your Mother Never Told You

Remember how, when you would get that really, really, really *bad* haircut, it seemed to just take forever to grow it out? Well, it might have *seemed* that way, but the truth is, regardless of most circumstances (including that bad cut) your locks usually continue to grow about a half inch per month, with each hair on your head experiencing a growth cycle lasting from two to six years. When an individual hair reaches its peak growth stage it "rests" for a short while on your head and then, believe it or not, falls out. Fortunately, the follicle from which it grew—the tiny "root factory" that's in your scalp—doesn't die. Instead, it begins rapidly growing a new hair to take the place of the old one. And so the cycle continues, well into your thirties and even your forties—or until your hormones begin to kick up a fuss. In fact, prior to menopause, only about 13 percent of women report a problem with hair loss, while after menopause that number jumps to 37 percent or higher. Clearly, part of the problem has to do with aging. As we grow older, many systems in our body simply slow down—including that which governs hair health. Much the way our skin cells turn over less frequently as we age, so too do we experience equivalent slowdowns in the cycles that govern the health of our hair. Depending on how much hair you had prior to perimenopause, you may notice this a little or a lot. For most women, however, the end result is a slight thinning—problems that usually show up as a lack of "body" or poor manageability.

However, for a growing number of perimenopausal women, the words "bad hair day" can take on a whole new and different meaning. The reason is a problem known as androgenic alopecia, or in women, "female pattern balding"—a genetic propensity that can rear its ugly head as we approach our middle years. What happens?

Normally, each hair follicle in your scalp contains a variety of hormones and enzymes, each of which plays a different role in the hair growth cycle. One of them is called 5-alpha reductase, an enzyme that converts testosterone found in your bloodstream to a slightly different and more potent hormone known as DHT, or dihydrotestosterone. If you have inherited the gene for hair loss, over time your follicles respond to DHT by becoming progressively smaller. This, in turn, shortens the growing cycle of each hair, which in turn causes more hairs to be shed as time goes on. When you are young—in your twenties and thirties—you hardly notice the change. That's because so few follicles are affected that the loss isn't noticeable. But as you age, and follicles continue to shrink, more and more hair is lost. Eventually, some of your follicles will die completely, while others will shrink to such a small size they can no longer foster the growth of new hair. All these problems can be further complicated by still another factor—your bouncing hormones. How do *they* affect the growth of your hair?

As you read earlier, in addition to estrogen and progesterone, your ovaries also make tiny amounts of testosterone. When estrogen levels fall, however, even this small amount can suddenly take on new importance. Without estrogen to balance its effects, it can begin to assert a more dominant effect on your body. That's one reason why many women approaching menopause begin developing facial hair—the classic "menopause mustache" over the upper lip, or sometimes "sideburns" along the edge of the face. All of that is thanks to testosterone. But while it might encourage hair growth on your face and body, it can have the exact opposite effect on your scalp. Indeed, the more testosterone you have in your bloodstream—and the less estrogen you have to balance it—the more DHT your body can make and, ultimately, the more exposure your hair follicles will have. If you are genetically predisposed to hair loss, this hormonal tango is enough to exacerbate conditions so that somewhere between age forty-five and fifty (or sometimes even younger) you begin to notice a profuse thinning throughout your scalp.

Complicating matters just a bit further: Another enzyme known as aromatase is also present in hair follicles, in much greater amounts in women than in men. The job of aromatase is to convert testosterone back to estrogen, which in turn keeps it from being converted to DHT. Some doctors believe that in women who are susceptible to hair loss, there may also be a shortage of aromatase—which means that the normal conversion of testosterone to estrogen in your hair follicle is just not happening. And that also means more testosterone and ultimately more DHT—and, in the end, more hair loss.

Because the study of female pattern balding is still in its infancy, even renowned experts confess they know far less about this problem in women than in men. But what is known is that, unless you take steps to change your fate, for those who are genetically predisposed, the years just prior to and following menopause can be one never-ending bad hair day.

Overcoming Hair Loss: What You Can Do

Although hair loss is often the result of the process I just described, sometimes it can also be caused by other factors. Autoimmune diseases such as lupus, or sometimes thyroid disorders (see "From the 'M' File: Is It Really My Hormones?" later in this chapter), can also cause you to lose your hair, as can certain nutritional deficiencies. So, if you are losing your locks, the very first thing you should do is find out why. And the best way to do that is to seek a consultation with a dermatologist. Although sometimes a very sophisticated or clever hairdresser may be able to make an educated guess about what is wrong, if your hair loss is significant you owe it to yourself to see a medical expert—and the earlier in the game you do that, the better off you will be. Why?

First, if there is another problem going on, obviously the faster it's diagnosed the faster you can begin getting your dream locks back in shape. In this respect, your dermatologist will not only perform a detailed examination of your scalp but also offer you a battery of blood tests that can help confirm the cause of your problem. But more importantly, even if your hair loss does turn out to be genetically linked female pattern balding, this same medical professional can put you on the right track to the treatments that can really make a difference. Fortunately, there are quite a few good ones from which to choose. Indeed, once your diagnosis is confirmed, you can begin almost immediately to make a real difference in how your hair looks and feels. In many instances some relatively simple scalp treatments can do the trick.

Among the most popular remedies for both male and female pattern balding is the FDA-approved over-the-counter topical preparation minoxidil (Rogaine). It works by helping to enlarge and lengthen the hair follicle. And while experts say it may do little to grow more hair on your head, it can extend the growth phase of the hair you do have, which in turn will help you to keep your locks a little longer. Although it's available in two strengths—a 2 percent solution for women and a 5 percent solution for men—experts say the weaker preparation is not likely to offer much help.

"If a woman wants results, she should use the 5 percent solution," says Dr. Michael Reed, a dermatologist and hair loss expert at New York University Medical Center. Indeed, in a head-to-head study of the 2 percent and 5 percent solutions published in the *Journal of the American Academy of Dermatology* in 2004, women themselves indicated the higher concentrations offered "superior" results. And this, say experts, is where your doctor can help. Although both the 2 percent and 5 percent solutions are available over the counter, according to the study, the higher concentrations appeared to cause some scalp irritation, itching, and dryness. In a few women this was shown to be not only extremely uncomfortable, but also make styling hair a lot more difficult. That problem, however, is often remedied by customized minoxidil prescriptions frequently available at your doctor's office.

"Most dermatologists treating hair loss do have custom formulations available combining higher concentrations of minoxidil with other ingre-

dients that can make the product easier for women to use," says Dr. Ted
Daly, a dermatologist and hair loss expert from Nassau University
Medical Center in New York.

If even these custom preparations don't help, you needn't be discouraged. Many experts say that "off label" use of certain other medications
(drugs prescribed for other problems or strictly for use in men) is also
likely to help many women. Among the most popular is the otherwise
"man-friendly" medicine finasteride—a drug originally developed to treat
prostate disease and, later, hair loss in men. Prescribed under the names
Propecia (the 1 milligram strength) or Proscar (the 5 milligram strength),
this medication works by interfering with the process that converts testosterone to DHT in the hair follicle. With less DHT hanging around to
shrink follicles, the longer those follicles will hang around sprouting
hairs—so the more hair you will keep. In some women, Reed reports, it
may even jump-start some dormant follicles and encourage new hair
growth. However, since both Propecia and Proscar should never be used
during pregnancy (they can be harmful to the baby), it's important for
you to be using birth control—unless, of course, you have already gone
more than twelve months without a period.

While side effects for both these medications are generally rare, you
could experience a heavier growth of hair around your hairline—a problem that automatically reverses once the drug is stopped, or sometimes
even when the dosage is reduced. Because both these medicines have the
potential to affect hormone levels, some women also experience a slight
reduction in libido, with a reduced desire for sex—though most doctors
say this is practically never severe enough to stop treatment.

What may turn out to be the (hair) saving grace for women is a
"cousin" of finasteride—a brand-new drug known as Avodart. Like
Proscar and Propecia, this medication was also originally developed to
treat prostate disease. However, doctors now say it may be especially beneficial for treating hair loss in women. Here's why: While finasteride
blocks just one enzyme involved in hair loss, Avodart blocks two—and
the second one is specifically involved in hair loss in women. Currently,
Avodart is being tested on women, in private doctors' offices in select
parts of the country. However, it could become available nationwide in
the very near future.

For those of you who don't find help from any of these traditionally "male" drugs, there is still another prescription your doctor can write—this time for the medication Aldactone (spironolactone). It works in a slightly different fashion, impacting the enzyme receptors in the hair follicle, and disrupting the cycle of testosterone-related hair loss. While it works well for some women, it can sometimes cause breast tenderness.

If some or all of these medications are helping your hair loss, but side effects—like a burning scalp or intense itching—make using them difficult, again, many dermatologists stock an arsenal of customized versions of popular drugs that can boost performance while reducing side effects. Some even take the time and trouble to custom blend milder formulations, mostly by suspending the key ingredients in kinder, gentler, though more expensive, preparations. If your dermatologist does not offer you these customized preparations—or if you've tried what he or she has to offer to no avail—do seek out a second opinion. Often, just going across town to a different doctor may net you a whole new bag of treatment options to try.

Finally, at least some women find hair loss help via the use of estrogen-dominant birth control pills such as Yasmin, Demulen, Desogen, or Ortho-Cyclen. These oral contraceptives work by overriding the excess testosterone and literally flooding the hair follicle with estrogen. However, because treatments for other perimenopause symptoms—like hot flashes and night sweats—generally involve very-low-dose estrogen pills (see Chapter 11) using these high-estrogen pills for hair loss may only be appropriate if you are on the "younger" end of the perimenopause spectrum—in your early forties. Also important to note: If you are at risk for breast or endometrial cancer, this is definitely not an option for you at any age.

And while a rumor has long persisted that birth control pills can actually cause hair loss in some women, doctors say this is definitely not the case. What they can do is cause a temporary change in the growth and shed pattern of your hair (similar to what occurs in pregnancy), and this, say experts, can sometimes aggravate hair loss already occurring due to another problem. So, if your loss seems to grow worse when you initially start the Pill, don't despair. Chances are the problem will clear in a short time, and then the help should kick in.

SHAMPOOS, CONDITIONERS, AND MASQUES FOR HAIR LOSS

Although true female pattern balding *won't* be affected by products such as shampoos or conditioners, if your hair is at all stressed, or even damaged from either bleaching, dying, perming, straightening, or sun exposure, or if it's starting to show the signs of age (dull, dry, and hard to style), there are a number of products that can help. There are even a few that might influence the rate at which your hair loss occurs, or give your scalp what it needs to encourage new growth.

Here are a few suggestions for products that could help—and be sure to visit www.yourmenopause.com for more detailed product information.

- *Lamas Hair Care:* This line of totally natural shampoos, conditioners, and styling aids was created by legendary New York City stylist Peter Lamas. (www.lamasbeauty.com)

- *J Beverly Hills:* Developed by world-renowned French stylist Juan Juan of Beverly Hills are shampoos, conditioners, and hair masques that literally infuse each strand with soy and other important botanicals. (www.jbeverlyhills.com)

- *Tova's Cactine Hair Masque/Shampoo:* Developed by the extraordinary skin-care/fragrance maven Tova Borgnine, try this amazing hair masque and volumizing shampoo duo. (www.qvc.com)

- *Olivarium Hair Fortifying Masque by Perlier:* This Italian-made hair conditioner reconditions and reenergizes even the driest, dullest hair in just five minutes. (www.hsn.com)

- *Jean-Marc Maniatis Shampoos and Conditioners:* Imported from France and now available in the United States, this line includes an Anti-Aging Shampoo and Anti-Aging Conditioner that can do wonders for graying or thinning hair. (www.ccb-paris.com)

From the "M" File

IS IT REALLY MY HORMONES?

Q: I am forty-seven years old and have recently started losing a lot of hair—a lot. I talked to my dermatologist about it, and he suggested that I probably have female pattern balding—a hereditary form of hair loss that he says gets worse at this time of life. But the problem is, I don't have anyone in my family—either male or female—who has hair loss problems, and I'm wondering if there could be another cause. He wants me to start minoxidil, but I'm hesitating—I'd like to know for sure if the cause is hereditary or something else. Is there a test I can take?

A: Although most of us think that "hereditary" means we can tick off a roll call of family members who share our problem, the truth is, a condition need not be obvious in others to be present in our genes. That's because it is the combination of genetic material from your mother and your father that comes together to create your uniquely personal gene profile, along with any specific hereditary conditions you may face.

That said, you are right in assuming that there can also be other reasons for hair loss—and that we shouldn't always jump to the "genetic conclusion," at least not before investigating other possibilities. Topping the list are certain autoimmune disorders such as lupus. These illnesses can result in a type of hair loss known as alopecia areata—an inflammatory condition that causes hair to come out in clumps or patches. Additionally, following childbirth, or sometimes as a result of crash dieting, surgery, or even a highly charged emotional event, a temporary hair loss known as telogen effluvium can also occur.

A third possibility links hair loss to a problem in your thyroid—a tiny gland located at the base of your neck that secretes a number of hormones involved in your reproductive and overall health. Problems related to hair loss can in fact be caused by either an over- or under-active thyroid—a gland that either overproduces or underproduces those hormones. And while doctors say that going through your midlife transition won't necessarily increase your risk of a thyroid dis-order, often the symptoms of perimenopause can mask the problem, simply because so many of the signs overlap—including hot flashes, sweating, insomnia, and nervousness. And while it's possible for peri-menopause and thyroid disease to exist simultaneously, according to endocrinology expert Dr. Richard Shames (author of *Thyroid Power: 10 Steps to Total Health),* when they do, thyroid abnormalities are bound to make perimenopause symptoms far worse. So, if you *are* experiencing a particularly severe perimenopause—with symptoms much worse than what many of your friends talk about—then it's pos-sible a thyroid problem may be the reason, as well as one possible cause of your hair loss.

You can also look to the rest of your body for signs. Has your pu-bic hair grown sparse—or do you find that you shave your legs or un-derarms less frequently? Is your skin exceptionally dry—and are you either very cold or very warm much of the time? If any of these sce-narios are true for you then a thyroid disorder may be at work. To know for sure, talk to your doctor about a simple blood test called TSH—short for thyroid-stimulating hormone. If results are borderline, or if other symptoms of a thyroid disorder exist, an ultrasound scan or even an X ray of your thyroid may help. In some instances, a be-nign tumor can be hiding on a section of your thyroid gland causing intermittent symptoms that can be hard to pin down with a blood test alone.

If ultimately your thyroid proves to be normal, and you have not been diagnosed with any autoimmune disorders, then it's likely your dermatologist may be right in assuming your hair loss is heredi-tary.

From the "M" File

LASERS FOR HAIR LOSS

Q: I've heard about a procedure that uses lasers to combat hair loss in women. I know it sounds a bit "Star-Warsy" but I've been diagnosed with female pattern balding, and the standard medications don't seem to be doing me much good. Do you think I'd have any better luck with this method?

A: First off, I hope you've given the medications enough time to work—you need several months before you really start to see measurable results. That said, yes, it's true, lasers are the newest weapons in the treatment arsenal for hair loss. Approved by the FDA in 2003, this treatment is currently being offered by an increasing number of dermatologists around the country. It involves sitting under a hair dryer–like device for about thirty minutes, during which time a laser scans your scalp. The idea here is to stimulate cell turnover and increase circulation. This, in turn, may help any dormant follicles to wake up and begin producing hair. In addition, a home device has also recently become available, making this treatment easier to come by. In this version, the laser is built into a device similar to a handheld hair dryer or electric comb. It's used twice a week for about five minutes. At least a few dermatologists believe the lasers work best as an adjunct treatment to hair transplants, encouraging the hair grafts to "take" and begin growing. It might be worth a try, but you should talk to your doctor about whether or not you can combine the treatment with the medication you are already using to "boost" the effects. The cost of a home-use laser comb is between $600 and $700. Laser treatments in a dermatologist's office vary widely depending on where they are done, and how often they need to be repeated.

COMBATING HAIR LOSS—NATURALLY

In addition to any traditional medical treatments your doctor can offer, there are also a variety of natural methods of encouraging hair growth. Although none can actually regrow your hair, at least some may be able to slow down the loss. In some instances, where thinning hair is strictly the result of the aging process and no genetic loss is involved, then natural treatments may be especially effective.

Among your best lines of defense is eating a healthy, nutritious diet. Because at least some hair loss may be caused by a lack of nutrients, the healthier your diet is, the healthier your hair will be. The foods that are good for your hair, say experts, are the same ones that are good for your body: high-protein, low-carbohydrate meals with a low saturated fat content. What is also important, however, is increasing your intake of omega-3 *essential fatty acids*—the "good fats" found in foods like walnuts, canola oil, flaxseed, fish, and soy. Although there is little in the way of scientific research, at least some nutrition experts believe that omega-3 fatty acids may play a subtle but important role in hair health and that even a subclinical deficiency may have dramatic effects on your mane.

In addition, if you have been plagued with heavy perimenopausal bleeding—particularly if you have fibroid tumors or polyps—then you may also have an iron deficiency, which can be a major cause of hair loss in women. According to New York University nutritionist and dietician Samantha Heller, even a slight deficiency can be powerful enough to trigger hair loss—or aggravate any loss that is occurring due to age, or even heredity. Adding more iron-rich foods to your diet, such as broccoli or brewer's yeast, may, says Heller, help reverse some hair loss.

Also important are foods rich in vitamin B_{12}, like eggs, meat, and poultry—nutrients that hair just "can't live without"! However, because so many women are prone to a B_{12} deficiency, experts say taking a supplement might be wise. And while you're shopping the vitamin aisle, you might also want to pick up a bottle of biotin, another B vitamin essential to healthy hair growth. In fact, this nutrient is so important to hair health that supplements are often recommended by dermatologists whenever traditional hair loss treatments such as Propecia, Proscar, or minoxidil are prescribed. According to clinical researcher and vitamin developer

From the "M" File

TRANSPLANTING A GOOD HAIR DAY

Q: My husband recently had a hair transplant, and it looks fantastic—so much so that I would like to get one as well. But my sister-in-law says that the procedure isn't done very often on women because the whole transplanting system is not appropriate for the way women lose their hair. Is this true? And if so, why don't they invent a hair transplant that is right for women?

A: Although medically speaking there is nothing that would stop a woman from getting a hair transplant, the reason it's rarely done—and yes, your sister-in-law is right on this one—is because results are not often cosmetically pleasing. Because hair loss in women is diffuse rather than confined to one area, the transplanting system tends to make hair look "clumpy" rather than full. That said, there are some who say these problems can be overcome. A report in the November 2003 issue of the *Journal of the American Academy of Dermatology* says that advances in the way transplants are being performed—including new methods that reduce scarring—*can* make it a viable alternative for some women, providing expectations are realistic. According to a group of doctors from Mount Sinai Medical Center in New York City who authored the new report, the key lies in a new technique that removes entire strips of hair. Those strips are then subdivided into very tiny sections, which are then surgically placed only where the hair is needed. In fact, this method can be so precise that the transplanted hair can even be relocated *between* hairs that are still growing, creating a totally natural look and feel. Still, many experts say that this should be a woman's last resort—after a trip to a dermatologist for a diagnosis, and at least one round of treatment with medication.

Andrew Lessman, "Biotin is a major component in the natural hair-manufacturing process—it is essential to not only grow new hair, but it also plays a major role in the overall health of skin and nails." While it's possible to get biotin from our diet in foods like liver and egg yolks, those foods are not necessarily healthy in the amounts we would need to eat in order to significantly boost biotin levels. So, most experts agree supplements are in order—and that they can help. Dr. Daly recommends up to 3 milligrams of biotin daily, while Lessman, who developed a healthy hair, skin and nails product, recommends 2 milligrams, which he believes is the minimum for healthy hair. The FDA-recommended intake of biotin is just 300 micrograms—and Lessman says even a very healthy diet usually doesn't contain more than 30 to 50 micrograms.

While some dermatologists recommend zinc along with biotin, both Lessman and Heller advise caution and say never to exceed the amount found in a good multivitamin. Although zinc can affect levels of androgens (male hormones) in the bloodstream, it can also impact copper levels. Since it's vital that copper and zinc remain in a precise balance, taking either one individually may eventually throw off the balance of both and, in some instances, exacerbate hair loss. What may be important for you to take, says Lessman, is the nutrient known as methylsulfonylmethane, or MSM—a sulphur-containing amino acid that is intrinsic to the structural development of hair. Lessman recommends 700 milligrams of MSM daily.

MOTHER NATURE HAD GREAT HAIR: THE NATURAL BUZZ ON OVERCOMING HAIR LOSS

Because there has been lots of buzz generating around the use of the herb saw palmetto for prostate disease in men, some experts believe that, like the prostate drug finasteride, this herb may also help hair loss. While there are no clinical trials showing it can, there is some research indicating it can impact the way androgens like testosterone react in the hair follicle—and that in turn may have an effect on hair loss. If this *is* true, you certainly don't want to take this herb without first consulting with your gynecologist—particularly if you are using any type of natural plant

From the "M" File

STYLING THINNING HAIR—WHAT WORKS

Q: My hair has been getting progressively thinner over time—not so much that I need a medical treatment, but certainly enough that it needs some style attention. Men have comb-overs to turn to—what can a woman do, style-wise, to make a difference? Are there hints or tricks that would help?

A: Because women generally lose hair in a different pattern from men—a diffuse loss as compared to a balding "spot"—it's true that comb-over techniques won't do you much good. As such, your goal, stylewise, should be to minimize the appearance of your loss—and experts say one of the best ways to do that is with a shorter, more layered cut. While it seems counterintuitive to cut hair that is already in short supply, in fact, leaving hair long only accentuates how little there is of it, compared to a natural "healthy" or "full" head of hair. Conversely, wearing a shorter style plays up the style and puts less emphasis on length, which ultimately take the focus off how much hair you have—or *don't* have. If your hair is dark, lightening it a few shades or adding highlights can also be a plus, since it will help blend your hair into your scalp—meaning you won't see the spaces in between as easily or readily. And that can make you look as if you have thicker hair. Remember, the darker your hair, the more obvious your scalp will be.

To give hair instant volume try one of the new powder volumizers, like "Brush & Ready." This product uses an ultrafine, vanilla-scented powder tinted in natural hair colors that allows you to literally "spray in" volume. Because the powder adheres to each hair strand, it auto-

estrogens, or even pharmaceutical hormones for other perimenopause symptoms. At least theoretically, if an herb is strong enough to affect androgen pathways in the hair follicle, it may also be strong enough to interact with other hormonal preparations, even those of the plant variety. What may be safer—and possibly more effective—for women is

matically poufs your pouf—and can give you the appearance of having almost double the amount of hair. By the way, it also works great between hair colorings, or to cover or blend in gray. It's sold online at www.hsn.com and versions from other companies may soon be available, so check your local drugstore or beauty supply shop.

Finally, don't overlook wigs or hairpieces as a possible solution for styling thinning hair. Very different from wigs of the past, today's styles use up-to-the-minute, lightweight, synthetic materials that are available in a wide range of colors and color blends that can look not only natural, but a whole lot better than what most women can accomplish stylewise, even at the hairdresser. Great sources for inexpensive but good-quality wigs include www.BeautyTrends.com, www.PaulaYoung.com, www.WigsInternational.com, and www.hsn.com (see the resource section at the back of this book for toll-free numbers and catalog information).

Also pay attention to hairpieces—partial wigs that can work to "fill in" a thinning top, or "clip-ons" such as buns, chignons, and ponytails that can add dimension and volume, making you look years younger, and as if you have more hair than you do. Among the best you can buy are the Toni Tails line of products sold on the Home Shopping Network. The brainchild of Oklahoma entrepreneur Toni Brattin, they are reasonably priced and yet extremely high quality, utilizing a unique color blending system that puts sixteen shades in each color wave. This makes it incredibly easy to mix their pieces into your own hair, without any "line of demarcation" between true and false! Check the resource section at the back for other sources for hairpieces, or visit www.yourmenopause.com.

green tea. Why? Research indicates it may influence the levels of at least one hormone linked to genetic hair loss—SHBG, or sex hormone-binding globulin. In one study published in the journal *Nutrition and Cancer* in 1998, a group of Japanese researchers found that drinking several cups of green tea a day can increase levels of SHBG in women significantly. And this in turn can impact the amount of testosterone in the bloodstream, and ultimately the amount that is converted to DHT in hair follicles.

Other natural approaches to hair loss include licorice extract (thought to prevent hair loss, but can also increase blood pressure); horsetail (which is a source of silica, a component in healthy hair); apple cider vinegar and sage tea applied directly to the scalp (thought to stimulate hair growth); psoralea seeds (a Chinese herb applied to the scalp); and ginger (either taken as a tea or applied to the scalp).

Common Sense and Your Midlife Hair

Although it may seem counterintuitive—at least it did for me—the surprising truth is that bleaching, coloring, or even perming your hair will not increase your risk of hair loss, at least not genetic hair loss. In fact, I was extremely surprised when not one, but numerous well-respected dermatologists told me that the kind of damage that occurs from overprocessing hair—as well as the overuse of blow-dryers and curling irons—*is not* the same kind of loss that occurs due to female pattern balding. So, by and large, color and perms are safe to use. In fact, many dermatologists say that coloring your hair during midlife can be a wonderful way to add thickness and body, and actually make your mane easier to manage. And even if you don't want to change your look in any kind of dramatic fashion (although that *is* what makes being a girl so much fun!), most hair colorings available today can simply add fresh new highlights without a major color change—and in the process help you and your hair look younger, healthier, and more vibrant. So if your hair is thinning—or even if you are losing a significant amount—don't automatically stop grooming or styling your locks.

At the same time, however, I can't help but point out that doing anything with your hair when it's in a less than perfect state requires a hefty dose of common sense. While a hot blow-dryer or curling iron might not cause you to lose your hair at the roots, it can certainly cause breakage of the hair you do have—as can overbleaching, overdying, or overperming.

So it's important that you not abuse your hair during any of these processes.

Also keep in mind that hair which is dry and brittle is also likely to snap off more easily when abused—or at the very least be difficult to manage. This may be particularly true if your hair is graying, since the very process of losing pigment can turn hair "wiry" and make it more difficult to style.

So, whether you seek treatment for your thinning hair or just try to cope on your own, make a few extra efforts to be "kind" to your tresses. Use gentle shampoos (the type recommended for dry or color-treated hair, even if yours isn't), apply lots of conditioners, and limit exposure to superhot dryers, curling irons, or electric rollers. In addition, don't skimp on what you pay for your hair-care products—buy the very best you can afford. While it's true that there are some low-priced products that offer excellent results on young, normal, or otherwise healthy hair, as we age, our hair demands and needs more from the products we use. So, consider purchasing salon-quality shampoos and conditioners. Most do contain a higher grade of ingredients as compared to what's on the supermarket shelf, and in many instances it can make an important difference in how your hair looks and styles.

Finally, even if you've always groomed your hair on your own, if possible treat yourself to a salon visit now and again. A good professional hairdresser can be worth his or her weight in diamonds in terms of advice, product recommendations, and an extra level of care.

7

Outsmarting Your
Menopause Metabolism

*Successful Weight Control and Exercise
in Your Middle Years*

At first the changes can be so subtle you barely know they have occurred—or at least you pretend not to. Your slacks fit a little tighter on the waistline, your blouses feel a bit snug in the sleeves. And if you're anything like me you're thinking, "water retention," right? Oh yeah, I've been there. I may not have had eight ounces of water to drink in seventy-two hours, but that tight snap on the top of my jeans? Definitely water retention.

Before long, however, that squishy feeling between your thighs, or that mushy feeling at the back of your arms becomes hard to ignore—though heaven knows, we try.

"You know, I think they're cutting clothes a lot smaller than they did a few seasons back, don't you?" my friend Nadine rationalized as we both struggled to zip up the fall collection in the dressing room at Barneys. I rolled my eyes and shook my head, indicating that no, that wasn't the reason we had both apparently gone up at least one size from the summer.

"The clothes are the same—it's us that's changing," I said, wishing I *could* blame it all on Calvin or Randolph or Ms. Karan.

"That's impossible—I think it's a conspiracy, one of those *Stepford Wives* experiments where men secretly change the sizes on women's clothing so we all begin starving ourselves into weakness and submission," she said with a certain conviction.

"Submission? Me? Have you ever seen how mean I get when I'm starving? I could kill for just one bite of a deep-fried Twinkie," I said, remembering just *how* miserable I made everyone, including myself, the last time I was on a diet.

As we headed out of the dressing rooms and back to the racks for a larger size I couldn't help but face the truth: My friend and I were getting older. And despite the fact that neither of us was eating any more or exercising any less, our bodies were changing. The reason? It's called midlife metabolism—the physiological system of hormones and other body chemicals that is responsible for how many calories we burn and how much energy our body expends on any given day. Studies now show that as we age, our metabolism changes—sometimes significantly. So while we may eat the same amount of food and get the same amount of exercise, we're just not going to stay the same size.

But what makes our metabolism change—and why at midlife? One reason is that we are simply losing certain biological and physiological functions that impact the number of calories our bodies burn in the course of a day. Among the first of those changes for women is a reduction in the activity of the reproductive system. Although you might not think of activities like ovulation or menstruation as burning calories, the truth is, every body function requires energy—and that means it burns calories. What's more, when that body function stops, those calories are no longer being burned. The end result: More of what you eat is now available to store as fat.

However, even more significant is that as we age, we also begin to lose muscle mass. And since muscle mass burns energy—even when you're just sitting on the sofa watching the Home Shopping Network—the less muscle mass you have, the fewer calories your body burns. The end result: You may be eating the same amount of food and exercising at the same rate, but you're gaining weight.

One more factor affects the way your body looks and feels—your hormones. In studies reported in the *Medical Journal of Australia,* doctors showed that estrogen can affect how quickly fat is burned in the body—and the less of this hormone you have, the more sluggish your fat-burning metabolism can be. Other research has suggested an estrogen deficiency may also interfere with the normal action of still another hormone known as leptin—a compound believed to play a role in controlling appetite and increasing the rate at which calories burn. When estrogen levels fall, leptin may not work as efficiently—so you end up hungrier *and* it takes less food to put on the pounds. Which is probably one of those facts you want to hang on to, so the next time your "I'm-just-naturally-thin" sister-in-law happens to mention that your jeans are fitting *a little tight,* you'll have an appropriate comeback that doesn't involve hair pulling or emptying the contents of the deep fryer into her skinny little lap.

Your Blood Sugar, Your Weight, and Perimenopause

In addition to changes in your reproductive hormones, there is another biochemical shift that can occur as you age—and it can play a significant role in not only weight control but also how you feel, and your level of energy throughout your perimenopause. I'm talking about insulin. A hormone that is manufactured by the pancreas, insulin is secreted into your bloodstream whenever you eat. Its main job is to shuttle nutrients—particularly sugar—from your blood into your muscle cells. Here the sugar is stored and then later released to meet your body's demand for energy. And, in fact, it is the presence of insulin that encourages muscle cells to "open up" and accept and store these sugars. You say you don't eat many sweets? You're still getting more sugar in your bloodstream than you realize. The reason is because much of what you *do* eat—including foods like a baked potato, an ear of corn, an apple, even bread—eventually gets broken down into *some* form of sugar. How quickly that happens is greatly reliant upon what is known as the glycemic index—which is essentially how quickly a food is metabolized (see "Trick Your Body," later in this chapter). So, when you hit the gym for that mid-morning workout, it's the sugars from your breakfast cereal and whole-wheat toast that are fueling all those rounds on the stationary bike. And when you work late at the office, it's the glucose left over from your fish and chips dinner that helps you burn the midnight oil.

In addition, by transporting sugar into your cells, insulin also helps *clear it* from your bloodstream—which is not only important for your overall health but also helps control your weight. This entire system of metabolic "checks and balances" is pretty much in place and working at full capacity from virtually the time you are born. And for most folks it functions pretty well, clear into the middle years. But at around age forty-five, things can begin to change. According to New York University gynecologist and researcher Dr. Lila Nachtigall, it is during this time that "some unknown, unseen switch turns the whole system off!"

Indeed, as we age, our muscle cells don't respond as readily to insulin. So instead of immediately opening up their "door" to accept and store the sugars that insulin carries, they resist. This causes two important things to happen. First, because your cells aren't getting the sugars they need they can't respond to your body's demand for energy. So, you start to feel tired and sluggish. Second, because sugar can't get into your cells as easily, much of it is left floating in your bloodstream. This, in turn, sends a signal to your pancreas to produce more insulin, in hopes of stimulating the cells to "open up" and let the sugars in. And for a while, this overstimulation signal works—your cells eventually *do* open up and the sugar *does* get in. Unfortunately, this can sometimes require insulin levels up to forty times higher than what is normally produced. When this overproduction and overstimulation goes on long enough, it creates another condition known as insulin resistance. When this occurs, your body becomes even more resistant to insulin, so less and less sugar gets into your cells after each meal—and more remains in your bloodstream. When this continues long enough, sugar levels in your blood not only rise, they remain elevated—and type 2 diabetes develops. In this disease your body is clearly making enough insulin, but essentially your cells are no longer responding at all.

Interestingly, research into this very phenonmenon has produced a new link between insulin resistance and middle-aged "spread." In addition to shuttling sugar into muscle cells, insulin *also* takes fatty acids into our fat cells. And the more insulin we have circulating through our bloodstream, the faster our fat cells are stuffed—and the fuller they get. When they can hold no more the body begins to manufacture *new* fat cells to take up the slack—and that's when weight gain can really take hold. But that's not all that's going on. Whenever your body is being primed to add more fat cells—which is what is happening as long as insulin levels remain high—it is impossible to *lose* fat cells. So, the longer your insulin levels remain elevated, the more difficult it becomes to lose any weight. At the same time, insulin resistance is also changing the way your fat cells function—making it harder for them to break down and burn their contents for energy. And that too influences how easily you can burn off fat—all of which is complicated even further the less active you are. While regular exercise can help your cells respond to insulin in a timely fashion, leading a sedentary life does the opposite.

The end result of all this: You not only *gain* weight, it also becomes much more difficult to *lose* weight, even if you watch what you eat.

Making matters just a bit more complicated, studies show that gaining weight around the midsection—your abdomen and waist area—actually increases your risk of insulin resistance. The catch-22 here: As estrogen levels drop, weight naturally shifts from your hips and thighs to your abdomen and midsection, thereby automatically increasing your risk for insulin resistance to develop.

The good news—it doesn't have to be this way! And yes, there are some brand-new ways to outsmart your midlife metabolism and keep your weight under control.

The Mysterious Syndrome W: The Riddle That May Provide the Answer

Although most doctors are aware of the hormone/weight/insulin resistance connection, it wasn't until just a few years ago that Dr. Harriette Mogul, an endocrinologist from New York Medical College, began to piece the information together in a brand-new way—and in doing so arrived at some startling conclusions about women and their midlife bodies.

It began when Mogul started noticing an interesting phenomenon occurring among the women who were coming to her office to discuss hormone therapy, ostensibly for perimenopausal or menopausal symptoms. While they were of differing ages, races, and sizes, and each was at a different point in her midlife hormonal profile (some in perimenopause, others already in menopause), Mogul noted that they all shared certain common traits. All the women were, for example, extremely health conscious, nonsmokers, and very physically active. And yet they were all complaining about gaining weight, particularly around their midsection. And they were each having great difficulty losing it. In addition, all of the women also complained of overwhelming fatigue—even though they were active and health conscious.

Among the first things Dr. Mogul tested was the women's blood sugar levels—obviously looking for signs of insulin resistance or even type 2 diabetes. If their sugar was high, she reasoned, it would be easy to see why they were gaining weight and why they were so tired. Mysteriously however, their sugar tests were "normal"—something many of the women reported was previously the case when other doctors had tested them in the past. At the same time, however, all of the women's blood pressure was intermittently high, and Mogul also noted elevations in blood fats, like cholesterol and triglycerides—indicating that something in their bodies was amiss. Working on a hunch, she decided to give the women one more test—to measure insulin levels. And the results were nothing short of astounding.

Although all the women had normal *sugar* levels, their insulin levels were soaring. Along with the intermittent elevations in blood pressure and blood fats, Mogul suspected that even though *most* of the sugar was eventually cleared from their blood, the elevated insulin level necessary to accomplish this was creating the same type of weight-gain and fatigue problems seen in patients with true insulin resistance—a condition marked by both high insulin and high sugar. Searching for a way to identify these patients, she called the problem "Syndrome W"—and she began recording other symptoms the women shared as well, including an increased appetite, food cravings, and a continued inability to lose weight, despite dieting and exercise. All this, she concluded, was the result of high insulin—even if sugar levels were normal.

Ultimately, Mogul began to believe that the symptoms of Syndrome W were really precursors to insulin resistance (signified by high blood sugar and high insulin) and, eventually, type 2 diabetes—when sugar levels hit an all-time high. The good news in her finding: Mogul says Syndrome W is relatively easy to identify and treat. And in doing so, she believes women can not only control their midlife weight problems, but also delay the onset of heart disease as well as insulin resistance or even full-blown type 2 diabetes.

Her solution: A low-glycemic diet—(see "Trick Your Body," later in this chapter). Essentially this is an eating plan that focuses on avoiding foods that cause rapid spikes in blood sugar—which in turn helps keep insulin levels from soaring too high. And, Mogul believes, not only is this key to helping you lose the weight you've already gained, but when followed early on in your perimenopause, it may actually keep you from gaining any weight at all, regardless of what your hormones may be doing at the time. Additionally, if your insulin levels still remain high, Mogul suggests the oral diabetes medication Metformin may help—even if your sugar levels are normal. This medication works by increasing a cell's sensitivity to insulin so sugars can be accepted and stored—which in turn helps keep the body from overproducing insulin.

According to Mogul, this combination has provided dramatic results for all the women in her study—with weight loss of forty or more pounds common. And in fact, a 1999 study conducted by doctors from Washington University in St. Louis verified at least some of what Mogul was saying. In their research, female patients who had gained fat around the midriff and had an apple-shaped body were at greater risk for insulin resistance—so much so that many doctors now believe this body type (rounded, with a larger middle) could be a "marker" for this problem.

Be that as it may, don't be surprised if your doctor is not so quick to embrace this explanation of your problem or the idea that insulin may be behind your midlife weight gains—particularly if your sugar levels remain normal.

"I think the reason that this wasn't previously diagnosed is that traditionally, thin, male physicians who never had to struggle with their weight said, 'Oh, you're just eating too much and not exercising enough,' and for many women this just isn't true," says Mogul.

As to why this propensity toward insulin resistance seems to occur at midlife, doctors aren't certain. Mogul believes genetics may play a role, along with some metabolic changes that occur around age forty, including a shift in hormones. Although all women are susceptible to this problem, those most vulnerable include women of Asian, Middle Eastern, and Hispanic descent, as well as Ashkenazi Jewish women. In addition, if you have been diagnosed with polycystic ovarian syndrome—a condition that is also earmarked by interplay between female hormones and insulin—you may also be at higher risk for insulin resistance when you reach midlife.

Fighting the Midlife Fat Cell— and Winning!

Whether your extra pounds are the result of your hormones, your metabolism, or even your insulin levels, the important thing to remember is that midlife weight control is not beyond your reach. Of course you'd know I was lying if I said dieting—at any time is life—is either fun or easy. It's not—you know that. And, in truth, if you had trouble controlling your weight in your twenties and thirties, doing so in your forties, fifties, and sixties is certainly not going to get any easier. On the other hand, science *has* provided us with an answer or two we probably didn't have when you were twenty-five or even thirty-five. Indeed, doctors now know more about a woman's body—and particularly her body at midlife—than at any other time in recent history. And for you, that means more answers *and* more options—as well as more opportunity to control your midlife weight *without* having to resort to the "Diet from Satan."

Of course, in the end, much of your success is going to come down to burning up more calories than you take in—because no matter how you cut the cheesecake, the biggest piece is going to end up on your hips *if* what you put in your mouth has more calories than what your body can burn. That said, there are some important food strategies that can help boost your metabolism, increase your ability to burn fat in your

From the "M" File

CRASH DIETS AND MIDLIFE CRISIS

Q: I know it's not considered very healthy, but for me, the best way to lose that extra five or ten pounds has been one of several different "crash diets"—the quick loss motivates me and I've always been pretty lucky in that the weight usually stays off, at least for a while. But I've just turned forty-six, and suddenly the "old reliable" diets don't work anymore. And the weight is really starting to creep up. I'm a little frantic—thinking that maybe nothing will work anymore. Can you explain?

A: While the so-called "crash" diets are never healthy, they may be the most harmful and the least likely to do you any good in midlife. One reason is because as we age, the body can't lose fat as quickly as it can when we are young, says exercise physiologist Bryant Stamford, director of the Health Promotion and Wellness Center at the University of Louisville in Kentucky. So, what you often end up losing on a crash diet, he says, is muscle mass. Since muscle burns calories, the more you lose, the slower your metabolism goes, which in turn actually keeps you from losing weight—even though you may be dramatically lowering your caloric intake. In addition, studies show that when you throw your body into the "starvation" mode, your metabolism shuts down further, which in turn increases your desire for fat and sugar—a craving that can make dieting even harder. The solution: Skip the crash diets and instead focus on healthy eating, cutting calories by about 20 percent—about 200 to 400 calories a day should do it. Also consume most of your calories during the day, when your metabolism is revved up and working at optimum speed. (Think: Bigger lunch, smaller supper.) This should help stabilize your weight and keep you from gaining any more. Then, if you add an aerobic exercise regimen to your weekly workouts, or step up what you are already doing (exercise a little longer each time or add an extra session a week), the weight should come off—though *slowly*. But in the end Stamford says that's more likely to give you lasting results.

midlife body, and generally work *with*—and not *against*—many of the hormonal changes you are experiencing right now. What follow are three such strategies. Based on a variety of research and some important medical studies, the following three plans not only work together to help you lose weight and control some of your "change of life" symptoms (including foods to reduce hot flashes!) but may also keep you from gaining weight now, and in the future. While on its own any one of these strategies will provide you with some results, I urge you to use all three together. This will not only give you the best shot at weight control but also benefit your health in myriad ways.

STRATEGY #1: CUT YOUR CALORIES

As simple a concept as this can be, you might be quite surprised to realize how effective a weight control system it really is, particularly at midlife. In fact, studies show that if you reduce your caloric intake by just 200 to 400 calories daily, you will generally compensate for the slowdown in your midlife metabolism—and the decrease in muscle mass—and practically guarantee that you won't gain any weight. If you also increase your activity level by just a small margin, you will not only prevent midlife weight gain, you will actually *lose* weight. This was something researchers discovered in the Women's Healthy Lifestyle Project, a major five-year study conducted by the National Institutes of Health. In their research, 535 premenopausal women were randomly assigned to either participate in a behavioral lifestyle group (which involved cutting calories and increasing physical activity) or continue their normal dietary and lifestyle habits.

The end result: Four and a half years into the study twice as many women in the calorie-cutting group were at or below their original weight, while the women in the control group (the ones who made no dietary changes) progressively gained weight.

And if you think you are going to rely on your normally "thin" metabolism to keep you as slim in your fifties as you were in your twenties, guess again, glamour puss. Unless you take action now, you won't evade those extra midlife pounds. In studies reported in the *Archives of Internal Medicine* as early as 1991, doctors found that women who were thin prior to menopause gained weight just as easily as women who were not.

So, how can you cut calories without feeling deprived, depressed, and otherwise doomed to a life of dieting? Experts say the simple art of substitution can make it easy—so much so that you may not even miss those extra 200 to 400 calories a day. Here are a few easy substitutions you can try:

Exchange two teaspoons of sugar in your tea or coffee for a sugar-free sweetener, while substituting two tablespoons of reduced-fat milk for the same amount of half-and-half—and save a total of 50 calories just on your coffee break! Adding a bagel to snack on? Leave off the two teaspoons of butter or margarine and instead try two teaspoons of nonfat cream cheese and save another 50 calories.

When lunch rolls around substitute mustard on your sandwich for mayonnaise—and save 85 calories—or use low-fat mayo and save 50 calories. Skip the high-fat salad dressing and opt for the low-fat variety—and you could save up to 70 more calories.

If you just love afternoon snacks (and I don't know about you but I'm convinced the four o'clock hour was *invented* for chocolate!), skip the candy and instead have a banana dipped in low-fat chocolate syrup and save up to 100 calories again. Have popcorn instead of potato chips in the evening—and save 60 or more calories.

At the end of the day, you've cut out almost 400 calories, and I'll bet your appetite—and your tummy—would never guess you were on a diet!

If you use a bit of imagination and what I like to call "creative food shopping," you can find many ways to decrease your caloric intake without depriving yourself of the foods you really like to eat.

STRATEGY #2: TRICK YOUR BODY

Although it's a tempting option, this suggestion does not involve papering your bedroom walls with "skinny mirrors" or using self-hypnosis to think yourself thin! What it does entail is recognizing that sometimes, a calorie is more than just a calorie—and *what* you eat can matter more than *how much* you eat. It's a philosophy that's based, at least in part, on what doctors now call the glycemic index, a way of rating certain foods according to how quickly they burn—and consequently, how much, and how rapidly, insulin is released into your bloodstream. Developed in 1981 by doctors at the University of Toronto, the glycemic index was originally intended to help folks with type 1 diabetes calculate how much insulin to take after eating certain foods. So how can this system help *you*?

Essentially, the glycemic index rates carbohydrates on a scale of 1 to 100, all based on how quickly your body breaks down each particular type into sugar. Those foods consisting of carbohydrates that break down quickly—like starches and some fruits—result in an immediate surge of glucose into your bloodstream, and a subsequent fast and sometimes overpowering release of insulin. They are considered "high" on the glycemic index. Those foods consisting of carbohydrates that break down more slowly—such as whole grains—are slower to release sugars, so insulin levels are not as likely to soar after eating. These foods are considered "low" on the glycemic index.

Initially doctors believed that simply sticking to low glycemic foods—and avoiding those rated as high—would be all that's needed to control insulin levels. And to some extent this still holds true. However, more recently researchers have taken the glycemic index concept one step further by defining what is called the "glycemic load." This is a way to calculate how much of a particular carbohydrate is found in a *single serving* of a food—and to take into account other factors that might also mediate sugar breakdown and release, such as fiber content. In short, while the glycemic index gives you a number that refers to how quickly a particular carbohydrate is converted to sugar, the glycemic load gives you a number that details the amount of that carbohydrate found in a *single serving of food*.

This is an important distinction because sometimes foods that are high on the glycemic index are okay if you eat them in moderation because the amount of carbohydrate found in an individual portion is not that high. Watermelon is a good example. The kind of carbohydrate found in watermelon breaks down very rapidly—so initially it's rated as high on the glycemic index. However, because of the water and the fiber content, there isn't actually a whole lot of that carbohydrate in a single serving, so experts calculate the actual glycemic load of watermelon to be just 4.32, which is considered quite low.

Why does all this matter? As you read earlier, the more insulin your body produces, the more likely you are to store fat—and the more you may be prevented from losing fat that is already stored in all those extra pounds. So, by focusing on foods with a "slow burn"—those with a low glycemic load or a low glycemic index—you will not only feel fuller longer, which will hopefully translate into fewer calories overall, but your body will not have to overproduce insulin. And that not only means fewer fat cells are being made, but also that what you do eat is more likely to be burned as fuel—and less will be stored as fat. Keeping insulin levels under control may also help you to ultimately ward off type 2 diabetes, which in turn can help protect your kidneys and your heart later in life.

You can find more information on the glycemic index in the resource section at the back of this book as well as at www.yourmenopause.com—including where to find complete glycemic index and glycemic load information on all major carbohydrates. In the meantime, however, you can use the following chart to help get you started in planning the meals that can keep you feeling fuller longer, while not adding to your waistline.

GLYCEMIC INDEX AND GLYCEMIC LOAD OF COMMON FOODS

The following chart is based on information published in the *American Journal of Clinical Nutrition*, July 2002. The first number following each food is the glycemic index. A number of 70 or more per meal is considered high, 56 to 69 is medium, and 55 is low, and it is your ideal number to shoot for. When calculating your glycemic load (the second number), 20 or more per meal is considered high; 11 to 19 medium; and 10 or less low.

The numbers are for "average servings"—one potato, for example, or one fruit; one-half cup of rice or vegetables or cereal. Whatever the standard measurement of one serving is for that food (and most will be listed on the label) correlates to the approximate values in this chart.

FOOD	GLYCEMIC INDEX	GLYCEMIC LOAD
All-Bran cereal	42	8
Apple juice	40	11
Apples	38	6
Baked potato	85	26

Bananas	52	12
Beets	64	5
Canteloupe	64	5
Carrots	47	3
Cheerios	74	15
Chickpeas	28	8
Corn	54	9
Cornflakes	85	26
Couscous	65	23
Fettucine	40	18
Grapes	46	8
Kidney beans	28	7
Life cereal	66	16
Macaroni	47	23
Navy beans	38	12
New potatoes	57	12
Orange juice	50	12
Oranges	42	5
Parboiled rice	50	12
Peaches	42	5
Peanuts	14	1
Pearled barley	47	17
Pears	38	4
Pinto beans	39	10
Popcorn	72	8
Red lentils	26	5
Shreaded wheat	75	15
Sourdough wheat bread	54	15
Spaghetti	42	20
Strawberries	40	1
Sweet potatoes	61	17
Watermelon	72	4
White bread	70	10
White rice	64	23
Whole-wheat bread	71	9
Wild rice	57	18

STRATEGY #3: FILL YOUR PANTRY WITH MENOPAUSE-FRIENDLY FOODS

In the past twenty years, and particularly in the past decade, researchers have finally begun to address the nutritional needs of midlife women. While we always assumed that a good diet is . . . well, a good diet, no matter what your age, more and more, doctors are coming to recognize that certain stages of your life present your body with unique and different challenges. In many ways, the foods we eat, as well as those we avoid, can play an important role in how well we meet those challenges and maintain our good health. Certainly, weight control is important, but it's not the only reason to eat a healthy diet. Reducing your risk of heart disease, breast and endometrial cancer, even osteoporosis, can all be accomplished by simply choosing the right foods, even if we don't start to concentrate on those foods until we are in our forties or fifties.

In addition, there is important new evidence to show that certain foods may even help us avoid some of the short-term consequences of whacky hormones—like hot flashes, fatigue, and even mood swings. By including certain foods in our diet—and, when appropriate, eliminating others—we may, in fact, not only better control our weight but also have a healthier, and even more pleasant perimenopause and menopause experience. Okay, so not really pleasant—but would you accept more tolerable?

So, what should you eat—and, more importantly, avoid? Well, truthfully, at least some of what's going to be on your shopping list will come strictly from you—as you begin to observe how your midlife body reacts when you eat certain foods. The same way you may have figured out what gives you a migraine headache or what aggravates your PMS, paying attention to links between what you eat and how you feel will also provide clues as to how your midlife metabolism is responding. But there are also some universal suggestions as to foods that both time and science have shown to have either negative or positive effects on midlife metabolism and overall health. Together with the glycemic index and your basic calorie-cutting strategies, incorporating or—when necessary—avoiding the following foods can go a long way in helping you devise meal plans that can work with your metabolism and your hormones.

MENOPAUSE-FRIENDLY FOODS: WHAT TO EAT

Estrogen Boosters

These are fruits and vegetables that contain a fairly good amount of phytoestrogens—plant estrogens that, while not nearly as potent as your own, can take at least some of the edge off your naturally dwindling levels. Best sources include fruits (apples, bananas, cherries, citrus fruits); whole grains (barley, oats, rice, rye, wheat); herbs and spices (fennel, parsley, red clover, sage, cinnamon); soy and soy products (tofu, miso, soy milk, soy flour); sprouts (alfalfa, mung beans); and vegetables (beetroot, broccoli, carrots, celery, garlic, green beans, potatoes, yams).

Vitamin E Boosters

At least anecdotally, I can tell you that foods high in vitamin E can be a real energy booster during perimenopause, increasing your sense of well-being and even helping to alleviate some symptoms such as hot flashes and vaginal dryness. Foods high in vitamin E include wheat germ, safflower, corn, or soybean oil; nuts.

Fiber Boosters

In general, foods high in fiber help move waste products out of your body more effectively while also slowing down the release of sugar into your bloodstream, which in turn helps keep insulin levels from soaring. Not only can this help keep you from storing fat, it may also help control your appetite, so you simply eat less. Fiber comes in two forms—soluble, which is more gentle on your stomach and can be found in fruits, vegetables, and oats, and insoluble, found in foods like brown rice, nuts, and fruit peels. While bran was once thought to be a good source of fiber, studies now show it can interfere with the absorption of zinc, magnesium, and calcium—all important perimenopause minerals. If you feel you are not getting enough fiber from the foods in your diet (or if your digestive system simply can't tolerate high-fiber foods) you might want to try fiber supplements—either in pill or liquid form or powders you can add to beverages like tea or juice. If you do take this approach, I caution you to go slowly—and start with far less than you think you need. Some high-fiber supplements can be hard on the stomach, so begin slow and build until you discover your personal level of tolerance.

Calcium/Vitamin D Boosters

It's no secret that foods rich in calcium and vitamin D can increase bone strength and improve your overall skeletal health. But now new evidence shows these same foods may also help calm jangled, hormonally harassed nerves and even reduce the risk of high blood pressure. According to the American College of Obstetricians and Gynecologists (ACOG) peri-menopausal women need 1,000 milligrams of calcium daily—and the closer you are to menopause, the more calcium you need. Women who have already stopped menstruating and are not taking estrogen require at least 1,500 milligrams daily. According to the ACOG, the top five food sources of calcium include:

- Yogurt, plain, low fat—one cup—425 mg calcium
- Skim milk—one cup—302 mg calcium
- Swiss cheese—one ounce—272 mg calcium
- Cheddar cheese—one ounce—204 mg calcium

UNFRIENDLY FOODS: WHAT TO AVOID

Processed/high-sodium foods

Some sodium is necessary to help regulate heartbeat and blood pressure and transmit certain nerve impulses from your brain to your body. However, consume too much and you not only increase the chance of water retention and subsequent bloating, you can also begin to pull calcium from your digestive tract before it can be used by your bones. And while you may think that simply avoiding the salt shaker at mealtime will do the trick, you may be getting more sodium than you think, hidden in a variety of foods. Hidden sources of sodium can be found in baking soda, baking power, canned and cured foods, prepackaged convenience foods like soups or frozen dinners, potato chips, condiments, flavor enhancers (MSG is almost pure sodium), sausages, smoked fish, ham, bacon, bologna, hot dogs, and packaged turkey or chicken roll. Aim for no more than 3,000 milligrams daily.

Caffeine
Not only can caffeine-rich foods increase your risk of hot flashes (see "Foods and Your Moods," later in this chapter), they can also increase breast tenderness, as well as leach calcium from your bones, increasing your risk of osteoporosis. Do be aware, however, that eliminating all caffeine from your diet too quickly can result in withdrawal symptoms including headaches, nervousness, insomnia, drowsiness, nausea, and constipation. The best way to quit is a gradual withdrawal, slowly replacing caffeinated beverages with decaffeinated ones.

Sugar
Whether or not your hormones are doing the tango—but probably more so if they are—sugar is going to stimulate your appetite and can cause cravings. In addition, sugar can suppress your body's ability to properly utilize calcium and phosphorus, both necessary for strong bones and healthy nerve transmission between brain and body. You can control cravings for sweets by keeping protein levels steady—eating frequent small, high-protein meals—and keeping sugar-laden foods to a minimum. Studies show the more sweets you eat, the more you may crave.

Fats and Cholesterol
In your twenties, thirties, and even your early forties, a steady supply of estrogen from your ovaries helps suppress fat buildup on artery walls. And that means eating high-fat foods is a lot less risky. But once estrogen levels start to tank, so too does your arterial protection. Cholesterol can start to rise, and sometimes blood pressure as well, as arteries begin holding on to fatty deposits. In addition, the older you get, the greater your risk of breast cancer—and there is at least some evidence to show that a high-fat diet could contribute to this problem. The solution: Reduce fatty food intake whenever possible by avoiding butter, rich sauces, gravy, fatty meats, whole milk, and ice cream.

Alcohol

It's true—I admit it: Sometimes nothing takes the edge off the midlife crazies like a relaxing glass of white wine at day's end. And while occasional alcohol won't harm you, overdo it, and you just might find your blood pressure rising to a dangerous level. Heavy drinking also increases your risk of osteoporosis, not to mention aggravating hot flashes *and* promoting weight gain with lots of empty calories. How much is too much? More than a glass of wine a day is pushing the envelope—and more than ten drinks a week is way too much. While everyone's tolerance levels are different, just know that whatever amount you drank in your twenties and thirties may be too much in your forties and fifties, so do yourself a big midlife favor and cut back when you can.

FOODS AND YOUR MOODS: THE HOT FLASH DIET

Is it hot in here? When you're having a hot flash, it's hot *everywhere*! The problem, as you read in Chapter 2, is falling estrogen levels, which in turn affect your body's internal thermostat and ultimately cause you to lose a whole lot of body heat all at once—thus resulting in a hot flash. While taking supplemental hormones was once believed to be the only way to control or eliminate flashes, many experts now believe that you can also influence their rate and severity based on what you eat—and sometimes what you leave on your plate. According to researcher and cookbook author Cathy Luchetti *(The Hot Flash Cookbook,* Chronicle Books, San Francisco), the key to controlling hot flashes lies in eating those foods which supply the nutrients that can impact some of the physiological mechanisms involved in the hot flash, including vasomotor functions. An extra bonus: Many of these same foods can also help quell other perimenopausal and menopausal symptoms including vaginal dryness, dry facial complexion, and lackluster hair.

According to Luchetti, foods that can help ease hot flashes include:

- Fish high in omega-3 oils and vitamin E including mackerel, bluefish, tuna, salmon, butterfish, pompano, and haddock.

- Fruits high in vitamin E and C, including apples, apricots, wild blackberries, blood oranges, oranges and lemons (particularly the citrus pulp and white membranes of these fruits), grapes (which may also help control bleeding), mangoes, papaya, and peaches.

- Whole grains including brown rice, corn, barley, buckwheat and millet, whole wheat, and rye.

- Nuts, including almonds, Brazil nuts, and walnuts.

- Oils like canola, hazelnut, olive, sesame, and wheat germ.

- Seeds such as anise, flax, and sesame.

- Spices including cayenne pepper (in moderation can cut hot flashes, but in excess might exacerbate them) and ginger.

- Soy foods including tofu, soy milk, and soy flour.

Exercise and Your Midlife Body: What You Need to Know

There is absolutely no getting around it, exercise at any time in your life, but particularly in your middle years, is one of the very best things you can do for yourself. What's that you say—you hate to exercise? You'd rather have your teeth drilled without Novocain than do twenty-five sit-ups? I hear you, muffin—you are talking to the woman whose sole purpose for learning to play tennis was the chance to shop for all those cute little white pleated skort sets. And even then, I think I spent more time sitting in the clubhouse sipping mint juleps in my cute little white pleated skort sets than I ever spent out on the courts. Be that as it may, midlife is upon us, dearies, and the consensus of opinion is in: Exercise *is* key to controlling our midlife weight, as well as setting the stage for a healthier, happier life for the next several decades to come. Truth is, studies show that beginning as early as age thirty-five we lose about seven pounds of muscle every decade, and often that is replaced by twice as much fat. Still hate exercise? Think about this: Unless you do *something* to change things in your life, your ability to do heart-pumping activities (including sex and shopping!) will drop a few percentage points every year. By some estimates by the time most of us reach age sixty-five, we can lose as much as 65 percent of our ability to do physical activity!

And those of you who already hit the gym with vigor three times a week? Don't be so sure you'll escape *all* the problems. Because the truth here is that not everything you did to stay in shape in your twenties, thirties, and even your early forties is going to have quite the same effect as you approach midlife. While any activity is certainly better than no activity, and almost any kind of workout is beneficial, there are certain types of exercises that are vital to include in your midlife regimen—and if you're not doing them you'll pay the price, even if your gams are in tip-top Tina Turner shape!

EXERCISE NOW—FEEL BETTER IMMEDIATELY

In addition to whatever long-term goals your workouts accomplish, there's also quite a bit of interesting research to show that certain exercises can actually have an immediate impact on midlife symptoms, helping to squelch even some of the most irritating of problems, including hot flashes.

While it may *seem* counterintuitive (wouldn't all that jumping around make you hotter than a pancake on the griddle?), the fact is, exercise can have a *calming* effect on your vasomotor system—the physiological "works" that set hot flashes in motion. A recent Scandinavian study found that women who exercise regularly have fewer hot flashes overall, and the ones they do get are less severe than those experienced by women who basically sit out menopause at the quilting bee! In other studies it was shown that circulating blood levels of estrogen actually increase after aerobic workouts—and they remain elevated for a significant number of hours afterward. And you know what that means—more estrogen in your bloodstream, fewer hot flashes on your face!

But that's not the only immediate benefit of working out. Other studies show it can help reduce the number of those hormone-related weepy moments (like bursting into tears during the Hallmark commercials, or because the bakery is out of rye bread), as well as taming those wild sleepless nights you're spending fighting with the sheets and pillows. According to Shan Mames, an exercise physiologist and manager of the Duke University Center for Living, when we work out (yes, even against our will!) our brain releases bucketfuls of endorphins—those same happy little hormones that circulate when we are in love! And do I have to tell you how great *that* feels? Bah-Bye mood swings and hello, smiley faces on all your e-mails.

On a more serious note, the American Council on Exercise reminds us that endorphins can also help relieve midlife depression and anxiety and, for many women, significantly patch the potholes on that winding road to menopause.

When it comes to caring for your body, certainly, the fat-burning potential of almost any activity is going to help ensure that you don't gain weight—or certainly not as much as you would if you were spending all your hours scrapbooking. But it's not only burning off calories that helps, it's also the strength-building power of certain types of workouts that increase your muscle mass. Since muscle burns more calories than, say, loose hanging flesh, your metabolism is going to work at a higher rate, even when you're resting. So, in a way—yes, you *can* burn calories while you sleep, if you take the time to build some additional muscle mass during your waking hours.

And then there's bone loss. Yes, it does occur as we age, and no, it's not your imagination, you probably *are* getting shorter as you get older. As estrogen decreases so too does our ability to make new bone mass—at least as easily as we did before. Why? Throughout your lifetime, your skeleton is maintained by an automatic system of bone cell renewal. As "old" cells die out, they are immediately replaced by new ones, which helps keep your bones healthy and strong. One of the ways new bone cells are made is through the use of calcium—which, in women, is brought into the bones primarily through estrogen. (In men, it's mostly testosterone that does this job, with just a small amount of estrogen). From a strictly evolutionary standpoint the estrogen connection is nature's way of ensuring that your pelvis and your skeleton as a whole are strong enough to bear children—one reason hormone levels soar so high during pregnancy.

As we age, however, and estrogen levels drop, bone doesn't receive or hold on to calcium as effectively. The end result: Fewer new bone cells are made, leading to a more fragile skeleton. For some women, the additional threat of the bone-robbing condition osteoporosis (see Chapter 12) looms

From the "M" File

AM I FAT OR FIT? HOW TO TELL!

Q: I've just turned forty-eight, and although I've never been involved in a formal exercise program, I am raising three children on my own and I'm pretty active—mostly running after the kids, but also doing laundry, vacuuming, cooking, all of which can be pretty strenuous at times. Now that my perimenopause seems in full swing I want to start doing aerobics—and I'd like to know if there is any way I can tell how fit I am, so I know where to begin? I don't have the money to spend on a gym or a personal trainer, so I'll be doing everything pretty much on my own.

A: I love the idea that you are recognizing just how much physical activity is involved with everyday living—and how things like housecleaning and laundry, and (bless you!) raising three kids on your own, can amount to substantial activity. Still, as you probably know, sometimes just moving around isn't quite enough to give you the protection your midlife body needs. So, it's also a good idea that you do get involved in some specific workout activities geared toward optimizing your midlife health. And aerobics is a great choice! Of course you should check with your doctor before starting any exercise program and get his or her input as to what level of activity might be right for you. That said, experts at *Health* magazine offer these tips for discovering your aerobic fitness level.

large during perimenopause and can make bone loss even more rapid and more devastating.

The good news here: On all fronts, exercise can help. Ironically, the more stress you put on bones and muscles the more you "force" your body to rebuild new bone—and the stronger your skeleton will be. This, combined with the benefits of flexibility that come when you are toned and buffed, means stronger supporting muscles and ligaments—which in turn can also help protect your bones in the event of a fall or other type of

AEROBIC CAPACITY AND STRENGTH TEST

You'll need a step that's about twelve inches high. You can use a stair step in your home or apartment, or a wood block or other solid, free-standing step that will hold your weight. You'll also need a stopwatch to time yourself.

To begin: Practice doing one complete round of stepping. This consists of right foot up, left foot up, right foot down, left foot down. Practice this pattern until you can do about twenty-four steps in about one minute. Once you have the pattern down, rest for about ten minutes, then do some stretches to limber up (calf, thighs, and hamstrings), and start a speed test, doing as many steps as you can within a three-minute time period. The second you finish, sit down and take your pulse for one full minute. Here is how to score your results:

- Ages 36 to 45: Pulse rate 98 or less—good shape; 98 to 112—average shape; greater than 112—below average shape.

- Ages 46 to 55: Pulse rate 103 or less—good shape; 103 to 118—average shape; greater than 118—below average shape.

- Ages 56 to 65: Pulse rate 105 or less—good shape; 105 to 120—average shape; greater than 120—below average shape.

accident (see "From the 'M' File: Bone Health and Exercise," later in this chapter).

Finally, it's also important to note that as estrogen levels fall, your risk of cardiovascular disease rises—placing your risk of a heart attack or stroke right up there with that of your stress-driven hubby. While doctors once thought that restoring estrogen levels through hormone replacement therapy was the answer, the Women's Health Initiative (WHI) study released in 2002 has shown this not to be the case. While doctors aren't sure why, one theory is that synthetic hormones don't have the same kind of positive effect on the heart as the kind our body makes naturally. Another theory says that HRT may need to be started earlier in life (the women in the WHI were, on average, sixty-three when they started) in order to have protective effects on the heart. As a result of these findings, exercise has once again been elevated to primary status as a way of not only protecting your bones but also reducing your risk of cardiovascular disease in much the same way estrogen did when you were younger.

Still not convinced to hit the mats and start that workout? Now hear this: Do the *right* exercises beginning in your forties and fifties and you might just reduce your risk of breast cancer later on. You can also stop worrying about spending your golden years in diapers, since regular exercise can help tone your entire pelvic area and cut your risk of incontinence by a wide margin. And how about great sex for some motivation? Studies show that exercise can boost some of the chemicals involved in your sex drive, make your vagina more responsive to stimulation, and generally help keep you looking and feeling like someone your partner may actually *want* to have sex with! (Okay, just kidding here—in reality, naked men over age fifty-five should be thankful we aren't running from the room screaming with laughter!)

In short, my dears, exercise can be your ticket to not only short-term but also long-term menopause relief, *and* make you the healthiest, as well as the best-looking, doll at the country club!

YOUR MIDLIFE EXERCISE PRESCRIPTION: THE WORKOUTS YOU NEED NOW

When it comes to the protective effects of midlife exercise, experts agree that your basic program should have a three-pronged approach, with three different and distinct types of physical activity to meet your needs. According to Dr. Mona Shangold, director of the Center for Women's Health and Sports Gynecology in Philadelphia, Pennsylvania, the "ideal prescription" for midlife workouts includes a combination of aerobic exercise (to increase energy and build cardiovascular health and strength), resistance training (to build new muscle mass), and stretching (to remain limber and flexible and reduce your risk of injury). All three can and should be individualized to suit your personal level of fitness. With this in mind, here is the regimen Dr. Shangold suggests.

AEROBIC EXERCISE

- *Activities include:* Brisk walking, stationary biking, swimming, rowing, dancing.

- *Experienced exercisers:* 7 days per week, 20 to 60 minutes per session, beginning and ending at a slightly slower pace to warm up and cool down.

- *Newbies:* If you have not exercised before, or have engaged in only minimal activity, start with 15 minutes of walking, 3 times per week, gradually increasing time, distance, and intensity. Gradually add more activities as your strength builds.

RESISTANCE EXERCISE

- *Activities include:* Lifting weights, using rubber resistant bands (like Body Flex), machines designed to cause your muscles to push against a force.

- *Experienced exercisers:* 2 to 3 days per week, 30 to 45 minutes.

- *Newbies:* Same frequency, but under the supervision of an instructor until techniques are mastered.

STRETCHING

- *Activities include:* Full body stretches and individual muscle stretches performed after each aerobic and resistance training session to improve and maintain flexibility.

Important note: It's a good idea to have a baseline physical exam, including cardiogram, before starting any exercise program, particularly if you are age forty-five or older. That said, your doctor will know what's best for you and whether this exam is necessary, so be certain to at least check in with her or him regarding your workout intentions before you start.

From the "M" File

BONE HEALTH AND EXERCISE

Q: My mother has osteoporosis, and so does my aunt—so it looks like I might be next in line. My doctor says I need to do more exercise, but he never gets specific about what I really need to do. Are there exercises just for bone health—or doesn't it matter as long as you are in good shape?

A: Although any exercise that helps strengthen supporting muscles and ligaments is going to help protect your bones from fracture, there are, in fact, some specific moves that can have a significant effect directly on your bone health. One of the major types of exercise recommended by the National Osteoporosis Foundation (NOF) is known as "weight-bearing workouts"—exercises that cause your bones and muscles to work against gravity, forcing your feet and legs to bear the brunt of your weight. How can these help? As you read earlier, bones go through a natural remodeling process that helps make new cells, which in turn helps increase their strength. One of the things that may stimulate more rapid bone cell turnover and the subsequent manufacture of new bone is this push against gravity, which creates a natural, healthy stress on the bone. Examples of exercises that accomplish this include

New Body—New Age—New You

If you're old enough to be needing the information in this book, you're probably also old enough to remember the now infamous TV commercial line "You're not getting older, you're getting better." If you're anything like me, at the time when you first heard it you probably thought of your mother—or even your grandmother—and you probably doubted if it could even be true. Now I hope you know that it is. In fact, if there was ever a generation that would figure out how to beat the aging game, it would most certainly be ours. And in many ways, we have done just

jogging, walking, stair climbing, and dancing. Studies show that just thirty minutes of brisk walking several days a week may be all you need to encourage bone growth. In fact, you don't even have to do all thirty minutes at one time: ten-minute increments three times a day should do the trick!

Resistance workouts are the second type of exercise recommended by NOF—activities that use pressure against muscles to build strength and improve muscle mass. Examples of these activities include weight lifting and isometrics. There are also a number of progressive resistance machines at many gyms and health clubs that accomplish similar results. While all of these exercises are considered safe and effective ways to increase bone health, if you are at risk for osteoporosis, and particularly if you have already been diagnosed with this problem, then it's important to exert extra caution when working out. In addition, make certain that you run all your exercises by your doctor before starting any workout program. Also important: If you are working with a personal trainer, or if you belong to a gym or health club, make sure your instructors know the condition of your bones—and be sure to remind them before each session. It's important that you avoid anything that might put your bone health in jeopardy, or push you beyond the limits of what your body—including your bones—can tolerate.

that—through diet, exercise, nutrition, and with access to better medical care (not to mention Botox, moisturizers, and Clairol).

But while this is clearly not "your mother's menopause," it's also not necessary to push yourself to distraction trying to prove that point, particularly in regard to how you look. Because while I firmly believe that controlling your weight at midlife—and keeping your body active—is not only important, but essential to your future health, too often, I fear that women—you, me, all of us—put just a little *too much* emphasis on our body image, particularly as we age. While we might not be the victim of an eating disorder, or even be a chronic dieter, it seems the older we get the more concerned we become with how we look—and the less tolerant we are of ourselves, and each other, when we feel we don't make the grade. In the same way our mothers and grandmothers caved to that "elderly" image at fifty, too often it seems we are driving ourselves hard in the other direction, forcing ourselves to compete with, and compare ourselves to, images that are quite simply impossible to achieve. Somehow, it seems, as soon as we hit middle age, we fall under some kind of all-consuming catatonic fashion spell that totally eclipses the fact that we are great wives, terrific mothers, wonderful friends, successful career gals—or all four— and instead leaves us searching for the meaning of life in the dressing room at Bloomingdale's. Suddenly, we wake up one morning and the only measure of our worth is the number on the bathroom scale—and the higher it is, the lower we feel.

Surely, there is nothing wrong in taking great pride in your appearance—and if you already have a body and a face like Diane Sawyer, Suzanne Somers, Sharon Stone, or Tina Turner, hey, you go, girl! But on the chance that, like the rest of us, you are, realistically a size 12 or 14 or more, and you have a few lines and creases to show for your years, don't feel you have to push yourself to an extreme just to meet somebody else's ideal of what you *should* look like or who you *should* be. By all means, push the envelope every chance you get—with your wardrobe and your hairstyles, with your verve and élan and your "yes I can" approach to the second half of your life. But at the same time don't be afraid or ashamed or embarrassed to *embrace* the changes that are part of this half of your life as well—and don't fight who you are, or all you have become. In the end, for every line on your face, for every inch on your waistline, for every extra pound you carry, there is a cache of wisdom, experience, self-confidence, accomplishment, and courage—so don't forget that. Enjoy yourself—and your life—no matter what your size. You've earned it.

8

Sex in Menopause City

A Hot New Guide to the Sexiest Time of Your Life

I'm flatlining," my friend Katy said as she stared into a slice of cheese-cake that she and I were sharing at a small Upper East Side bistro.

"Flatlining? What, like your cardiogram—your brain scan—your spending limit at Bloomingdale's?" She shot me a glance that told me this was no laughing matter.

"No," she finally said, as she continued pushing the cheesecake all over the plate with her fork. "I'm flatlining in sex—don't want it, don't need it, don't like it—I'm just turned off," she said, heaving what seemed like a huge sigh of relief over just getting the words out.

"And . . . this is a bad thing, right?" I said, only half joking.

"Yes, it's a bad thing, it's a terrible thing," she said, clearly in no mood for humor and showing more emotion in her voice than I'd heard in quite a few weeks. "I love my husband, I want to be close to him, I want to be around him all the time—I just don't want him to touch me—and most of all I'm really frightened that it might always be this way."

With just a little more prodding I found that Katy's problem was not only one of a lack of desire, but that even during the times when she thought she felt that old "spark" coming back, her attempts at physical intimacy were not pleasurable—and some were even painful. Further, the longer the period of time between intimate moments, the less physically gratifying and, sometimes, the more uncomfortable sex became for her.

By the end of our conversation she was very nearly in tears, convinced that something dreadful was wrong and feeling too embarrassed to talk to her doctor about what it could be.

As unusual as Katy's problem seemed to her, I tried to explain that she wasn't alone. At age fifty-one she was just about easing her way from perimenopause into menopause (or, as Katy likes to put it, she has one egg left and it can't decide whether it wants to be fried or scrambled), and the kind of sexual problems she was experiencing were far more common than many women realize.

Certainly, sexual dysfunction, or "flatlining" as Katy put it, doesn't happen to every one of us—nor is the extent to which it does occur the same for every woman. But unfortunately, one way or another, there's no getting around it—there *are* going to be *some* temporary changes in this area. One reason is because so much of our desire for and enjoyment of sex is wrapped around our hormones. So, when they change, it's only natural that those things that are linked to hormone function—like our sex drive—are going to change as well. Still, it's important to remember that even though we all experience these changes, the way in which we are affected is as individual as we are.

For some of us the differences are so slight, we may barely even notice anything is different. My pal Suzanne—now fifty-two—recently confided that with the risk of pregnancy behind her she felt more uninhibited and more sexually charged than she had in a long time—in spite of whatever her hormones were doing. For my friend Judy, recently divorced, saying good-bye to sexual desire came as a welcome surprise—one that significantly lessened the tension of no longer having a partner with whom she could share her marital bed. And certainly, at least some of you reading this book will be like my friend Janet, using her midlife time as an opportunity for great personal discovery. She has focused her energies on so many new and exciting things right now, she's almost glad to put her sex drive on the back burner. If this is how you feel as well, follow her lead and don't feel guilty or obligated to search for the holy grail of midlife orgasms.

If, however, like Katy, you *are* concerned and even upset by changes in your sex life, or your sensuality, it's important to realize that things don't have to remain this way forever—and that there are answers. While it's true that our physiology plays a key role in our sexual functioning, you probably already know that a woman's libido involves a lot more than a handful of hormones. In fact, unlike men, whose Speedos are permanently droopy if they lose even a thimbleful of testosterone, women are much more complex. Our desire for and enjoyment of sex goes far beyond a chemical reaction. So even if your hormones are running amok, other factors involved with your sexual responses—like your thoughts and your emotions—are still in place. Learning how to channel those sparks into a sexual response can help bring all those lusty feelings you're missing back into your life. Add to this the now booming erotic medicine chest, with a number of treatments aimed specifically at moving some of those hot flashes from your cheeks to below your belt, and the possibilities for improving your sex life—even at midlife—can be pretty amazing.

The key to making it all work, however, is knowledge. By learning a little more about what your body is going through right now, and how that's affecting the way you feel about sex, you'll be better able to understand just how to compensate for the changes. If you do have a regular partner, I invite you to share this chapter with him, so that together you can work toward a happier and more satisfying midlife sexual experience for you both.

Sex, Hormones, and Desire: What Every Midlife Goddess Needs to Know

If you're like many women, from almost the moment you set eyes on "the one," your libido went into overdrive. While initially this might have happened on an unconscious level, I'm certain that before long your heart was pumping and your sexual response was kicking in. Indeed, when you are turned on, circulation to your erogenous zones increases—particularly to your breasts and vagina. For most of us, the number one physiological sign that our sexual interest is peaking is lubrication, a distinct sensation of "wetness" that begins flowing from the walls of the vagina. This, in turn, readies your genital area for intimate activity, exciting sensitive nerve endings and filling you with a desire for not only more stimulation, but also gratification. And while lubrication clearly increases your desire for intercourse, it also makes it more pleasurable, which further increases your body's sexual response to your partner. The end result—your hormones orchestrate a powerful interplay between your mind, your heart, and the right partner!

But as a woman ages, and particularly as she enters perimenopause, things don't go quite the same way. When estrogen starts to decline, for example, at least some of the initial feelings of stimulation can be dampened. With less of this hormone available, your entire vaginal ecosystem is compromised—so you don't produce as much lubrication. Certainly, what you do produce can also take a lot longer to get going. Whereas before you might only have had to think of an intimate scenario or experience a light touch from your partner in order to feel some sense of wetness, now you may find that without significant physical stimulation, for an increased amount of time, you have little or no lubrication. This, in turn, not only means that your vagina and clitoris are less responsive, particularly to intercourse, it can also make the friction of intimacy feel extremely painful. In addition, because this lack of estrogen also influences circulation—reducing blood flow to all your erogenous zones—you may also experience a change in the acid level of the other fluids in your vagina. Not only will this increase your risk of certain problems—such as yeast infections—it may cause you to feel a burning in your V zone after your partner ejaculates.

Complicating matters just a bit more: The phrase "use it or lose it" was clearly born in the perimenopause lab. Speaking from a strictly physiological standpoint, the less you have sex, the more your vaginal tissue will atrophy, and ultimately, the more painful and difficult sex will become. So, the more you avoid intimate relations, the harder it can be to

From the "M" File

**THE FIVE MOST COMMON MIDLIFE SEX
PROBLEMS REPORTED BY WOMEN:**

1. Lack of desire

2. Decreased sensation and inability to be stimulated

3. Dry vagina (lack of lubrication)

4. Painful intercourse

5. Inability to have an orgasm

have them, even when you want to. Ultimately, many women simply stop having sex altogether and, like my friend Katy, feel as if they are "flatlining" when even the thought of intimacy crosses their mind. And that can have more impact on how you feel during this time than you might realize. Why?

Unlike men, women see sex as more than just a hormonally charged physical encounter. For us, sex is also a bonding experience with our partners—a way of establishing and holding on to feelings of intimacy that figure heavily into many other aspects of our lives. So, losing our desire for sex not only means a loss of physical pleasure, for many women it's also the loss of the emotional closeness that we need in our lives, particularly at this time. Often, that loss can have an effect that goes far beyond the bedroom, touching our psyches and tugging on our self-esteem in many ways. Unlike *choosing* not to have sex—a sometimes "freeing" decision and every woman's right—not being *able* to have sex, or more importantly, feeling as if you no longer have the *choice*, can have a completely opposite effect. Instead of feeling free, many of us end up feeling trapped by our lack of desire—and it's a feeling that can overwhelm us in many areas of our life.

The Way to Do the Things You Do

For those of you who choose to try some form of hormone therapy during this transition time, many of the sex-related problems you've read about thus far will automatically abate. While doctors clearly no longer recommend HRT if sexual dysfunction is your major midlife complaint (see "Once Upon a Time . . ."), if you are taking it for other reasons, then your intimate life will clearly benefit. In fact, studies show that when estrogen levels are restored—even pharmaceutically—your sex organs will begin responding in a more natural, normal way. As estrogen receptors in your vagina and breast are once again satisfied, much of your intimate sensitivity will return. Lubrication will be back as well, and your entire V zone will begin responding much the way it did when you were young. For some women similar results can occur with certain natural therapies— including herbal preparations that can impact hormonal activity and also help get your V zone back on track (see "Sex in the Garden," later in this chapter).

For many women, however, the best place to begin is with a variety of different *topical* preparations—including some hormones—all of which have the ability to compensate for many of the problems caused by a drop in estrogen within the vagina itself. This includes adding back the lubrication that can make sex more pleasurable and, in some instances, even impact desire. Sometimes these products can be so effective, it's all you will need to rev up your sex drive and bring the blush of desire back into your cheeks.

To help you decide which of these options may be best, do talk to your doctor—but also use the following guide to steer your conversation in the right direction. You can also read more about vaginal dryness and its overall effects on vaginal health in Chapter 3.

The Sex Helpers: What Really Works

Lubricants: These are topical preparations specifically developed to add more moisture to your vagina. The goal is to reduce friction during intercourse and keep delicate, estrogen-low vaginal tissue from becoming irritated or inflamed. Some women also say that when their vagina feels moist, it duplicates somewhat the wetness they feel when sexually aroused—and that, in turn, can send a message to the brain that revs up that "gotta have it now" feeling of desire. Good examples of lubricants include KY Jelly, Astroglide, ViAmor, and Replens, all of which can be bought in your local pharmacy. Results are usually immediate and can improve further with extended use. For additional help have your partner use the lubricants on his penis before attempting intercourse.

Lubricants Plus: These products not only provide moisture to the vagina but also contain other, nonhormonal ingredients designed to encourage the body to make more lubrication on its own—including plant estrogens, herbs, and polysaccharides. These extra ingredients may help improve the overall health of your vaginal tissue, as well as helping to ease the discomfort of dryness during intercourse. Used in the same way as more traditional lubricants, products in this category include Transitions For Health Vaginal Lubricant, Multi-Gyn LubraCare by Multigyn, and Vagisil Intimate Lubricant with vitamin E and aloe. Some are available in drugstores, while others can be ordered through specialty catalogs. See the resource section at the back of the book for more information.

Vitamin E or Vegetable Oil: For a totally all-natural increase in sexual pleasure, and to keep your vagina feeling good overall, try a natural oil including a vegetable-based product such as olive oil or vitamin E oil. Although neither one will offer the same kind of wetness you would get from traditional lubricants, there is some evidence to show these oils can encourage vaginal tissue to produce lubrication on its own. To use vitamin E place several pinpricks in a liquid capsule and squirt it into your vagina at bedtime. You might want to put on a sanitary napkin, or at least some beat-up undies, since it will leak and can stain. You can also try a vitamin E suppository, made specifically as a vaginal lubricant and available from the mail-order and Web catalog As We Change (listed in the resource section). It contains no petroleum or mineral oil, so it's safe to use with condoms. The vitamin E capsules are recommended nightly for two weeks, after which time you may only need one every seven to ten days. To use olive oil—or any vegetable oil—pour a few drops onto clean hands, warm by rubbing your palms together, and use your fingers to apply.

Topical Estrogen—Compounded Products: These creams and gels contain significant amounts of estrogen and are applied directly to vaginal tissue. Not only can they can help with moisturization, but because they are attaching directly to the estrogen receptors within the vaginal walls—the way estrogen in the bloodstream would do—they can also help counter vaginal atrophy or tissue shrinkage that can make sex uncomfortable. There is also some evidence these products can help halt the thinning of vaginal tissue that can also cause discomfort. Although estrogen creams are usually most helpful to women who have already entered menopause, some can be safely used by those who are in the tail end of perimenopause—no longer menstruating regularly, but have not yet gone twelve months without any bleeding. Most women—and most doctors—are familiar with the commercial forms of these creams—products such as Estrace or Premarin, which are manufactured by large pharmaceutical companies. They contain the most common form of estrogen, known as estradiol (see the following section on commercial products).

What you may not realize, however, is that there is another option: creams created by a compounding pharmacy. This is a drugstore that uses "raw" ingredients to create each individual prescription product from "scratch." (It's like the difference between buying a prepackaged frozen lasagna and making your own from fresh ingredients.) Frequently these pharmacies use a totally different form of estrogen, known as estriol. Although somewhat less potent it is nonetheless equally effective for vaginal complaints, and possibly safer. In studies where estriol was used topically in amounts of 2 to 4 milligrams per week, vaginal complaints were resolved without any thickening of the uterine lining, commonly seen with other forms of estrogen. Indeed, studies show it would take up to five times this amount in order to bring about unfavorable changes. Dosing for estriol cream is up to 1 milligram applied to the vulva or, using an applicator, directly to the vagina nightly or every other night for one to two weeks, followed by a twice-weekly maintenance program. Although some estriol is absorbed into the bloodstream, because the amount needed for the vagina to respond is so tiny, an increase in the blood level is minimal—so small, in fact, that some doctors feel it's safe even for women who have had breast cancer. However, it's important to point out that no long-term studies have been conducted, so you should make your decision to use this product in conjunction with your doctor's advice. To learn more about the different forms of estrogen, see Chapter 11.

Topical Estrogen—Commercial Products: Among the most traditional topical estrogen preparations for women already in menopause are prescription-only treatments such as the cream forms of Premarin, Estrace, and Ortho Dienestrol. These contain "active" estrogen, in the form of estradiol, and they *are* absorbed into the bloodstream, so they *do* contribute a significant amount of this hormone to your body. If used regularly, they constitute "unopposed estrogen therapy," which could carry significant health risks for women who have not undergone a hysterectomy, particularly the risk of endometrial hyperplasia, a precursor to uterine cancer (see Chapter 3). To help balance these risks, these treatments should be used in conjunction with progesterone therapy, the hormone that can balance the estrogen and keep your cell lining from building up. Progesterone can be used in cream or pill form, with the natural type among the most popular (see Chapter 11). Your exact dosage will depend largely on your symptoms, and the more vaginal atrophy you are experiencing, the more you will require for results. Most products come with applicators that allow direct application to the vagina, and they should be used at bedtime for best results. You may need to wear a sanitary pad to bed and one the next day, since some of these preparations can be drippy or messy.

The Vaginal Ring: Currently there are two forms of these devices, both of which contain estrogen.

> • *Estring:* The first of its type on the market, this prescription-only device is a tiny, hormone-filled flexible ring that is inserted into the vagina. Most women prefer their doctor do this, at least for the first time. The ring contains 2 milligrams of the synthetic version of estradiol, the most common form of estrogen produced by the ovaries. It works by releasing a consistently low dose into the surrounding skin and tissue for up to ninety days, at which time it must be removed and replaced by a new ring. Most women find they can do this on their own. Because the amount of estrogen in the ring is so small, and because most remains localized in the vaginal tissue, there

is little risk of tissue overgrowth in the uterus. So, there is also no need to take progesterone. Another benefit—Estring has also been shown to help urinary incontinence, mostly by providing estrogen to the urogenital system as well. Providing your doctor agrees, this device is considered effective to use during perimenopause. In clinical studies, the most common side effects were headache, vaginal or uterine discharge, back pain, and genital yeast infection. Although hormone absorption is low, this product should not be used if you have any abnormal genital bleeding, if you are pregnant, or if you have breast cancer or any estrogen-related abnormal cell growth, unless directed by your doctor.

- *Femring:* Approved for use in the United States in July 2003 by prescription only, this version of the estrogen ring also contains estradiol, in fairly concentrated amounts. It was approved not only for the treatment of vaginal dryness, but also for hot flashes and night sweats, so you know it's pretty potent stuff. As such, it's primarily recommended for women who are already in menopause—again, no menstrual cycle for at least twelve months. A flexible ring similar to Estring, it is inserted into your vagina (usually by your doctor), where it remains for up to three months, after which time it is replaced with a new one. Most women find they can do the replacement insertion on their own. In a study of 5,150 women, nearly 93 percent said Femring did not interfere with intercourse and their partners couldn't feel it. Since Femring does contain a substantial amount of estrogen, if vaginal dryness is your primary symptom this product is not advised as your first line of defense. It should also not be used if you have dysfunctional vaginal bleeding or blood clots, have had a recent stroke or heart attack, or if you are pregnant or trying to conceive. Side effects include headache, irregular vaginal bleeding, spotting, breast tenderness, and abdominal cramping. You should also avoid this product if you are at risk for breast or uterine cancer, unless your doctor specifically recommends it.

Important Warning: Both types of vaginal rings are readily available on the Internet through online prescription services, requiring only that you answer a few questions before being allowed to purchase the drug. I strongly warn you not to buy or use these products unless prescribed to you by your personal physician, in conjunction with regular gynecological exams. These products contain hormones that under some circumstances may not be right for you. They should never be used without the consent of your doctor.

Vaginal Tablets: One of the newest entries into the vaginal health market is an over-the-counter estrogen "vagina pill" called Vagifem. Containing a natural form of estradiol derived from plant sources, it is inserted into the vagina twice a week with a thin, easy-to-use applicator. It usually begins working within two weeks, but it can take up to twelve weeks before full results are realized. Because the estrogen is contained within a capsule, it is not messy and won't leak. If used twice weekly, in the recommended dosage, it is considered safe, even for women who have had breast cancer. It also does not require progesterone to balance the effects. If it is used in higher doses, however, or for an extended period of time, progesterone supplementation may be required. Also, check with your doctor before trying this product if you are still having dysfunctional bleeding. Side effects are mild and rare, but in some women they can include headache, abdominal pain, back pain, upper respiratory tract infection, vaginal itching, and vaginal yeast infection. Among the latest studies, research published in the *American Journal of Obstetrics and Gynecology* found that placing an estrogen tablet in the outer third of the vagina (rather than deeper inside) provides greater symptom relief and is safer in terms of potential effects on the uterine lining.

When the Desire Dies: What You Can Do

While for some women simply increasing the body's physiological responses to sex can help, for still others there remains a gaping hole in their sex life. I'm talking about the *desire* for intimacy, which may not always return, even if the vagina seems ready, willing, and able. Many doctors now believe the reason has less to do with estrogen and more to do with what is being called the "other" sex hormone—the one most women know little about. I'm talking about testosterone. Although it's known as

From the "M" File

HOT STUFF FOR HOT SEX

**Q: I've heard of certain "warming" lubricants that can in-
crease sexual desire. I'm a little bit afraid of using them—
because no one explains what they do. Are they safe? Will
they cause burning—and how long will the effects last?
Most important, can they really help me enjoy sex again?**

A: It sounds as if you are referring to one of several topical products
that work to provide both lubrication and a temporary sensation of
warmth when topically applied to the vagina. Although these kinds of
products have been around for years—mostly sold through mail-order
sex-toy ads or in erotic boutiques—you are right in assuming there has
been little in the way of safety or efficacy testing of these products.
More recently, however, KY Brand Jelly has come out with a warming
liquid that is not only tested for both safety and efficacy, it's also the
first such product of its kind to receive FDA approval. And it has clinical
studies to back up its claims. Like the original KY Jelly, it works to provide copious lubrication. At the same time, however, it also provides

the typically male hormone, the virtual "juice" that fuels a man's aggressive, competitive, and even sexy side, you may be surprised to learn that
women's bodies also manufacture this hormone. Because even at its peak
concentration our supply of testosterone is very small, for decades doctors didn't believe it could play a very important role—or even that it had
any influence at all on a woman's sexual response. Now, however, that line
of thinking has changed.

"We now know testosterone is intimately involved in a woman's sexual response, in her ability to be aroused by stimuli triggers . . . and in her
appetite for being sexual," says Dr. Rosemary Basson, an internationally
known researcher at the Center for Sexuality, Gender Identity and
Reproductive Health in British Columbia. Some research has shown
testosterone may even increase sensitivity of both the nipples and the clitoris—so this hormone can affect not only desire, but pleasure as well.

the added benefit of a gentle warming sensation that research shows can be quite stimulating for some women. In the clinical studies conducted by the company, 72 percent of couples who tried the warming jelly reported their sex lives were more enjoyable. Seventy-one percent said the product enhanced sexual arousal.

The consistency of the new KY Brand Warming Liquid Personal Lubricant is similar to that of the original jelly, but a little less thick than their Ultragel formulation. And unless you have a sensitivity to the product, there should be no "burning" sensation—only a gentle warming feeling that lasts for anywhere from fifteen minutes to an hour. Ingredients include propylene glycol, glycerin, acacia honey Type O, and methylparaben, with the honey being the operative ingredient responsible for the warming. But in case you're thinking of bypassing the drugstore and using natural honey as a lubricant instead, don't. The sugars present in natural honey can dramatically alter the natural chemical environment of your vagina and may increase your risk of yeast infections and other problems. KY Warming Liquid sells for about $6 for a five-ounce bottle—but you can get a free sample by visiting the company's website at www.k-y.com.

More recently, in May 2004 Procter & Gamble released the results of a clinical trial conducted on Intrinsa, their new experimental testosterone patch. The twenty-four-week controlled study involved 562 women whose ovaries were surgically removed and were already taking some form of HRT who were assigned to either a testosterone patch or a placebo. The end result: Those using the testosterone patch showed a 56 percent increase in sexual desire; among those who engaged in sex, the women saw a 74 percent increase in satisfying sexual activity.

In addition, says Basson, testosterone plays a role in bone growth, bone density, the production of red blood cells, and muscle development, and it even influences our memory and our mood—not coincidentally, all functions that can decline as a woman enters menopause. In one study published in the *New England Journal of Medicine* doctors found that when testosterone levels were low, supplements were able to increase a woman's overall health and her sense of well-being as well as increasing her desire for sex.

Although about half of the testosterone in your body is made by your adrenal glands, the other half is made by your ovaries—one reason levels decline as you head toward menopause. In fact, by the time you reach age forty, the amount of testosterone being made in your body is roughly half of what it was in your twenties. If you have your ovaries removed the drop is sudden and can be severe, causing you to feel the "bump" in the road with even more intensity.

In research presented at the eighty-fifth annual meeting of the Endocrine Society in June 2003, Dr. Susan Davis of the Jean Hailes Foundation in Melbourne, Australia, presented new evidence of how dramatically testosterone can decline as a woman ages. In this extremely detailed study researchers not only measured the level of free testosterone in a woman's bloodstream (the amount that's available for immediate use), they also calculated levels of other hormones that could be converted to testosterone on demand—including DHT (di-hydrotestosterone), DHEA-S (dehydroepiandrosterone sulfate), and androstenedione. In doing so they discovered that not only do levels of testosterone decline as a woman ages, so too do all the functions linked to testosterone production. By and large, the closer you get to menopause, and the more your ovarian function declines, the lower your level of testosterone may go.

This appeared to be the case for my friend Eileen. She had been using a form of natural hormone therapy (see Chapter 10) to quell her menopause symptoms and, at least in the beginning, was quite satisfied with the result. Initially she said she felt terrific, crediting soy supplements and flaxseed for lifting her midlife depression and sending her on shopping sprees with a renewed sense of vigor and energy. But after Eileen had bought pretty much all the shoes and handbags her closet could hold, she slowed down enough to realize that as good as she had been feeling, she'd rather shop than have sex. Now I realize that at least some of you may be asking, "So what's wrong with that?" But as Eileen put it, it would be nice if she had a choice! And her husband Bob, though quite understanding of his wife's problems, was very quick to agree. Because as good as Eileen was feeling in other areas of her life, in the bedroom her interest was less than she could ever have imagined it would be. And both she and her husband agreed that without the intimacy that sex provided, their relationship was starting to suffer.

After numerous trips to her doctor yielded no helpful suggestions, Eileen read about testosterone therapy. She brought me some of the articles she collected, and together we began sifting through some of the scientific literature. Although there wasn't a great deal to be found on the subject, one of the first things we learned was that certain HRT formulations—including the popular Premarin prescription—can impact the hormones that bind testosterone, thus reducing the amount that is circulating in your blood. According to hormone specialist Dr. Jeannie Alexander, the end result can be a significant decline in the desire for sex. We also found at least several clinical studies suggesting that tiny amounts of testosterone supplementation on a regular basis could revive a woman's sex drive, increase her energy level, and offer a renewed sense of well-being that even traditional estrogen/progesterone therapy could not provide. As Eileen remarked, "What's not to love?"

And many experts agree. According to Dr. William Regelson, author of *The Superhormone Promise,* "For many women who are not quite themselves, the ingredient missing from the blueprint is testosterone."

In studies conducted at McGill University in Canada, doctors found that adding just a "dollop" of testosterone into a traditional HRT formula not only increased a woman's interest in having sex but also increased her sensual enjoyment and her rate of orgasm.

The more we read the more we began to realize that the same hormone that keeps sex and action films on the minds of men 24/7 can, surprisingly, increase *romance* in a woman's life—and my friend Eileen was certainly ready and willing to try it.

Choosing a Testosterone Supplement: What You Should Know

If you are intrigued by the promises of testosterone and want to give it a try, don't be too surprised if your doctor isn't initially in favor of this supplement—and some of his or her concerns are likely justified. Among the most common issues cited by many doctors is a lack of long-term data proving either safety or efficacy. Which could mean that taking testosterone is a lot like (if you'll excuse the expression) poking around in the dark when it comes to enhancing your sexual satisfaction. Moreover, of the studies that have been done, at least some have reported a potentially dangerous change in blood lipids, increasing a woman's "bad" cholesterol and decreasing the "good" cholesterol—both of which can set the stage for heart disease.

Other problems can be seen with certain forms of testosterone supplementation—including the pill form, which has been linked to liver damage. And while many women do well on one oral form of testosterone known as Andriol (at dosages of about one-tenth what men normally take), doctors are still frequently hesitant to prescribe it. Fortunately, other, ostensibly safer options exist. Compounding pharmacies (those that "compound" or make your prescription from scratch using raw ingredients) frequently offer testosterone in various forms including lozenges, gels, creams, ointments, patches, injections, and even a sublingual pill (which immediately dissolves under the tongue). See the resource section at the back of the book for more information. Although a bit more expensive than mass-produced medicine, each testosterone prescription can easily be customized in a variety of ways to match your specific needs. In this respect, you can not only get the exact right amount your body requires, you can also get it in the form that is best and easiest for you to take. (By the way, most compounding pharmacies offer a variety of medications and most types of hormones, so they are an excellent resource anytime you need a customized medication.)

Ultimately, Eileen and her doctor chose a customized topical cream formulation that she applied directly to her vagina. And the first few weeks of using it were, she said, definitely filled with some surprises.

"The first dosage turned me into a virtual 'porn goddess,' which Bob thought was kind of fun for a little while, but eventually we both agreed it was becoming just a bit harrowing and, for me, somewhat annoying," she says. Eventually, however, the dosage was adjusted, and now she says her desire is at a comfortable and more normal level. Her sexual spontaneity has returned as well, in full bloom.

"If the situation presents itself I can easily get turned on—but it's not like I'm walking around thinking about nothing but sex all day long," she said, also indicating she is grateful the therapy hasn't interfered at all with her occasional need to put hubby on hold and attend a designer shoe sale at Saks!

CAN THIS SEX HORMONE HELP YOU? HOW TO TELL

Although many women find success with testosterone supplements, there can be a downside. For some, the supplements can increase anxiety, mood swings, and bouts of anger and dramatically increase stress. Side effects can also include masculinization (a deepening of the voice and growth of facial hair) as well as acne and oily skin. In addition, if your dose is too high, you could experience an intense increase in your sex drive. And while "doing without" for a while can make *this* reaction feel welcome, as Eileen pointed out earlier, the novelty of it all gets old *really* fast. By making some simple adjustments in the dosage, however, most women find they can customize their prescription to just the right balance of desire and interest.

But can testosterone really help you? Experts say that if your sex drive has waned significantly, and if your sense of overall well-being is diminishing, then testosterone might be what the doctor ordered. However, before you decide for sure, it's important to remember that other problems not related to testosterone—including low thyroid function, or even depression—can cause similar symptoms. That's one reason why it's so important to have a full physical and blood screening before any hormone therapy is prescribed.

While there *are* tests that can specifically measure your testosterone levels, don't be surprised if your doctor is reluctant to offer them to you. One reason is that there is no one "baseline" level of this hormone that is considered normal for all women. Indeed, the amount we start out with as young adults can vary significantly from woman to woman. So, what would be considered low in one gal might be quite normal in another. Remember, what you are looking for here is the *drop, or decrease* from what was present before your symptoms took hold. If you don't have a baseline level from your twenties or thirties to which you can compare levels now, testing may not help much.

If you decide to try a test anyway, recent research has yielded a few guidelines that can be applied. According to Dr. Nisha Jackson, a special-

ist in natural hormone therapy from Medford, Oregon, "normal" blood
levels of free testosterone—the amount that is in your system and available for use—lie between 2.2 and 8.0 nanograms per deciliter (ng/dl).
However, she says most women feel best when "free" testosterone registers somewhere between 3.0 and 6.0. (If your doctor measures total
testosterone, readings should fall between 40 and 60.)

In addition to testing your *blood* levels of testosterone, testing your
saliva may prove to be even more helpful. Studies show it can be the most
reliable way of all to determine the true amount of usable testosterone in
a woman's body. While the most efficient form of saliva testing calls for
numerous samples to be taken over a twenty-eight-day period, it's also
possible to get some benefits from a one-time testosterone saliva test. It
can be ordered by your doctor, or you can check the resource section at
the back of this book for laboratories that arrange testing directly with
consumers. Because each laboratory uses a slightly different scale to measure testosterone in saliva, there is no way to generalize what a "normal"
level might be. However, laboratories will usually advise you if your levels
fall within their "normal" range, as well as if your test results indicate a
problem. Be aware, however, that saliva samples can sometimes degrade
without proper storage, so for the most reliable use of this test the sample should be sent to the laboratory as soon as possible—and the closer
you are to the destination, the more reliable the results may be.

THE DHEA OPTION:
TESTOSTERONE WITHOUT THE WORRY

In lieu of using testosterone supplements, some experts are now recommending another steroid hormone known as DHEA (dehydroepiandrosterone), an offshoot of another hormone known as DHEA-S (sulfate).
Manufactured by the adrenal glands, as you read earlier, DHEA and
DHEA-S are precursor hormones—natural chemicals that the body converts into testosterone as needed. Studies show that as we age levels of
both these compounds drop, which some doctors believe may further
contribute to a woman's decrease in testosterone.

Available as a cream or in pill form, the natural form of DHEA can
be purchased without a prescription. And this over-the-counter version

is said to increase testosterone levels to one and a half to two times what-ever is already present in your body. Although the therapy can take up to four months to kick in, for many women this is the most natural way to boost testosterone gradually.

Because, however, DHEA is also a precursor to estrogen, it is not rec-ommended if you are at high risk for breast cancer. And because it is metabolized by the liver, if you have any history of liver function prob-lems—including a history of hepatitis—you should be monitored closely by your doctor when taking DHEA. Although it can be purchased with-out a prescription, most experts say that because there is so little data available on either safety or efficacy, it should not be used unless your doc-tor agrees to monitor your health while you are taking this supplement. Although rare, side effects can include acne, oily skin, and unwanted hair growth, most of which can often be controlled if dosages are kept under 50 milligrams daily.

Moving to the Groove: Exercise for Better Sex

Of all the benefits that I know you know exercise can provide, I'll bet you don't know this one: It can impact your sexual response and turn you on! While in the past sex therapists often advised warm baths and candlelight to get a woman's juices flowing, today many are advocating vigorous activity, particularly aerobics, to set the libido on fire! One rea-son, say experts, is that after you work out, blood flows generously to all your erogenous zones, opening the floodgates of sexual response and making it easier for your body to respond to touch and stimulation. In a breakthrough study conducted at the University of British Columbia, psychologists put two groups of women to the exercise test. The first group said they had a healthy libido and normal sex drive; the members of the second group reported sexual dysfunction with a low sex drive and little interest in their partners. Each of the women in both groups was fitted with a tampon-like electronic device designed to measure sexual stimulation inside her vagina and then told to work out on an exercise bike for about twenty minutes. Afterward, they watched a short erotic film.

From the "M" File

THE FEMALE SIDE OF VIAGRA

Q: I've heard that Viagra is now being used to increase sexual desire in women. Is this true—and if so, how does it work? And can I just pop one of my husband's pills or do I need some special version of this?

A: It's true that there have been some limited studies on the use of Viagra in women. In at least one trial of thirty-five women conducted by sex therapist Dr. Laura Berman and her sister, urologist Dr. Jennifer Berman, at the Women's Sexual Health Clinic at Boston University, results were promising. The women in the study, all of whom had undergone a hysterectomy, reported problems with vaginal sensation and the inability to achieve orgasm in the months following their surgery. After being treated with Viagra twice weekly for six weeks, however, 85 percent reported major improvements, particularly in regard to orgasm. While no one is certain what caused their sexual dysfunction to begin with, the Bermans theorize that nerve pathways leading to the vagina may have been severed or in some way disrupted during their operation. This, in turn, may have reduced circulation as well as sensation to the genital area, thus resulting in the dysfunction. Since Viagra works by increasing circulation to the genitals, it makes sense that the drug would offer these women relief. However, to assume that this is the cause for your lagging libido requires a huge leap of faith—with little in the way of additional evidence to show this drug could help

The end result: The electronic devices showed *both* groups of women experienced similar levels of sexual stimulation—something that was not achieved in an earlier study that involved watching the movie without benefit of exercising first. The theory, say researchers, is that exercise causes a woman's nervous system to reach an excited state, with an increase in blood pressure, heart rate, and muscle activity. When this occurs, circulation to the genitals increases—and it doesn't matter much

you. Further, taking your husband's pills without a doctor's okay is not a good idea, since dosages can vary greatly between men and women. And, of course, the same coronary precautions apply to women as to men, so if there is any risk of heart disease in your health history, this is probably not a drug with which you should experiment on your own. This is particularly true since there is little in the way of short- or long-term evidence of either safety or effectiveness in women.

The good news is, there are some drugs in the pharmaceutical pipeline—medications being specifically developed for female sexual dysfunction. Among those under consideration right now is a medication based on the amino acid L-argenine, which also increases blood flow to the vagina and can impact nerve stimulation. Another experimental treatment is apomorphine, which also stimulates blood flow to the vagina. A vaginal suppository containing the chemical phentolamine is being studied for its potential to relax vaginal muscles linked to sexual response. And there are also two new vaginal creams under investigation—one containing the male impotence treatment known as prostaglandin E-1, and a second version known as Alprostadil cream. Both are thought to improve arousal as well as increase lubrication, while bringing more blood flow to the genitals. For now there are no oral prescription medications specifically approved for the treatment of sexual dysfunction in women. There are, however, some all-natural products that claim to offer good results (see "All-Natural Sex Pill for Women").

what is causing that to happen. Some researchers say any stimulating activity that makes your heart pound—like watching a horror movie or an action flick, for example, or even having a pillow fight or a tickle session with your partner—could have a similar influence on genital circulation. Even anger can get your emotions up and, for some women, ignite a sexual charge—one reason why "make-up sex" can be so dramatic and exciting for some couples.

From the "M" File

ALL-NATURAL SEX PILL FOR WOMEN?

Q: I've been seeing all these advertisements for a new "sex pill" for women known as Avlimil. Can you tell me something about it—how it works, what it contains, and most importantly, does it work? Are there any downsides—like the kind of dangers associated with Viagra?

A: There's no question that Viagra has changed the lives of tens of thousands of men—and their partners. And ever since the "little blue pill" hit the market, women have been clamoring for their own version—a "little pink pill" that can offer similar benefits. While there are a number of such drugs in the pharmaceutical pipeline right now, the pill you are referring to—Avlimil—is actually an all-natural supplement that contains no synthetic or natural hormones. Instead it uses a proprietary blend of herbs and other ingredients to, as the company says, "enhance libido, sexual feeling, and sexual response," in women. It contains plant substances such as sage leaf, raspberry leaf, red clover, licorice, black cohosh, ginger, valerian root, and damiana, many of which have been used traditionally for their various effects in the female reproductive system. Whether or not combining them in any special way can provide increased benefits—or any benefits at all—is still a matter of some debate. Although the manufacturer has conducted a multicenter clinical trial revealing that Avlimil increased arousal, de-

Interestingly enough, while the electrical devices used in the study revealed that exercise was capable of turning a woman on—at least physiologically—the women themselves didn't report *feeling* any more turned on. In short, while their bodies were saying, "come and get me, I'm ready," their psyches were saying, "What, are you kidding—I'm all sweaty!" And that response validated what researchers have suspected for a long time—namely, that mood, feelings, and emotions must *also* be present in order for a woman's sex drive to really kick in. Indeed, although

sire, the rate of orgasm, and overall satisfaction for the majority of women, to date the results have not been published in any peer-reviewed medical journal. However, within one year of marketing, nearly a half million women have tried Avlimil, and currently, a more expansive clinical trial, with a larger sampling of women, is under way. So, more results are likely to be available in the near future. Another plus: Avlimil is manufactured to exacting pharmaceutical standards, ensuring the ingredients remain consistent from bottle to bottle—which is not always the case with all-natural products.

Unlike Viagra, which produces results directly after taking it, Avlimil requires up to four weeks of daily use before you will begin to see any changes, and up to twelve weeks for optimal changes. In terms of safety, the only reported side effect was mild gastrointestinal upset. That said, because, at least theoretically, anyone can be sensitive to anything, it's difficult to say if you will have any adverse reaction to any of the herbs used in the product. Additionally, if you are taking medication for any other problem, or if you are taking any other herbal preparation, particularly for menopause-related symptoms, check with your doctor before adding Avlimil to your regimen. The cost of Avlimil—which you can buy without a prescription—is about $140 for a supply of 120, or $240 for a year's supply. But you can get a free thirty-day supply by visiting the company's website at www.4avlimil.com or by calling 800–AVLIMIL.

the body may be in motion, a woman's brain still needs some cues in order to get lubrication—and interest—going.

According to Eileen Palace of the Center for Sexual Health in New Orleans, what can be gleaned from these findings is that women should use exercise to pump up their physiological drive for sex, at the same time paying attention to their body cues so they know when they are capable of being "turned on." In her clinic Palace uses a combination of exercise and biofeedback mechanisms to help demonstrate to women how and when

From the "M" File

YOGA, SEX, AND PERIMENOPAUSE

Q: My best friend swears yoga is better than hormones for increasing her sex drive. I can't see how it could work, since I thought yoga was supposed to relax you—not exactly the state of mind for sex. Is there any truth to the idea that yoga can impact your sex drive?

A: The studies are in and the answer is yes, yoga can do it—but it works in an entirely different way than traditional exercise to turn your body on. Rather than concentrating on exciting your system and pumping up brain chemistry, yoga and tantra (a form of yoga) work instead through various postures designed to specifically impact certain sexual problems. One way is by increasing blood flow to your nether regions—your pelvis and your vagina. Other exercises concentrate on toning muscles specifically linked to sexual satisfaction or even sexual function. Some yoga moves simply help you to focus, which in turn can aid you in blocking out distractions that alter the spontaneity of your natural sexual response. Yoga also teaches us to be in tune with our body—and that, say sex experts, can make it easier to recognize when we are feeling turned on so we can communicate that to our partner. In addition, the added flexibility that your body gains via yoga may boost your sexual self-esteem—just knowing what your body is capable of achieving can help you release physical inhibitions and allow you to go for the brass O! If you have any back or neck problems, however, do consult a doctor before trying any yoga poses.

their body responds to sex, and then teaches them to identify that feeling and act on it, launching whatever personal fantasy or thought pattern can put the rock and roll in motion!

In addition, there are some studies to show that exercise helps release endorphins—brain chemicals responsible for things like a "runner's high" or the exhilaration of skiing down a mountain. It turns out these same chemicals are also necessary for us to perceive pleasure, *and* they appear to be linked to the release of certain hormones that power up our sex drive. It's not surprising that studies show that women who exercise regularly report a better sex life and more satisfaction—including more orgasms—than those of us who'd rather nap than move.

Sex in the Garden: Blooming in Mother Nature's Bedroom

Rumors notwithstanding, there are many women who swear by the power of Mother Nature to help them do what comes naturally—make love. One of the most popular treatments hails from the Brazilian Amazon—where we all know the women are fabulously sexy well into their golden years! It is known as muira puama (mo-ra poo-AH-ma), and both its bark and roots are considered worth their weight in aphrodisiac gold, increasing a woman's sex drive by driving up levels of testosterone. It's probably no coincidence that this very possibility would catch the eye of a group of French researchers who conducted two separate studies on the effectiveness of this herb. Both proved it did have some important effects. According to Dr. Jacques Waynberg, when 262 patients used 1.5 milligram doses of muira puama daily for just two weeks, 62 percent found it improved their libido, while 51 percent said sexual performance was greatly enhanced. The findings were presented at the First International Congress of Ethnopharmacology in Strasbourg, France, and the product was launched worldwide. Sold in capsules of 1 milligram and 1.5 milligram strengths, as well as in tincture form with dosages from 10 to 60 drops daily, it should be used every day for about two weeks, followed by two weeks off, according to experts. The cycle can then be repeated as often as needed. And here's the really good news—you won't have to wait long to see results: It's said to take effect within twenty-four hours! Although there are no reported side effects, do consult your doctor before trying this herb, particularly if you are using a testosterone supplement or any other hormone treatment.

And ooh la la, leave it to the romantic French to improve on love! In a separate study conducted at the Institute of Sexology in Paris (I promise I am not making this up!), doctors found that combining muira puama with the herb ginkgo biloba worked even better. In their study, 65 percent of the women reported significant increases in sexual desire and fantasy, and more frequent intercourse after using the herb combo. Their ability to reach orgasm and the intensity of their orgasms were also said to increase (and you thought it was all about the champagne and pastries!)

With just a little less "ooh la la" but the spirit of Gracie Slick to inspire them, researchers at the University of California at San Francisco found that when used on its own, ginkgo biloba could have some pretty impressive effects on a woman's sex drive as well. In their study just 40 to 60 milligrams daily reversed lagging sex drive caused by treatment with antidepressant medications such as Prozac and Paxil. The San Francisco gals also reported greater levels of desire, more lubrication, and better orgasms. (Champagne and pastries optional, of course!) Before taking this herb, however, check with your doctor—particularly if you are using any heart medications or taking aspirin daily. Ginkgo acts as a blood thinner.

Still one more popular herbal approach involves phytoestrogens from sources like black cohosh, red clover, licorice, and ginseng that alone, or most often together, have been known to restore the sex drive in some women. Anecdotal reports also claim that licorice can increase vaginal lubrication and make all your erotic zones a bit more sensitive to the touch. Normally, it takes from two to four weeks of daily use of any of these herbs before you can begin to see results. When you do, however, the bedroom might not be the only place you feel a difference. A few studies have shown that these same herbs can tame hot flashes, mood swings, and other symptoms of perimenopause (see Chapter 10). While most traditional Western doctors have little information about how these herbs work—or if they do—it's still a good idea to run the idea by your doctor before starting this therapy, particularly if you are already using HRT. Some of the ingredients—including licorice and ginseng—could impact your blood pressure and may interfere with hypertensive medications.

Finally, for the most immediate herbal result you may want to try a presex "cocktail" of damiana liquor. This is an alcoholic beverage formulated from the herb damiana. While no one is certain just how it affects libido, at least one recent study on the herb itself showed it may affect desire by binding to certain receptors linked to the sex hormones. And you won't have to wait long to see if it works. Results are said to be apparent in about an hour. Yikes! Damiana is also available in health-food stores as a liquid supplement or in capsules, though these may take longer to work.

Mind Over Sex Matters: How Fantasy Can Put You in the Mood

One of the many differences between men and women lies in the forces that control our sex drive. While men are pretty much slaves to their hormones—not to mention a blood supply that is either above the neck or below the waist and almost *never* in both places simultaneously— women are far more multidimensional. *We* have the glorious ability to think *and* have sex at the same time—a fact that takes on increasing importance as we age. Why? While it's true that our hormones are going to slide, because our desire for sex can be mediated by many other factors— including our thought processes—we are not dependent on hormones alone to fan the flames of desire. For women, sex and intimacy take place as much in the mind as in the vagina. And sometimes, increasing desire may be as simple as a few mind–body visualizations—thought patterns and relaxation exercises that can send the circulation to our genitals in much the same way as hormones do when we are turned on. The key lies in our ability to get in touch with those thoughts and then learn how to use them to our sexual advantage.

"One important way to focus on eroticism is by tuning in to your body's response to sexual stimulation," says Dr. Dennis Sugrue, past president of the American Association of Sex Educators. While a man frequently has visual proof of how his body is responding to stimulation, a woman's response is more subtle, says Sugrue. As such, it may require a bit more effort and concentration before we can fully identify or even appreciate just what happens when we are feeling turned on.

Is it a great romance novel or film that gets your heart pumping? Or how about a daydream involving sex with a mysterious stranger you meet on a deserted beach? Or maybe it's all about a naughty film or fantasy starring you in any role you've always wanted to play—French maid, Wonder Woman, Nurse Nancy? The point here is to identify the factor or factors

From the "M" File

GOOD MEDICINE AND BAD SEX

Q: I'm fifty-one years old, still in perimenopause (with irregular periods), and I was recently diagnosed with high blood pressure. My doctor put me on a beta-blocker and a water pill to reduce the pressure and it's working. But after several weeks of taking these drugs I noticed that I began losing interest in sex—not only did my desire take a dip, but I don't really enjoy it even when it happens. My doctor says it's my hormones—but I swear I was just fine until I started on this medication. Could there be a connection?

A: While your doctor is right in mentioning that the hormonal changes of perimenopause can certainly impact your desire for sex, you are also right to make the connection between your medication and your intimate life. There is ample evidence to show that blood pressure medications, as well as many different types of drugs, can cause the kind of drop in libido you describe. The problems often stem from the fact that at least some of these medications work on the same brain circuitry necessary to process aspects of our sexual functioning. It's almost like having three electric cords to plug into the wall, and only two outlets: Something has to remain unplugged—and with many drugs, that can be your libido.

The good news here: According to sex education expert and psychologist Dr. Dennis Sugrue, oftentimes a change in your dosage, or even the time you take your medication, can alleviate or at least lessen the impact on sexual desire. In other instances, you may be able to switch to a drug that has less effect on your sex drive. You can also add certain medications to your regimen that can alter the sexual side effects of the drug you have to take. Broach the subject with your doctor

that *you find erotic*. Once you do, says Sugrue, your mind can set your body in motion.

"Sexy thinking and imagery can help a woman maintain the erotic focus that is critical for sexual arousal," says Sugrue.

again—and discuss all the possibilities. Certainly, never alter or change your medication regimen without your doctor's okay—and make certain to get his or her approval before stopping any prescription, particularly a blood pressure drug. If your doctor refuses to at least consider the possibility that your medication may be the cause of your sexual distress, seek a second opinion.

In the meantime, here is a partial list of medications with known sexual side effects:

Blood Pressure Drugs: Aldactone (spironolactone); Aldomet (alpha-methyldopa); Catapres (clonidine); Digoxin (lanoxin); Hygroton (chlorthalidone); Inderal (propranolol); Ismelin (guanethidine); Lopressor (metoprolol); Minipres (prazosin); Oretic (hydrochlora thiazide); Prinivil, Zestril (lisinopril); Serpasil (reserpine).

Cancer Medications: Nolvadex (tamoxifen).

Tranquilizers: Ativan (lorazepam); Tranxene (clorazepate); Valium (diazepam); Xanax (alprazolam); Compazine (prochlorperazine); Haldol (haloperidol); Mellaril (thioridazine); Navane (thiothixene); Prolixin (fluphenazine); Risperdal (risperidone); Thorazine (chlorpromazine).

Antidepressants/Mood Disorder Drugs: Anafril (clomipramine); Effexor (venlafaxine); Elavil (amitriptyline); Eskalith (lithium); Nardil (phenelzine); Paxil (paroxetine); Prozac (fluoxetine); Tofranil (imipramine); Zoloft (sertraline).

Sedatives: Dilantin (phenytoin); Luminal (phenobarbital).

Stomach Medications: Tagamet (cimetidine); Zantac (ranitidine).

Social Drugs: alcohol; cocaine; methadone; narcotics.

It is equally important, experts say, to share those erotic visions with your partner and help turn these thoughts into opportunities for seduction. If that's not possible, at least remember them—and bring them up when the situation is right. Likewise, Sugrue says if you've ever had a really thrilling sexual adventure or experience in the past—even with a different partner—try to recall it in vivid detail, even writing about it in a journal. If you want to share it with your partner, you don't have to admit it took place with someone else. Instead, take just a little liberty and fib this one time—and present it as sheer fantasy! The point is to take advantage of the fact that your mind is as sexual as your body!

Sex in the Kitchen: Eating Your Way to Ecstasy!

Since almost the beginning of time, food and sex have been intimately entwined. Not only have certain dishes earned an anecdotal reputation for having some sexual punch, but the whole idea that "good food equals good sex" has some solid science behind it. It seems the area of the brain that controls both our lust for pasta and our desire for sex is one and the same. Add to this some interesting data linking the nutrients in certain foods to hormone production, and you have the makings of a menu for desire—or at least a little lusty encouragement! While it's not likely that any one dish is going to send you on a bus ride to nirvana, when food is combined with other natural approaches, including exercise, herbs, and fantasy, it can kick your sex drive over the edge and stir at least a small fire in your libido.

So, what should you eat to get your love lights burning? Experts say a diet high in protein and complex carbohydrates will generally give you more energy—so your sex drive is less likely to fight fatigue for a place in your life. In addition, complex carbohydrates, like whole grains and fruits, may influence brain chemicals linked to hormone production—though this is more likely to happen over an extended period of time and not give you that immediate cause–effect reaction. For more help in the bedroom try eating small, high-protein meals about every three hours. This can stabilize blood sugar, fight fatigue, and help keep mood swings under control—all of which can contribute to a temperament that is at least conducive to any sexual stimulation that might come your way.

In addition, there *are* a few foods that may actually offer you that one-two punch and nudge your libido up a notch. Here's what you can try:

- **Chocolate:** There's a reason why chocolate is the valentine food of love—and it's not just that it comes in those pretty red satin boxes! The natural chemicals in this candy not only induce relaxation—lowering your inhibitions in somewhat the same way as a glass of red wine—but also tempt your olfactory senses, sending a message from your nose to your brain that stimulates hormones linked to desire. Chocolate also contains high levels of phenyl ethylamine, a natural chemical that encourages a sense of well-being and feelings of anticipatory excitement, all conductive to lovemaking. To test the theory: Arrange a bedroom picnic with berries dipped in chocolate and see what happens!

- **Chili, cayenne pepper, ginger, or any hot spice:** The key here is circulation—and like exercise, which revs up your body and speeds blood to your erogenous zones, so too can hot and spicy foods. Be forewarned and try them first when your paramour is not around. These same foods can also increase hot flashes in some women—which, as you probably know, is not to be confused with hot desire.

- **Lobster, oysters, or shrimp:** With or without a Mai Tai and a Hawaiian sunset, shellfish can help set the mood. The reason is it's packed with zinc—a mineral that is intimately linked to testosterone production in both men and women. Load up on these foods—along with other zinc-laden fare such as pumpkin seeds, brown rice, cheese, eggs, and turkey—and you might jump-start your own supply of testosterone . . . and your desires.

- **B$_6$-rich foods:** This vitamin works with zinc to impact testosterone levels, so toss some potatoes, bananas, chicken, tuna, or avocados into your daily menu.

- **Sex fruits: strawberries and raspberries:** Potent sources of antioxidants, these sexy little fruits are thought to increase circulation *and* help the heart—which not only means more blood flow to all the right places, but also lots more energy and stamina to boot.

- **Phytoestrogen-rich foods:** These are estrogens that come from plants—and cherries are highest on the list. Tomatoes, red onions,

From the "M" File

ELECTRONIC SEX: NO COMPUTER REQUIRED

Q: I'm fifty-four and single, and my sex life is in the dumps. I don't feel like giving any, getting any, or doing anything with anybody, mostly because I just don't seem to enjoy sex anymore. However, I've recently heard about some kind of computer mouse type device that can help women like me. Is it really therapeutic—or just another silly sex toy?

A: It sounds like you are referring to the Eros/CVD—a clitoral suction device approved by the FDA in 2000. About the size of a computer mouse—and kind of shaped that way—it comes with a suction cup attached and runs on a battery. And of course, no computer required! To use the device, you place the soft, pliable cup over your clitoris and turn the tiny machine on. Different from a vibrator, which only provides stimulation, this device creates a vacuum-like suction that pulls on the clitoris. Clinical studies have shown this can increase blood flow and in turn increase sensitivity, improve lubrication, and increase your chance for orgasm. Some users report it also enhances the overall sexual experience. It can be used with a partner, or on your own, as a kind of therapy that helps restore sexual responsiveness in your vagina. While it may not do much to increase your desire for sex, experts say that when your genitals are stimulated, desire is frequently rekindled. While some women report a noticeable change almost right away, others say they required several weeks of therapy with Eros before they could see a difference. Eros, which is available only by prescription, is approved for female sexual dysfunction related to decreased vaginal lubrication or wetness, decreased clitoral sensation, difficulty experiencing orgasms, or inability to have an orgasm. In your case, the real bonus is that you can experiment on your own and see if your sex drive returns before going out and seeking a partner.

soy products, oats, and celery are also rich sources of the plant estrogens that can encourage your own estrogen production as well as some activity below the waist!

Sex, the Pill, and Midlife Pregnancy: What You Must Know

Although I've spent most of this chapter helping you learn new ways to revive your desire for sex, it's also important to touch on another subject that's linked to the time you spend in the bedroom—pregnancy. Clearly, at our age, there's no question that the chance of conceiving isn't anywhere near what it was when we were thirty or even thirty-five. Still, it can happen, and often when we least expect it. According to figures recently released by the National Survey of Family Growth, 51 percent of all pregnancies in women over age forty are *unintended*!

While your menstrual cycle may be highly irregular—indicating you are ovulating only a few times a year—unless you have not had any bleeding at all for a minimum of twelve months (and are thus considered officially in menopause), you can still get pregnant, at least theoretically. If this is not something you want at this time in your life, then it's important that you take steps to prevent it from occurring.

For many women, the answer is the low-dose birth control pill. According to Dr. Ronald Burkman, professor and deputy chairman of obstetrics and gynecology at Tufts University School of Medicine, in addition to protecting you from getting pregnant, it can also help reduce some perimenopausal symptoms—including hot flashes and even some forms of sexual dysfunction. So in this respect, you are getting more than one benefit from using oral contraception.

In terms of safety, Dr. Burkman says there is good news here as well: Studies show that if you are basically healthy, and a nonsmoker, you can safely use the Pill well into your mid-fifties with very little risk of problems. Although some very early studies indicated an increased risk of blood clots, strokes, and even heart attacks for older women on the Pill, virtually all of that research involved very high-dose estrogen formulas—with as much as 150 micrograms per pill. This is far different from the low-dose Pills routinely offered to older women today—with most containing just 30 micrograms of estrogen per dose.

That said, many of you may also be concerned about recent information on the risks of hormone replacement therapy. However, it's important to realize that these studies do not include the same kind of hormonal formulations found in birth control pills. Although HRT and the Pill *are* both hormone-based preparations, they affect the body in different ways. While HRT works by *adding* hormones to what your body is already producing, birth control pills *shut down* your body's natural hormone production and replace it with a small, metered amount of hormone. In this way, levels can be more closely controlled. Studies show that regular use of oral contraceptives, even during the perimenopause years, *reduces* the risk of both ovarian and endometrial cancer—and the protection continues for up to thirty years after you stop. There is also mounting evidence the Pill can protect you against colorectal cancer as well. A new Swedish study found that using oral contraceptives in your forties reduces your risk of hip fracture later in life by up to 30 percent, mostly due to an increase in bone density, which is also linked to pill use. While there is some research indicating the Pill might slightly increase the risk of breast cancer in some women—particularly those at high risk—there are equal numbers of studies showing no increased risk at all.

The bottom line: If you are at all sexually active, and interested in birth control, taking a low-dose Pill makes good sense—at least until you reach twelve full months with no menstrual period and no vaginal bleeding. If you are still concerned about safety issues, talk to your doctor about the benefits of *ultra low-dose* pills such as Loesterin, Alesse, Mircette, or Levlite, which contain just 20 micrograms of estrogen per dose. They can still protect against pregnancy. (For more information on the use of low-dose birth control pills in perimenopause, see Chapter 11.)

If you are absolutely convinced you don't want to use oral contraceptives, still consider other forms of birth control—either a diaphragm or an IUD, or have your partner use a condom. In fact, condom use should be routine anytime you are not in a completely monogamous relationship, regardless of whatever type of birth control you are using. Also remember that while the Pill can protect you from pregnancy, it offers no protection against sexually transmitted diseases—the risk of which may be even higher in midlife.

Sex, Your Body, and Your Partner: Making It All Work

Perhaps the most important thought you can keep in mind while you are thinking about your sex life is that any angst you may be feeling now is not going to last forever. Remember, menopause *does not* automatically correlate with a decrease in sexual desire—and certainly not a lasting one. According to research published in *Menopause: The Journal of the North American Menopause Society* in 2004, factors far more likely to impact our sex drive include our overall physical health, our mental health, smoking, and the quality of our relationship with our partner—all situations that are definitely under our control!

The best news of all is that while some aspects of the "change of life" can certainly influence sexual dysfunction, studies also show that a good deal of our dissatisfaction with sex is actually linked to aging problems found in our partners! (And for *this* they needed a study?!) In fact, research shows one of the *best* antidotes for a sagging sex drive *is* a new partner—no matter what your age! While I don't advocate dumping your sweetie just to ensure your next orgasm, what's important to recognize is that if all it takes is a new pair of slippers under the bed to get your libido moving, then that's all the proof you need that desire is not dead—just resting for while! With the right attitude, some good partner communication, a few nifty pharmaceuticals on the nightstand, and a Steve Tyrell CD on the stereo, you and your soulmate can rekindle both your desire for intimacy and your passion for each other. What's going to make it all happen, however, is recognizing when something *is* amiss, and then making a commitment to fix it—not just on your own, but along *with* your partner. As any therapist can tell you, very few sexual problems occur in a single bed—it not only takes two to tango, it takes two to tangle. So, it's also going to take both of you to untangle the crossed communications that can contribute significantly to sexual dysfunction on both sides of the mattress.

For this reason I advise you strongly to share with your partner what is going on with your body during this time of your life and whenever possible to explain that, for the moment, your hormones may be overshadowing your heart and even your desires. Also make certain that he knows your body is going to require just a little bit more attention than perhaps was necessary in the past. If your partner knows and understands this, then he'll also know it's not him you're rejecting when you choose folding laundry over making love. Ultimately that realization should make it infinitely easier to work together to maintain your relationship until you can both rediscover the joy of sex in your lives.

At the same time, I urge you to share your feelings about midlife sex, and particularly any symptoms or problems you may be experiencing, with your doctor, and ask his or her advice on what you might do to improve your situation. Although it can be a bit embarrassing for some of you to broach this subject, particularly if you don't have a very long or close relationship with your gynecologist or family doctor, I can still promise that talking about the problem will not only help you feel better, it may actually bring you closer to a solution—be it pharmacological or otherwise. To help start the conversation you can simply say, "I'm not feeling quite the same in the bedroom as I did a few months ago, and I'm wondering if there aren't some medical tests I should take?" Putting the problem in the context of health rather than sex might make it easier for you to ask a question—plus, it allows you the opportunity to discuss some additional testing that might just get to the root of your problem.

The bottom line: Your sex life is here to stay! While it may seem, at times, that this couldn't possibly be true—or even that you wish it weren't true—the reality is, how you feel today is not a blueprint for how you will feel tomorrow. The really good news in all of this is that even with absolutely no treatment, no attention, and no effort on your part whatsoever, it's highly likely that this phase of your sex life will pass. You may be surprised at the confident, newly secure woman that emerges from the ashes—with a sex life that takes on a whole new meaning.

Until then, smile, and remember . . . there's always shoe shopping!

9

Your Brain on Menopause . . . Or, Why You Cry When the Bakery Is Out of Rye Bread

~~~~~~

How to Cope with Mood Swings and Memory Loss, and Reduce the Stress in Your Life

I was barely past my fortieth birthday when my beloved and I were sitting in our den one Sunday evening reading the *New York Times*. It was then that I became convinced that he must have learned some brand-new way of breathing down at that gym he just joined because suddenly every breath he was taking was annoying me beyond belief. Honestly—there I was trying to do the *Times* crossword while he was making this little rattling noise each time he inhaled—I can remember it sounded like a small train was screeching off the tracks with every breath he took—and it was driving me *crazy*!

"Stop that," I finally chided him in a tone normally reserved for cataclysmic conversations involving his mother.

"Stop what?" he said, as he sat back relaxed and comfy in our suede loveseat—the most comfortable seat in the house, I might add, reading the *Times Book Review*.

"That breathing—STOP IT," I said even more defiantly—and loudly.

"You want me to stop breathing?" he asked innocently, momentarily looking up from his page.

I thought for a minute about how silly my demand must have sounded, but then answered him anyway. "Yes, stop breathing—if that's the only way to stop that rattling noise coming from your nostrils every time you inhale," I said quite matter-of-factly, clearly having one of my finest diva moments.

He rolled his eyes, closed the paper, and got up. He leaned over and pecked me on the cheek. "If you need me, I'll be in the home office— breathing," he said with a wink and a smile.

Now—now I was *really* irritated. How dare he humor me this way? But a few curses under my breath later I thought—oh well, who cares? He's gone and I've got the comfy loveseat—and the *Book Review*—all to myself.

But no sooner was I settled in, pillow squished behind my back and feet up on the hassock, when I began looking around the room. That's when I realized he was not the only thing irritating me that day. The carpeting was also getting on my nerves. Why hadn't I ever noticed how ugly it was before? I thought for a minute and jumped up from the comfy love seat, convinced of what I must do.

I headed straight for the kitchen and retrieved the utility knife. What a great idea, I thought to myself—I'll just rip it all up and tomorrow I'll call in a carpet salesman and order something new.

I came back into the den and knelt down near the far left-hand corner of the room. With total free-spirited abandonment I began hacking away, pulling the carpet back from the wall tacks, strip by strip. Slice, rip, slice, rip—I wasn't even sure where I was finding the strength, but I did know the activity seemed to ease at least some of my irritated feelings. Then suddenly, there was a crackling sound and all the lights went out— except, of course, for these sparks spewing just inches from where I was kneeling. Holy moly—I remembered the electrical cable that was running along the baseboard. I had sliced it, knocking out power to half the house and nearly setting myself on fire in the process.

I think that's the precise moment when it hit me: "You have finally gone off the deep end," I told myself. "You *are insane*." And as I sat there, in the dark, covered in carpet scraps, utility knife still in my hand, I burst into tears.

Fortunately, what I found out soon afterward was that my sanity was in pretty good shape after all. My hormones, however . . . well, that was another story. Welcome to my perimenopause—a time, I was soon to discover, that was destined to become the carnival ride of my life. Ups. Downs. Twists. Turns. And, much to my beloved's distress, death-defying screams when least expected. Hot flashes, I soon learned, would be the least of my problems when compared to this seldom discussed "netherworld" of emotional highs and lows—feelings that seemed to overtake me without rhyme or reason and usually without warning.

And while my doctor could quote me chapter and verse on the physical symptoms I might experience—hot flashes, dry vagina, fatigue, insomnia, even weight gain and thinning hair—never did he, or anyone else for that matter, warn me, or God forbid explain why, my emotional life would turn upside down. Or, more importantly, tell me what I could do about it.

Well, if this story is starting to sound a little too familiar, take heart— there is, I found out, some good news to report. First . . . no, you are not wigging out, even when you continually burst into tears every time the bakery is out of rye bread. And no, you will not be seen wearing a dribble bib and absentmindedly snapping your fingers to an accordion rendition of "Stairway to Heaven" anytime soon! More importantly, yes, there are things you can do to ease the difficulties and smooth out the transitions from high to low. Not only that, but there are also ways to avoid at least some of the emotional turmoil and actually get through this time of your life without the need for a criminal trial attorney—or a divorce lawyer.

For me, the first step in taking control of my midlife crisis was understanding a little something about what was going on in my body as it related to my emotions, and to some extent even my thought processes.

Your Midlife Emotional Crisis:
What's Really Going On in Your Brain— And How to Fix It!

For most women, menopause—and particularly the period leading up to menopause—is all about the ovaries. As egg production winds down and hormone levels start to drop, our reproductive era slowly closes, and soon, menopause is upon us. And while your ovaries certainly play a huge part in this aging process, your brain is every bit as involved. One reason is because estrogen not only stimulates your ovaries to produce eggs, it's also intimately linked with the release and utilization of a variety of neurotransmitters—brain chemicals that control everything from your appetite to your emotions and a whole lot in between. While it may seem that your brain is just one great big organ orchestrating all this activity from a single source, it's actually divided into three specific layers or parts—your brain stem, your limbic system, and your cerebral cortex. These parts interact with each other, as well as with your hormones, to set the stage for how your emotions play out at any given time in your life.

Now if all this is starting to sound a bit too "heady," just think of your brain as kind of a jelly roll—with one layer of cream, one of jelly, and one of cake! The innermost "cream" layer—your brain stem—is the area that controls all of your involuntary actions, like breathing, digestion, and heart rate. Surrounding it is the limbic system—or the "jelly" layer—command central for processing not only your emotional feelings, but your appetite, your sex drive, your aggressive impulses, all your biorhythms including your sleep–wake cycle, and even the timing of your menstrual period. Last comes the "cake" layer of your brain, the cerebral cortex. It kind of wraps around everything, controlling your thought patterns, your language skills, and your problem-solving abilities.

Like cake, cream and jelly, each layer of your brain can function somewhat on its own. But in order for there to be a "jelly roll," all three areas must work together. And fortunately, most of the time this is the case. What makes it all work is a finely tuned network of naturally released chemicals known as neurotransmitters. The rhythm with which these compounds are released by cells in your brain, and their ability to find their way to specific areas (called receptor sites), is what is largely responsible for the way we feel *and* the way we function, particularly in regard to our moods. There are several different neurotransmitters involved in these processes—including norepinephrine, dopamine, and acetylcholine—but by far the most influential, at least in terms of our midlife emotions, is serotonin. When levels of this neurotransmitter are normal, we feel good and our moods are stable. When there is not enough to go around, or when what we have can't get to its proper docking station, or receptor site, that's when our moods begin to shift out of control. Depending on how far off the mark our serotonin levels are, and for how long, largely determines how "wild" our mood swing might be. If, in fact, levels remain disrupted and out of balance for a long enough period of time, serious depression can even develop, at midlife or any time.

So, right about now you're probably asking yourself how in the world estrogen fits into this picture. Well, in the not-too-distant past, doctors didn't think that it did. The consensus of opinion was that a woman's moods during this time of transition were pretty much mandated by her other symptoms. Hot flashes, for example, lead to sleep deprivation, which leads to fatigue, which leads to yelling at your partner for breathing, and then ripping up the den carpet! In the last decade, however, and particularly in the last several years, researchers have painted a whole new picture of the female brain. Part of this new "blueprint" includes never-before-seen receptor sites for not just neurotransmitters but also hormones—particularly estrogen and progesterone. What's more, we learned that the greatest concentration of these receptor sites is located in the limbic system—the "jelly" layer, or "command central" for processing our feelings and our moods. As such, it's not hard to see how, when estrogen levels go down and progesterone is no longer being made, these receptor sites are going to react—and when they do, the way we feel is going to change. And it does. Mood swings, temper tantrums, depression, surprising highs followed by unexpected lows, even lapses in memory and poor concentration all paint a pretty accurate picture of the way many women feel during this time of life.

"The constant change of hormone levels during this time can have a troubling effect on emotions . . . leaving some women to feel irritable and even depressed," reports the American College of Obstetricians and Gynecologists.

To give you some idea of just how dramatic these changes can be, just compare the average hormone levels before and after perimenopause begins. During the reproductive years, for example, most of us have about 100 picograms of estrogen coursing through our bodies at all times. But cross that threshold into middle age, and estrogen can soar as high as 300, 400, or even 500 picograms—and then just as quickly drop down to

50–80 picograms—all with little or no warning. Each time these hormones take a jump—up or down—brain chemistry has to compensate, mostly by altering the number and function of the receptors that process estrogen. Sometimes, when changes are slight or gradual, the brain makes its adjustments with nary a symptom. That's why some women experience only mild emotional highs and lows during this time. However, when changes are abrupt, as they are for most women, the brain has a much more difficult time stabilizing neurotransmitter function. This also explains why so many women experience at least some short-term depression after childbirth—the sudden drop in hormones that occurs after giving birth sends serotonin and other brain chemicals into a temporary tailspin.

These same wild hormonal swings are the reason why, for many women, the most frustrating part of their midlife transition is the instability: the ups and downs, the crying spells, temper flare-ups—even the unexplained anger that can be prompted by something as benign as the sound of your husband breathing!

"Your ovaries are failing, and trying to keep up estrogen production—some days they overshoot it, other days they can't produce enough," says Dr. Darlene Lanka, assistant professor at the University of California San Francisco.

Of course the good news in all of this is that the overwhelming majority of scientific studies confirm that *menopause is not just another term for "nervous breakdown."* Studies published as early as 1994 in the *British Journal of Psychiatry* verified that long-lasting despair, extreme irritability, even complete emotion-driven fatigue generally affect only a very small number of women. So keep in mind that whatever you are feeling, no matter how terrible, it is very likely going to pass.

Even better news: Studies also show that it is not so much the decrease in hormone levels that influences your mood swings as it is the *fluctuation.* In research published in 2003 in the *Harvard Study of Mood and Cycles,* experts verified that it is the *abrupt* alterations in hormone levels that interferes with mood and behavior most. As time passes and those levels begin to *stabilize*—even at a much lower concentration—emotional balance should return as well.

For many women—myself included—just knowing that there was a sound biochemical reason behind my weeping at the mere thought of a Hallmark commercial, or biting off my loved ones' heads with little provocation was enough of a comfort to help me get through at least the initial wave of perimenopausal influences.

I also discovered a war chest of both natural and pharmacological treatments that can be of enormous help. In fact, many of the same therapies that can help you overcome other symptoms of perimenopause—including hot flashes and night sweats—frequently have an impact on your mood swings as well. In the two chapters that follow you'll find many of these solutions.

Hormones and Your Car Keys: Tripping Down Memory Lane

I can remember talking to my friend Jeannie—who, by the way, is several years and several liters of hormones ahead of me in this whole midlife process—when her symptoms were just beginning. A typical conversation would go something like this:

Jeannie: So I went to this new restaurant called . . . um . . . you know.

Me: Rao's?

Jeannie: No, that's not it, they didn't serve Italian food, they served um . . . um . . . I had . . . um. . . .

Me: Chinese? Indian? Mexican?

Jeannie: No, no . . . It tasted like . . . um . . . but not, you know . . . it was like from . . . what's that place where what's her name went on vacation when she was married to that guy, you know, the one who was married before to that blonde—now what was her name again?

Before long I always found myself shouting out answers like I was on some kind of quiz show. Spicy! Mexican! Brazil! Maryellen! Roger! Blonde Rita! Somehow I always felt I should win a washer and dryer after every conversation Jeannie and I had.

As frustrating as it was at the time, I knew that memory loss was part and parcel of a woman's midlife changes, caused, or at least exacerbated, by the same fluctuations in estrogen that were behind so many of our other symptoms—including hot flashes and mood swings. That's because normally, estrogen plays several very important roles in our ability to remember. First, it helps bring more blood to the brain—and that in turn can literally "light up" our memory cells and stimulate them into action. But it also helps in other ways—playing a role in organizing memory data, for example, and transporting certain neurotransmitters, along with our thoughts, from one area of the brain to another. Estrogen also aids in the production of several very important brain chemicals specifically linked to memory, particularly acetylcholine. It even helps to regulate some functions in an area of the brain known as the hippocampus, which is where key activities involved in memory take place—like recalling where you put the car keys! Some research shows that estrogen may also play a role in the manufacture of a natural substance known as apolipoprotein E (apoE), a decrease of which is now believed to play a key role in the development of dementia. In one study conducted by Dr. Barbara Sherwin of McGill University in Montreal, women who were deprived of estrogen for any extended period of time lost at least some ability to recall verbal information. Other research published by a group of British doctors in the journal *Clinical Experiments in Pharmacological Physiology* in 1998 found that across the board estrogen appears to influence production of a good many of the brain chemicals involved in memory, cognition, and emotion.

Certainly, it's possible that *some* midlife memory loss is due to an early onset of dementia, or even just the aging process itself. When this is the case you may not recall the face of someone whom you have met or have known for a while, or you may fail to remember even simple directions five minutes after you receive them. For the most part, however, if your memory problems involve things like not being able to find the right word to express your thoughts, or if you find you can't recall a name, if you walk into a room and forget what you went there to get, or you make a call and suddenly can't remember who you dialed—chances are your memory problems *are* hormone related, and mediated by this transition time in your life.

The good news here: The effects are temporary. Experts agree that while the drop in estrogen may precipitate memory problems, again, it's really the fluctuations and not the low levels that matter most. So, once your hormones stabilize and the dancing comes to a halt, many of the memory problems you are experiencing will clear—and your thought patterns and levels of concentration will return to normal. Even better news: Many of the same therapies that can help you stabilize your hormone levels and improve your mood swings will improve your memory problems as well.

Perhaps the most important thing is to not become too stressed about either your mood swings *or* your failing memory. As you are about to discover, at least some of the ways in which you handle these and other problems in your life can go a long way in impacting how your hormones will function—and consequently how you will feel through much of your transition time.

Double Jeopardy: Stress and Midlife Hormones

The idea that stress can affect the way we feel, both physically, and especially mentally, is certainly not new. Doctors have long known that when we are emotionally challenged, our bodies respond. Blood pressure goes up, heart rate increases, and a flood of stress-related chemicals begins surging through our bodies, mostly aimed at creating a "fight or flight" response. In short, our minds are helping supply our bodies with the biochemical energy to either face the source of our stress or run from it. Either way, the operative goal is to eliminate the stressful situation. Once this occurs, our vital signs return to normal, brain chemistry calms down, and within due time we are back to feeling like ourselves.

But what happens when, for whatever reason, we can't either "fight" or "flee" the source of our stress? A boss who is never pleased no matter what we do; a spouse who is always ungrateful or unappreciative of our efforts; teenagers who, while just being teenagers, seem to be raging out of control; deadlines and traffic jams; burned dinners and broken vacuums—and all the while hormones are flaring and mood swings are raging. The end result: Your biochemical reactions to stress are ongoing—and your physiology almost never has the opportunity to return to normal. Because many of the same hormones involved in the stress response—like serotonin and dopamine—are also capable of impacting hormones like estrogen, when stress becomes chronic, perimenopausal symptoms can worsen, sometimes dramatically so. According to Harvard University stress expert Dr. Alice Domar, the effect of stress on hormone activity can be so profound, it's capable of inducing hot flashes. Domar reports that, on a strictly physiological basis, hot flashes look very similar to the "fight or flight" response to stress— your heart pounds, your breathing gets faster and more shallow, and stress hormones begin coursing through your veins.

But that's not the only midlife symptom made worse by stress. According to Joan Borysenko, a researcher at the Mind-Body Clinic of Harvard Medical School, chronic midlife tension can also cause an increase in headaches, anxiety, and mood swings. Other experts have linked stress to insomnia, which can also become a real issue during this transition time (see "To Sleep, Perchance to Dream," later in this chapter).

By the same token, taking steps to reduce or eliminate some of the stress in your life can have a dramatic effect not only on your hormone balance but, more importantly, on the severity of your symptoms, something Dr. Domar recently proved in an intriguing new study. In this experiment she compared the menopausal symptoms of two groups of women—those who practiced relaxation exercises and those who did not. More specifically, she gathered together thirty-three women who were experiencing at least five hot flashes a day—none of them taking hormones. She divided the women into three groups. One group was asked to set aside twenty minutes each day for reading; a second group was asked to put the same amount of time into listening to relaxation tapes every day; and a third group was asked to do nothing special and just live as they normally would if they weren't in a study. After seven weeks' time, the women listening to the relaxation tapes saw the greatest reduction in symptoms—a more than 30 percent reduction in their hot flashes, as well as a significant decrease in their levels of tension, anxiety, and even depression. They also reported having fewer mood swings and more stable emotions overall. Although this particular group was small, three other research teams subsequently followed larger groups of women using various relaxation techniques to reduce stress. Their finding: Up to 70 percent of the women were able to reduce the number and the severity of hot flashes.

Additional research backed up these findings. In a study conducted at

Guy's Medical Hospital School in London, women who took relaxation classes over a ninety-day period ended up with 50 percent fewer hot flashes compared to those who did nothing to reduce stress levels, or even those who turned to hormone replacement therapy for relief. Twenty-five percent of the women in the relaxation group said hot flashes completely disappeared.

Borysenko reports that many of the women she studied—most already in menopause—were able to control hot flashes with regular deep-breathing exercises (covered later in this chapter). Sometimes, they could even stop a hot flash from escalating by simply taking a deep "sigh of relief." The science behind the cure: Experts say controlled breathing short-circuits the fight-or-flight response, sending a message to the brain that all is well and you can relax. Not only does this make you feel better physically—your heart rate and blood pressure return to normal—but the deep breaths may also reduce the duration and the intensity of any hot flash you do experience.

COPING WITH YOUR PERIMENOPAUSE STRESS: WHAT YOU CAN DO

Right about now you're probably wondering if I'm about to suggest we all run away to Woodstock for a nice long weekend of candle making and chanting. Not that it wouldn't be a nice change of pace from the traffic jams, lousy bosses, crabby spouses, and crazy kids, you understand. Be that as it may, I am fully aware that it's no longer 1972—and as much as we might need it, I know we just can't while away an entire day listening to Joni Mitchell records and pondering the future of Greenpeace.

What I am going to suggest is taking *some* time out of your day, every day, to bring down your level of stress and give your body a chance to "chill out." Doing so will help you to cope with some of the perimenopause symptoms you are experiencing right now and, in the long run, help your blood pressure and your heart. According to some experts it maybe even protects you from cancer and other catastrophic diseases, all of which have been linked to chronic stress.

Still not convinced you need to relax? Okay, then think about this: According to the American Institute of Stress, the biochemicals linked to long-term anger and chronic stress—particularly cortisol—can be a leading cause of obesity, especially in older women. It can even influence where you gain your weight, significantly increasing the development of the "apple shape," which, as you read earlier, can increase your risk of heart disease. Conversely, reducing both stress levels and anger may make controlling your weight easier, impacting a whole series of hormones linked to those excess midlife pounds. Now I ask you—where else would you find someone to tell you that sitting by the pool and reading fashion magazines for an hour every day is good for your health?!

Relaxation: It's Strictly Personal, Baby!

It's always been my theory that relaxation is a highly personal experience—as witnessed by the fact that no two friends of mine *ever* agree on the subject. My best friend Dee, for example, finds maximum, soul-releasing relaxation while gardening, while for me, just the thought of sticking my hands in the dirt is enough to send me screaming to the manicurist. My other friend Sheila says nothing calms her stress like a long drive on the freeway, while for me, anything more than a twenty-minute road trip is a chore (unless of course I'm going for a manicure, in which case I'll make the exception!). The point is that most of the time you know what it is that helps you to relax—and you know what it takes to calm you down. Of course what we want, or even need, to do is not always possible, or practical. Let's face it, there are only so many opportunities in a lifetime for me to spend hours walking along a moonlit beach in San Diego, when I live in New York City. Nevertheless, experts report that there are a number of "universal" stress-busting activities that can work as well in New York City as San Diego or Paris—or anywhere you are. While not every activity will be right for every woman, what most have in common is the ability to relax your mind *and* temper some of the physiologic responses to stress directly linked to hormone function. What follows is a short guide to some of those activities. Based on information provided by a number of expert organizations, including the American Women's Medical Association and the National Institute of Stress, they are what I like to refer to as the keys that open the gates of hormone hell—and finally let you out!

Remember, don't overlook *any* activity that you suspect might help *you* relax, whether it's on my list or not. As long as it's legal (or you don't get caught!) and your children and husband won't be embarrassed if the photographer from the local paper catches you doing it—well, I say go for it! Relax, and have a great time! Even if your hot flashes and night sweats don't go away, at least you'll be doing something you enjoy while you're having them!

EIGHT WAYS TO REDUCE YOUR MIDLIFE STRESS

I. BREATHE DEEPLY

This is not just one of those pop psych suggestions that sounds like it should work but has no real effect. Some very impressive studies have shown that learning to control your breathing can go a long way in reducing the rush of biochemicals linked to the stress response—and it can have an impact on your hot flashes.

How to Do It: Inhale through your nose slowly and deeply and count to ten. Push out your tummy as you inhale, but keep your chest from rising with the breath. Exhale through your nose slowly to the count of ten. Repeat the breathing, concentrating on the sound of your breath only, zoning out other distractions in the room. Repeat five to ten times, several times a day.

Emergency Hot Flash Deep Breath: When you feel a hot flash coming on, stop what you are doing, close your eyes, and take a deep breath; hold for a count of five and release. Repeat several more times to help offset the flash—or shorten its duration.

2. LEARN TO MEDITATE

Now, I promised, no Woodstock mumbo jumbo, but that's not what this is. The concept here is something called "mindful mediation"—quite simply, a way of quieting the mind while concentrating on your breathing.

How to Do It: Sit upright on the floor, legs crossed, or just put your butt against the back of a firm chair with both feet on the ground uncrossed. With your eyes closed, begin paying attention to your normal breathing patterns—and if you want to, try visualizing your breaths on each exhale. If your mind wanders, don't stress about it—just keep bringing yourself back to the breathing exercise. If this is just too boring for you (and quite frankly, it was for me—I kept opening my eyes and finding all these little spots on the wall that the painter missed, and that was making me more stressed), try the Transcendental Meditation technique that adds a word or sound to your exhaling. Repeat the word silently over and over, for ten to twenty minutes, letting your thoughts go with each repetition. Pick a word that means something to you—in my case it was "diamonds." Very effective and not a bad image to conjure up, I might add.

3. TRY SENSORY PERCEPTION RELAXATION

This is about the best relaxation technique I could find for busy women—mostly because it allows you to do what you have to do anyway, and thus turn even the most mundane of household or work chores into an opportunity to relax. In this technique you simply heighten the awareness of your body during whatever activity it is that you are doing—the goal being to redirect your brain away from your worries, which in turn disrupts the stress response, blocks the flow of harmful brain chemicals, and allows you to relax.

How to Do It: If, for example, you're washing dishes, concentrate on how the water and soapsuds feel on your hands—how your skin responds to the changes in water temperature, and even how the surface of each dish feels to the touch. You can also concentrate on the smell of the dishwashing liquid (if you get one of those yummy new aromatherapy scented Palmolive dishwashing detergents it can be a real bonus). Or concentrating on any sight or sound in your immediate vicinity will do. If angry, stressful, or upsetting thoughts get in the way, bring your mind back to the sensory perceptions and feel the tension release.

4. CHANT

I know, I know, I promised nothing weird. But the research is there and for many of you, chanting can be a wonderful way to control symptoms. In truth, repetitive rhythms of any kind promote a sense of relaxation similar to yoga and meditation—and you don't have to put your body in any weird positions (or buy any new workout clothes) to do it! Chanting also promotes deep breathing, and believe it or not, studies show that the sounds produced during this activity can actually penetrate muscles, bones, and organs, causing cells to adjust to the frequency! It also stimulates the secretion of stress-reducing hormones and pain-relieving endorphins—and may even modify brain waves. So, as long as you are not chanting the name of your cheap ex-husband or your nasty boss, your experience should be a positive one!

How to Do It: Sit in a comfortable, relaxed position—many people find sitting up in bed or on the floor leaning on a heap of pillows does the trick. If possible wear unrestrictive clothing—or at least not something that is squishing your waist or thighs. The key here is to feel as physically unrestricted as you can. Then choose a phrase that feels comfortable for you to say—it can be the line of a song you like, a positive affirmation, or even just a string of sounds that feels good when you utter it. Close your eyes, clear your mind of thoughts, and begin repeating or "chanting" the phrase, speaking as rhythmically as possible. You can start slow and speed up, or keep your tempo even. You can also speak your chant as loud as you like (providing there's no one around who's going to question your sanity) or as softly as you like *(much* better idea). Try to "feel" the motion or the rhythm of your phase and let your body move to the beat if you feel it. Ten to fifteen minutes of chanting could leave you feeling like a new woman!

5. DO NOTHING (MY PERSONAL FAVORITE)

Light a candle, put on a CD, or just lie in bed and stare at the ceiling or out the window or at your favorite painting, and try not to think about anything that upsets or worries you. The key here is to give yourself *permission* to do absolutely nothing for ten to fifteen minutes, once a day.

How to Do It: Oh come on now . . . I don't really have to teach you how to do nothing, do I? But I will give you this advice: *Don't feel guilty* about doing nothing. Make it a necessary part of your day—something that you must do in order to increase productivity and work harder and better at everything.

6. GET TOUCHED

Another personal favorite! Be it a massage, a facial, a new haircut and styling, a makeup session at your favorite salon, a pedicure, a manicure, or just twenty minutes spent petting your dog or cat, the goal here is to touch someone, or have someone touch you, for at least a few minutes as often as possible. Massage, as well as other forms of therapeutic touch (where someone is doing something to make *you* feel better), has been shown to reduce cortisol, the key hormone involved in the stress response. It can also lower blood pressu e and boost your immunity—and many women report that weekly massages can keep hot flashes under control.

How to Do It: Schedule a *regular* de-stressing touch session once weekly—a massage at your local health club, a facial or a manicure/pedicure, for example—and don't let anything get in the way of taking this time out for yourself. If it's really and truly not possible to get away, arrange for you and your partner to swap body rubs on alternate nights. If all else fails, cuddle your pet for twenty minutes a few times a week—or if need be, visit a pet shop that allows you to play with friendly pups and kitties. Anything that allows you to touch or be touched can lower your stress levels.

7. MOVE AROUND

I'm talking about your body! It can be a brisk walk, a yoga session, an hour of shadow dancing by yourself to your favorite golden oldies—the activity is up to you, but the key is to move your body to move stress out of your mind. Not only will movement help free your physical tensions, it can also help you short-circuit some nasty stress-related chemical reactions while raising the level of endorphins and other chemicals that make you feel good.

How to Do It: Regardless of what activity you choose, move around for about thirty minutes per session, about three times a week.

8. STOP AND SMELL THE ROSES

No, really—*smell them!* This stress remedy is called aromatherapy, and it relies on the scent of various natural fragrances—including roses—to reduce tension and induce a sense of calm. While I know it sounds a little hocus-pocus, in reality, the nose is one of the quickest routes to the limbic system of the brain—the area that, as you know, controls your emotions. In addition to roses, the essences shown to have the most relaxing properties are lavender, vanilla, and lemongrass, plus essential oils like ylang-ylang, geranium (which helps ease depression and can help balance hormones), and clary sage (another hormone balancer).

How to Do It: Aromatherapy can come in many forms, including candles (just light it, and let the aroma waft through your room), essential oils (same principal as burning a candle but a bit more potent), soap, fragrance, body lotion, or shower gel, all of which you can use any way you like. For "emergency" stress relief try keeping a hankie that has been doused with your fragrance of choice in a plastic bag in your pocketbook. When stress starts to get you down, take out the hankie, take a few whiffs, and you should feel an almost immediate sense of calm and balance return.

To Sleep, Perchance to Dream—Or Perchance to Lie Awake All Night Sweating: How Hormones Affect Your Sleep Cycle

You're exhausted. You put in a ten-hour day at work; got stuck in a two-hour traffic jam; spent the next two hours at a parent–teacher conference where you heard less than good news; you came home to find your husband and son used every pot in the house to cook two plates of spaghetti—and the dishwasher is broken. By the end of the evening, all you can think about is hitting the mattress and falling into dreamland. And you do. For about three hours. Then, as if you'd been struck by some annoying bolt of lightning (and only a truly exhausted woman could classify a bolt of lightning as "annoying"), you wake up drenched in sweat and hotter than a sun reflector on the beach.

So you get out of bed, you change your PJs, maybe splash some cool water on your face and chest, think about putting some ice cubes in the bed, nix that idea, and get back in the sack. You close your eyes—still feeling exhausted, mind you—and you wait. The ticking of the clock becomes unbearably loud—dwarfed only by your partner's snoring. Before long the sun is coming up and you're facing another day on three hours of sleep—your third this week. And you wonder why people actually have to question the reason fifty-year-old women are crying at the drop of a hat one minute and screaming like there's no tomorrow the next. That's when you also probably also realize—Holy moly, I don't need hormones, I just need some sleep!

Well, if that is what you're thinking, you're at least partly right. Because yes, it's true, sleep deprivation does make us do wild and crazy things—and the older we are when we start losing sleep, the worse the consequences can be. There are still some physicians who insist that most if not all of the emotional symptoms of midlife are directly related to sleep deprivation—and for some women, this may be true. Certainly, whatever hormone-related problems you are experiencing can be made worse when insomnia enters the picture. More important, perhaps, is the idea that sleep deprivation in and of itself is really one more symptom of midlife change, as much hormone related as hot flashes or mood swings.

That's precisely the conclusion drawn by a group of Finnish researchers in October 2000. After recording the sleep habits of some 3,400 women they discovered that among those aged forty to fifty, nearly half who were not taking hormones reported sleeping problems. Among the most common concerns was what doctors call "nocturnal waking"—you know, getting jolted awake by something other than your husband's spontaneous romantic notions, or the boombox your teenage daughter and her new college boyfriend are blasting in the driveway. And once you're awake—there seems to be no turning back, at least not for that night, anyway.

While this particular study didn't cite a reason for midlife sleep problems, other research has. The going theory: Just because you're sleeping it doesn't mean your estrogen is. Indeed, as your hormones continue to dance through the night, they can interrupt the production and function of neurotransmitters essential to healthy sleep, such as serotonin. In addition, many experts believe that hot flashes can actually occur in our sleep as well—and not only will the sensation of warmth wake you (many women commonly refer to this as "night sweats"), but hormonal comings and goings linked to the flash itself can impact our sleep–wake cycle. In addition, fluctuations in hormone levels can delay your ability to fall asleep—even when you feel dead tired.

The very latest research also links those dancing hormones to an increased risk of sleep apnea, a potentially dangerous disorder that causes breathing to halt momentarily throughout the night—which often results in extreme fatigue upon waking, or throughout the day. In the new research, conducted at Penn State College of Medicine, some two thousand women between the ages of twenty and one hundred were studied over a five-year period. The finding: Postmenopausal women who did not use hormone replacement therapy were five times more likely to develop sleep apnea than women who used HRT. The Penn doctors suggest that the drop in estrogen and progesterone seen at midlife may influence the brain chemistry involved in sleep apnea.

Regardless of what is behind your nighttime problems, you *can* improve the quality of the rest you do get, as well as increase the length of time you are able to *remain* asleep. While hormone therapy can help, it's definitely not the first line of defense—nor should it be considered if that's your only reason for taking it. A better solution is to talk to your doctor about over-the-counter or even prescription sleep aids, or simply try some of the natural, alternative methods described below. Either way, if you are experiencing a bounty of midlife symptoms, there's a good chance that getting more sleep, or improving the quality of the sleep you do get, will go a long way in helping you cope.

SLEEP SOLUTIONS: WHAT TO TRY

Herbs: Many experts believe that one of the most natural ways to nod into dreamland is via the use of botanicals—plants and flowers that have a sedative property and can help you relax and unwind. At the very least they can help decrease the amount of time it takes you to fall asleep once you do get into bed. According to Dr. Susan Lark, an expert on natural therapies, among the most useful herb teas for insomnia are valerian root (150–300 milligrams forty-five minutes before bedtime); passionflower (tea made from 1 teaspoon of dried leaves before bed); and chamomile (steep 2 to 3 heaping teaspoons of flowers in one cup of boiling water);

or kava root capsules (140 milligrams before bedtime). Some or all may also be available in tea bags and are often sold at health food stores. Other natural treatments suggested by Lark include 50–100 milligrams of 5-HTP (an amino acid that helps promote serotonin production) before bedtime and 1 milligram of melatonin, a chemical involved in the sleep cycle, taken at bedtime.

Relaxation: According to Cornell University sleep expert Dr. Samuel Dunkell, taking twenty to thirty minutes out to relax and unwind before going to bed can go a long way in helping you fall into a deep sleep faster and easier. And that may mean you will stay asleep longer. Wind-down activities can include reading, watching nonstimulating TV, listening to music, taking a warm bath, or even playing solitaire—anything that you find personally relaxing. The key is that the activity not be stimulating or exciting. Dr. Dunkell also recommends progressive relaxation techniques, the kind often used to combat stress. One of the most popular forms involves lying in bed and concentrating on muscle groups, starting with your toes. Let your mind instruct your muscles to relax, concentrating on each group of muscles—like calves, thighs, and hips—until you feel a loosening of the tension in that part of your body. A second technique involves tightening a specific muscle group—like your toes or calves, for example—and holding the position until you feel a strain or a "burn," then releasing it. Progressively work your way up your body to each muscle group until you feel a total sense of relaxation—and, hopefully, sleepiness.

Sleep Cool: If getting to sleep seems easy, but you find yourself waking after only three or four hours of rest, one reason may be hot flashes occurring while you are asleep. Stimulating your central nervous system, the jolt can wake you and keep you awake for hours. To help cut down on the chance of nocturnal hot flashes, dress exceptionally lightly at bedtime. Avoid nylon nighties (which can increase, and hold, body heat) as well as all-cotton nightgowns or PJs, which will hold sweat and leave you feeling moist and wet, another potential "wake-up" call. The best sleepwear is a 50/50 cotton-polyester blend, or any fabric with a loose weave. You can also try a down comforter, which can work as a kind of an environmental "adaptogen," keeping your body temperature regulated. The best sheets are also 50/50 cotton-poly, but make certain to wash any new ones you buy. Many sheets advertised as "permanent press" are actually treated with the chemical formaldehyde, which can make some sensitive folks hot and sweaty while they sleep.

In Asian cultures, doctors believe that keeping the head cool during the night will help induce a deeper sleep and reduce your chances of waking mid-cycle. While you don't want to put an ice pack on your head, you might want to try a product called "Chillow"—a pillow that you fill with cool water before going to sleep. It remains remarkably cool (not cold) throughout the night and can help absorb heat from your head and neck, keeping your whole body cooler (see the resource section at the back of the book). And, of course, the old "standby" is to simply sleep with a window open—even a half-inch can help, since it allows some circulation of fresh air. Finally, don't eat any hot or spicy foods after seven or eight in the evening. They can rev up your metabolism and make you warmer while you sleep. If nighttime bathroom breaks disrupt your sleep cycle, don't drink anything for at least three hours before going to bed.

Menopause and the Power of Girlfriends . . . Or, How to Use the Buddy System to Beat the Midlife Crazies

The kids are driving you nuts, you're convinced your partner is having an affair, your boss has just told you that he doesn't think you're doing a good enough job, you found a lump in your breast . . . the litany of situations and conditions that can cause a woman stress are seemingly endless. And while some of us clearly cope by reaching for the chocolate—and quite honestly there is absolutely nothing wrong with that—when times are rough a great many of us reach for chocolate *and* something, or should I say some*one*, else—our best girlfriend. And sometimes more than one. As my dear friend Tina just wrote me in a note card recently, "A good girlfriend is like a great pair of shoes—they're always comfortable, they offer great support, and they never make you cry. Men, on the other hand, are like cheap shoes: never comfortable, never give you any support, and at the end of the day, always make you cry."

While I'm not sure I agree with all the card had to say, her point is well taken—girlfriends can be a gal's saving grace. But can hangin' out with your pals actually help you control your hot flashes, keep you from having night sweats and insomnia, and even chase away your perimenopause blues? Some new research says this might well be the case. The surprising discovery was made when a group of researchers began noting the different ways in which male and female colleagues responded to stress.

Let me explain. Although there is a great deal that doctors know about how stress affects the body, not surprisingly, much of what was learned about women was gleaned from research on men. Until 1995—the year the U.S. government mandated that all federally funded research projects include women—just 17 percent of the participants in stress-related studies were female. Even animal studies included mostly males. Thus, it's not surprising that, for a long while, everyone pretty much believed that the physiological response to stress was nearly identical in both men and women. That reaction primarily involved the concept of "fight or flight"—the classic stress response that triggers a cascade of hormonal activity that prepares our bodies to either face an aggressor or flee. As you read earlier, it is this fight-or-flight response that can initiate, or certainly exacerbate, many of the frustrating symptoms of perimenopause—including hot flashes and mood swings.

Interestingly, however, a group of female scientists from UCLA began examining the idea that perhaps men and women don't respond to stress in the *exact* same way. Rather than view the stress response as black or white, they found not only shades of gray, but clearly "pink" and "blue." In short, they postulated that while we all initially go through the classic flight-or-fight response, what happens shortly afterward might represent a significant gender bend in the road. To prove their theory they rounded up all the stress studies they could find that included women, or even female animals. And they began looking at the research with gender foremost in mind. What they found: Not only did men and women respond to stress differently on *a psychological* level, their *physiological and biochemical reactions were vastly different as well.* While it's true that men and women produce at least *some* of the same chemicals under stress—including the hormones involved in the fight-or-flight response—women, it seems, secrete greater amounts of another hormone known as oxytocin. Those of you who have delivered a baby may remember oxytocin as the hormone that is secreted when you are in labor to help you stay calm. ("Oh no, sweetheart, what makes you think pushing a ten-pound watermelon through an opening the size of a lemon is stressful?") Not coincidentally, however, oxytocin *also* encourages the mothering, nurturing, *bonding* instincts that are frequently so prevalent in women after birth.

While men, too, produce oxytocin in response to stress, when under the gun they also pour out testosterone, which researchers now believe overtakes oxytocin and more or less cancels its calming effects. If you want some proof of this little biochemical tango, just think back to the way your man acted the last time he came home from a particularly stressful day at work. If he's like most guys, he headed for the nearest bat cave, wanting to be left alone. Or worse still, he bit off your well-coiffed little head in an effort to blow off the day's steam. By comparison, think about your own stress-laden times. Chances are, at the end of a day filled with angst you're likely to turn to your children or your friends for comfort or, sometimes, try to work off your tension doing typical "nesting" activities, like vacuuming or dusting or cooking or laundry. The reason, say experts, is that in women, estrogen tends to *encourage* the production of oxytocin during stress. Now don't get excited, it's not a political statement—just a biochemical reaction that often sends us scurrying back to our "nesting" or "mothering" or "homemaking" roots in order to evoke a sense of calm in our lives. In fact, I recently realized that almost every time I get an urge to redecorate my bedroom it follows some particularly stressful event.

But oxytocin does something else for women as well—it fosters bonding among sisters and friends. *This* action—which is actually called "befriending"—causes even more oxytocin to be released, in both the women who are in need of the calming attention and those who are supplying it. The end result here: When we gals are under stress, we unconsciously seek to counter our tensions by bonding with other women, as well as with our children. And this, say experts, can have a *profound* effect on our health. According to the Harvard University Nurses' Health Study, the more female friends a woman has, the more likely she is to live a joyful life. In fact, the researchers concluded that not having enough female friends could be as damaging to your health as smoking or being obese. In studies of women who lost spouses, researchers found those with at least one close female friend were more likely to get through the experience with their health intact than those who didn't have a "sister" with whom to share their woes.

So, how does this all tie in to your hot flashes and mood swings? Well, the very stress hormones that can exacerbate some of the most troubling midlife symptoms are the same ones buffered by the effects of oxytocin—which, as you just read, may actually increase over cheesecake, hot chocolate, and a good round of gossip! In addition, if your relationship with your gal pals is such that you feel comfortable actually discussing your menopause symptoms, you may be surprised to learn how sharing your complaints can diminish their effect on your life—not to mention netting you some nifty coping advice from pals who may have already experienced what you are going through. While lunch with your best friend won't guarantee you'll be hot flash–free for the rest of the day, it *can* help you relax and definitely feel less alone—and that, say experts, can go a long way in helping you cope with symptoms and eliminate negative feelings.

The bottom line: Girlfriends are good for the body, mind, and spirit—not to mention fashion advice, beauty tips, and that all-important shoulder to lean on when the going gets rough. If you ever have any doubts about that, just tune in to Meredith, Star, Joy, Barbara, and Elizabeth, the ladies of *The View* on ABC—the show that has elevated the power of girlfriends to a whole new level!

10

Mother Nature Never Had a Hot Flash

Plant Estrogens, Herbs, and the Truth About Soy

I can remember quite well the afternoon I finally got my friend Elaine into a health food store. Of course the shopping trip didn't exactly start out that way—we had intended to spend the day at a Saks Fifth Avenue beauty expo, at the Stamford Mall. But it was there that Elaine went into full menopause mode, taking the entire fourth floor of Saks by surprise. It all started, believe it or not, over a *face cream*. It was a very expensive anti-aging treatment that both Elaine and I had been dying to try—but neither one of us was willing to pay the $200 price. When Elaine heard they were going to be giving away free samples at the expo, she insisted we drive up for the event.

Unfortunately, it was only after we got there that we found out Elaine got the day wrong—and all the samples were gone. As the clerk behind the counter tried to explain how our timing was off, I watched my friend melt into a puddle as she sat down on the floor and started to cry. The more the sales clerk tried to apologize, and the more I tried to get her to see how silly she was acting, the harder Elaine sobbed. When I noticed two burly security guards coming our way, I knew it was time to take action. Grabbing her by the elbow I pulled my friend to her feet and hustled her into the nearest ladies' room. Once inside she dropped down on a leather divan, and looking terribly Garbo-esque, held one hand over her forehead while fanning away an apparent hot flash with the other. I was the first to speak.

"Are you out of your mind—it's face cream, not money they were giving away!" I screamed in a loud whisper. She had stopped sobbing now but was still visibly shaken.

"I . . . I know . . . but I, I just couldn't help it—I don't know what came over me," she said, starting to sob again. But as strange as her actions probably seemed to everyone at Saks that day, Elaine's behavior was nothing new to me—or to her. You see, this wasn't the first time my friend was "overcome" with emotion over something as seemingly unemotional as a jar of face cream—even an expensive one. Elaine had, indeed, been regularly experiencing intermittent crying jags, as well as temper outbursts and hot flashes, for quite some time now. (In fact, we can no longer even go into Bergdorf Goodman when the weekend security staff is on duty—but that's a story for another time). Today, however, I decided *something* had to be done.

"Elaine," I said in a quiet voice, so as not to arouse her further, "we have to talk."

"About what?" she asked almost innocently as she stared into a compact mirror trying to wipe the raccoon-eye mascara stains from her face.

"About your hormones, dear." She heaved a big sigh—and gurgled—and then pulled herself upright on the divan and looked me straight in the eye.

"I told you before—no hormones," she said quietly but defiantly, referring to a previous discussion where she had made it quite clear that she was not interested in anything that came out of the back end of a horse—even a pregnant one. Estrogen, she said, was out of the question. And with a mother who died of breast cancer and heart disease on both sides of her family, I can't say I blamed her. On the other hand, I also hated to see my friend suffer—and besides, we were fast running out of stores that didn't hang out the "closed" sign when they saw us coming!

"I don't mean hormones as in chemical hormones, I mean some kind of natural treatment—something that, oh, say, grows in the ground and bears a nice pretty flower or maybe some fruit—could you handle that, do you think?" I asked, gently nudging her off the divan and out the ladies' room door.

As we made our way out of Saks and back into the mall, I slowly herded my friend down the walkway, toward a health food store where I knew we'd find a large assortment of natural products that could help her. Reluctantly she went along, but as we approached the entrance to the store, Elaine stopped in her tracks.

"Are you going to force me to buy something brown that tastes like dirt? Because you know, almost everything they sell in these places *is* brown and *does* taste like dirt," she said quite convincingly.

Of course she was just a little bit right—you *can* certainly find some pretty unappetizing things in a health food store, particularly when you're used to buying pastries and hot chocolate in a French bakery. On the other hand, I also knew that when it came to menopause symptoms, particularly mood swings and hot flashes, research *did* show that a woman can very often do as well spending her menopause dollar in the health food store as in the pharmacy. And I was convinced that Elaine was going to have to give it a try.

Within less than half an hour I loaded her cart with an assortment of herbs, nuts, seeds, and soy, and we headed for the checkout line. "I can't believe I'm letting you talk me into this," she said, opening her wallet to pay for the items. "Next thing I know you'll be putting Jimi Hendrix on the CD and convincing me that tie-dye is back in style," she said as we headed out of the mall and to the car.

"Tie-dye *is* back in style," I quipped, as I yanked my sweetie's Jimi Hendrix album from the glove compartment and treated her to a surround-sound version of "Purple Haze."

As reluctant as my friend was that day in the mall, it wasn't a month later when she came to my house bearing a tiny package under her arm, and a big smile on her face. I opened the bag, and inside . . . a tie-dye T-shirt.

"You were right," she said, grinning from ear to ear, "about the tie-dye—and the natural treatments. I have never felt better!"

Gloating is not in my nature, but I admit it was a little difficult not to be smug. Elaine suffered far longer than she had to, and went through much more angst over the decision about hormones than was necessary. Because the truth is, even if you never want to spend a dime on menopause-related pharmaceuticals, there are definitely ways to ease your symptoms and make your transition smoother and easier to bear. No tie-dye or Jimi Hendrix required!

Understanding Natural Treatments . . . Or, I Didn't Know My Begonia Had Ovaries!

Arguably, one of the most important natural treatments for menopause-related symptoms comes in the form of what experts call "natural estro-gens." Although you may have heard the term bandied about, used to describe a number of different types of products, in essence, a natural es-trogen is a phytoestrogen—a compound that contains an estrogen-like substance garnered from plants.

Now, if you're anything like Elaine you're probably thinking, "Hmmm . . . that rosebush out front doesn't seem to have any ovaries, so where's the estrogen coming from?" Good question. The answer is that all plants manufacture an estrogen-like hormone—a natural compound they need for growth and survival. Fortunately for us, on a molecular level some of those compounds are very similar to at least one type of estrogen produced in a woman's body. (Think of plant estrogens as a great copy of a pair of really pricey designer shoes—they're not exactly like the origi-nals but who would know?) In fact, once inside your body phytoestro-gens have the ability to behave somewhat like your own natural estrogen—in particular, the most potent form of natural estrogen, known as estradiol. Although much weaker than what is secreted by your ovaries—by some estimates, between a hundred and a thousand times weaker, depending on the source—phytoestrogens have at least some abil-ity to function like your natural hormones, particularly in regard to es-trogen receptors. As you read earlier in this book, a woman's body is loaded with these little hormone "docking stations"—and receptors are, in fact, found everywhere, but particularly in the breast, uterus, brain, heart, and bones. When these receptor sites receive the proper amount of estrogen stimulation, we feel great. But when they don't, well, that's when a variety of menopause-related symptoms begin to take hold—from hot flashes to night sweats, insomnia, mood swings, forgetfulness, and even a decrease in bone and cardiovascular health.

And here's where phytoestrogens can help. Although weaker than your own natural estrogens, they still have the ability to bind to estrogen receptors—putting the key in the lock, so to speak, and satisfying, at least to some degree, your cells' need for estrogen stimulation. The end result: Your body may begin to function just a little more the way it did before estrogen levels started to fall.

But that's not the only thing that makes a phytoestrogen so remarkable. In many ways, these plant compounds also work like "designer estrogens"—mimicking the effect of estrogens in some receptors (like those in the bones) while working as anti-estrogens in other receptors (like those in the breast). If, for example, you have a lot of estrogen in your system—the way you might during your reproductive years, or perhaps at the start of perimenopause—then these plant compounds will begin exerting anti-estrogenic effects. This in turn helps ensure that you don't experience a potentially dangerous estrogen overload. At the same time, should your natural estrogen levels drop—as they do when you are officially in menopause—then the phytoestrogens have the ability to change gears, functioning more like an estrogen, binding to receptor sites and filling the gap left by your own dwindling hormone supply.

The end result: When consumed regularly, in high enough amounts, phytoestrogens can be helpful during many stages of your midlife transition, from the very beginning of your perimenopause clear through to the time when your period officially ends, and beyond. If the men in our lives were as reliable as these plants . . . well, need I say more?

Why All Phytoestrogens Are Not Alike

Want to make your head spin? Think about the fact that, all told, there are over a thousand plants containing phytoestrogens. And even if you're a woman who simply can't buy enough shoes, in my opinion this is still way too many "phytos" for one shopping trip. So how do you narrow it down and know exactly which of these sources will help you most? The answer lies in how the whole concept of plant estrogens—and their link to menopause—came about.

Although researchers have long known about these compounds, their treatment potential kind of snuck onto our menopause radar screen quite by accident. It began when a group of epidemiologists (the medical number crunchers who look for health trends around the world) realized that Asian women living in their native countries experienced far fewer menopause symptoms than Western women living in the United States and Europe—in fact, about 90 percent fewer symptoms, by some estimates. (There isn't even a *word* in the Japanese language for "hot flash"!) At first doctors believed the differences were deeply rooted in genetics. Then a second curious observation was made: Asian women living in the Western world for one or two generations were experiencing the same kinds of menopause symptoms—and sometimes at similar rates—as their Western sisters. Genetics, it seems, was not the only key.

On to plan B: understanding what it was about the lifestyle of Asian women *in their native land* that seemed to shield them from so many otherwise common symptoms. Eventually, a very obvious answer began to emerge: their diet. More specifically, researchers began to recognize that Asian women living in their native lands were consuming a great deal of soy—far more than what Western women, or even Asian women living in a Western culture, were eating. While a typical Japanese diet included between 10 and 50 milligrams of soy a day, the American woman was lucky to consume between 1 and 3 milligrams daily. Why was soy so important? As we were soon to discover, soy plants contain three of the most potent phytoestrogens available—compounds known as genistein, daidzein, and glycitein. Collectively they fall under a category known as isoflavones—a "buzz" phrase you may be somewhat familiar with already. It wasn't long before these compounds, along with another other class of phytoestrogen known as lignans (found in flaxseeds and some legumes), were among the most studied natural, alternative treatments for midlife symptoms around. Ultimately, we came to recognize not only the importance of these compounds in reducing the symptoms of menopause, but also the important role they could play in protecting the many aspects of a woman's health—including our hearts and our bones.

PUTTING THE THEORY TO THE TEST ON SOY

Although the theories revolving around the importance of phytoestrogens, and particularly soy, seemed plausible, the time had clearly come to put the pedal to the metal and know once and for all if these plants could play a significant role in a woman's changing biology. A number of studies were launched to see if, indeed, soy could live up to its promise—at least in terms of menopause-related symptoms. The results turned out to be more encouraging than anyone anticipated.

In one sixteen-week study of seventy-five women published in the journal *Menopause* in 2000, nearly 61 percent found relief from up to seven hot flashes daily by including soy extract containing 70 milligrams of genistein and 70 milligrams of daidzein in their daily diet. This was compared to just 21 percent in the group that found relief on a placebo pill. In a second study, also published in *Menopause* later that same year, 177 women with five or more hot flashes a day took a slightly lower dose—an isoflavone extract containing just 50 milligrams of genistein and 50 milligrams of daidzein daily—and they too saw a significant improvement in about twelve weeks. For many, the relief kicked in after just two weeks of treatment. Most importantly, ultrasound exams of the uterus done before and after this study showed there was no increase in the endometrial lining—indicating that the soy did not have an estrogenic affect on uterine cells, the way traditional chemical estrogen therapy could.

These results backed up those from an earlier study, this one published in *Menopause* in 1999. Here researchers compared women who ate soy protein to those who ate a diet high in complex carbohydrates to see how symptoms fared. In this clinical trial fifty-one women with hot flashes ate 20 grams of soy protein daily (containing 34 milligrams of isoflavones) while the other group ate 20 milligrams of complex carbohydrates daily. Six weeks later the soy group reported a significant improvement in hot flashes, while the carbohydrate group saw little change. What's more, those who split their soy intake over two meals saw the greatest decrease in symptoms. This suggests that consistent levels of phytoestrogens may be better than one higher dose. Although only a limited number of studies have been conducted looking at the effects of isoflavones on vaginal dryness, those that have been done also show encouraging results.

As time went on, study after study began turning up similar results: Whether in supplement form or from a food source, soy had the power to reduce at least some menopause-related symptoms. At the same time, studies published in the *New England Journal of Medicine*—and elsewhere—began reporting that soy also appeared to lower cholesterol and, in some instances, even blood pressure. Other studies found it could decrease the risk of clot formation as well, thereby also reducing the risk of heart attack and stroke. In one 1998 Japanese study, tests on nearly five thousand women found that the more soy a woman consumed, the greater the overall health benefits.

A total of thirty-eight separate studies validated that as little as 47 milligrams of soy protein daily from soy-rich foods was all it took to achieve these important health advantages. But there was still more good news: In one small but significant study published in the *Journal of Clinical Nutrition* in 1998, sixty-six postmenopausal women consuming just 40 grams of soy protein daily (containing 2.25 milligrams of isoflavone per gram of protein) were able to *increase the bone density* of their lumbar spine by more than 2 percent in just six months. More recently, a review published in the journal *Menopause* in 1999 looked at all available soy studies and concluded that a diet rich in soy may actually counteract some of the detrimental effects of estrogen loss on bone.

SOY SORRY: THE DOWNSIDE YOU MUST KNOW

As impressive as the studies have been, not everyone is convinced that soy is the menopausal magic bullet—or even a particularly healthy alternative during this or any other time of life. Writing in the *Archives of Internal Medicine* in May 2001, Dr. Gina Glazier of the University of Pennsylvania School of Medicine says the effects of soy on menopause symptoms may be limited at best—sufficient only for those women with extremely mild symptoms.

"Although studies have statistically suggested [certain] results, the clinical significance remains unclear," she says. For example, Glazier points out that a 15 percent reduction in hot flashes would equate to only one less hot flash per day in women experiencing ten to twelve flashes daily. "This would be of limited practical benefit," she says.

Perhaps more importantly, there still remain many unanswered questions concerning the safety of soy supplements, particularly when used on a long-term basis. One concern is that high doses may in fact act as an endocrine disrupter, increasing concentrations of other hormones including thyroxin (a thyroid hormone), as well as insulin and glycogen.

According to Glazier, we don't even know the true potential for adverse effects, particularly when large doses of soy supplements are consumed over a long period of time. Also unknown: whether or not unopposed estrogen, even from a natural source, could have a cancer-causing effect in women who are susceptible.

Throwing more fuel on the skeptics' fire is the fact that studies conducted on all these issues thus far have produced conflicting and somewhat inconclusive results. While epidemiological data suggests soy may be protective against breast cancer, researchers who did the study say this may only be true in younger women, *and* if soy consumption begins at a very young age. And while Japanese women, in general, have lower rates of all estrogen-sensitive cancers, including breast and endometrial cancer, the key may lie more in the foods they eat than in dietary extracts in supplement form. The reason? In at least one laboratory study, breast cancer cells responded positively to phytoestrogens—growing more rapidly in much the same way they would when exposed to estradiol. Additional research showed that even limited exposure to low concentrations of some isoflavone supplements stimulated cell growth in both estrogen-positive and estrogen-negative tumors.

In addition, a study published in 1999—a headline heard round the world—concluded that even *eating* too much soy might have a potential downside, possibly increasing the risk of dementia. While this study involved nearly four thousand Japanese men who ate a diet high in tofu—and no women—still, the possibility that the findings may not be gender specific can't be denied. In fact, two experts at the National Center for Toxicological Research—Daniel Sheehan, Ph.D., and Daniel Doerge, Ph.D.—were so concerned about this finding, they wrote a letter to the FDA citing the potential for neurological effects when large amounts of soy were consumed by women as well by men.

MAKING THE SOY DECISION:

Currently, the debate over the safety and effectiveness of soy continues to rage. While many continue to uphold its natural health-giving properties, others point to studies that indicate the potential for problems. Currently the Food and Drug Administration has come out in *favor* of soy foods, allowing manufacturers to use the claim that soy *can* decrease cholesterol as well as reduce the risk of heart disease. As to the menopause-related effects, waters remain a bit murkier, with strong evidence on both sides of the issue. Most medical experts believe more research is needed before we can either offer a blanket recommendation or a clear-cut warning against the use of soy as a treatment for menopause-related symptoms. At the same time, most also agree that if you want to give soy a try, choosing soy foods over isoflavone supplements may be your best and perhaps safest alternative, particularly if you are at risk for breast cancer. As a mainstay of the Asian diet for centuries, the power—and safety—of soy foods in mitigating midlife symptoms can't be ignored. Whether or not consuming soy beginning in midlife will have the same effect as growing up eating a soy-based diet, as Asian women do, remains to be seen. But in the meantime, trying certainly seems worth the effort.

According to Dr. Daniel Carusi, a menopause expert at Brigham and Women's Hospital in Boston, until there are a series of head-to-head clinical trials comparing the benefits and risks of soy supplements to soy foods, "The best guarantee for total menopausal benefits may come with whole soy foods rather than isoflavone extracts."

But how much soy should you be eating to get the healthful effects? According to Mark Messina, a soy expert who serves as an adjunct associate professor of nutrition at Loma Linda University in California, a "safe" amount would contain no more than 100 milligrams of isoflavones per day (see the soy food chart later in this chapter).

"One hundred milligrams is like three servings of soy-rich food a day, and maybe 5 to 10 percent of the Japanese population consume that much," Messina recently told the *Washington Post*. Most, he says, have one serving of soy food daily.

While experts say there is no data showing more than 100 milligrams is harmful, some believe less is more when it comes to soy, recommending between 35 and 50 milligrams of isoflavones daily—an amount closer to what was used in many of the studies on menopausal health. If you are at high risk for breast cancer or have already been diagnosed with this disease, the recommendation is no more than about 30 milligrams of isoflavone two or three times a week. Further, if you are taking Tamoxifen or any of the bone-building SERMs like raloxifene (see Chapter 12), experts say consider limiting your soy intake even further. Since these drugs and isoflavones compete for the same estrogen receptors, if the soy gets there first, your medication may be rendered less effective. Also important: If you are using soy powders or supplements check the label for the percentage of isoflavones per serving. Some products contain a high level, others a much lower amount.

GETTING ALL THE GOODNESS FROM SOY

When choosing which soy foods to include in your diet, it's important to note that not all sources are equally rich in the much-sought-after isoflavone compounds. In addition, while the two primary isoflavones in soybeans are daidzein and genistein, the ratio of one to the other can vary greatly from food to food. Generally speaking, however, raw soybeans contain between 2 and 4 milligrams of isoflavones per gram. Soy-based food compounds such as tofu, soy milk, or miso contain about 30 to 40 milligrams of isoflavones. More potent sources include roasted soybeans with 61 grams containing 100 milligrams of isoflavones, while 75 grams of green soybeans will yield the same. So will 70 grams of texturized vegetable protein. If you're baking with soy flour, you'll get 50 milligrams of isoflavones with every half cup you use.

If you're looking for the highest concentration of isoflavones, be wary of foods made from soy protein *concentrates,* often found in frozen soy burgers and some soy snack bars. They may or may not contain significant amounts of isoflavones per ounce, depending on how the product was processed and packaged. To know what you're buying, be sure to check the label. You might also want to think twice about spending your money on what are referred to as "second generation" soy products—

those using soy as a minor ingredient, like soy dogs or soy desserts. The more ingredients other than soy the product contains, the less likely it is to contain significant amounts of isoflavones.

The soy chart that follows is designed to help make your food choices a little easier. It is based on data that was distributed at the American Dietetic Association's eightieth annual meeting, as part of a presentation by James W. Anderson, M.D., a professor of medicine and clinical nutrition at the University of Kentucky. According to the information presented, these values were gleaned from both published databases and individual analyses. Also important to note: Isoflavone content can vary widely depending on how the soy food in question is grown, where it is grown, and now it is manufactured.

FOOD	SVG SIZE g [a]	SVG SIZE	PROTEIN g/100 g	GENISTEIN ug/g prot [b]	TOTAL ISOFLAVONES ug/g prot	ISOFLAVONES mg/g prot [c]	ISOFLAVONES mg/svg
Mature soybeans, uncooked	93	½ cup	37.0	1,106	1,891	5.1	175.6
Roasted soybeans	86	½ cup	35.2	1,214	1,942	5.5	167.0
Soy flour	21	¼ cup	37.8	1,185	2,084	5.5	43.8
Textured soy protein, dry	30	¼ cup	18.0	472	928	5.2	27.8
Green soybeans, uncooked (edamame)	128	½ cup	16.6	301	548	3.3	70.1
Soy milk	228	1 cup	4.4	30	56	2.0	20.0
Tempeh, uncooked	114	4 oz	17.0	277	531	3.1	60.5
Tofu, uncooked	114	4 oz	15.8	209	336	2.1	38.3
Soy isolate, dry	28	1 oz	92.0	1,100	2,174	2.2	56.5
Soy concentrate, dry	28	1 oz	63.6	111	195	0.3	12.4

[a] grams.
[b] micrograms per gram of protein.
[c] milligrams per gram of protein.

Lignans: The "Other" Soy

Along with isoflavones, another potent source of phytoestrogen is "lignans." They are found in the outer portion of certain fibrous plants and contain compounds that also mimic the effects of estrogen. Although less studied than soy compounds, lignans have been shown to have similar estrogen-balancing effects, as well as antioxidant activity. Some studies have even shown certain anti-cancer benefits, particularly within the breast.

Like soy, phytoestrogens from lignans can be modified by intestinal bacteria, so if you are taking antibiotics you may not get the full effect. In addition, all lignans are rapidly excreted from the body in urine, so you will need to consume them pretty much every day in order to maintain enough of the therapeutic value for continued control of your symptoms.

Among the most potent source of lignans is flaxseed. While ground flaxseed meal appears to be the most beneficial form, flaxseed oil can be helpful as well, and both can go a long way in managing menopause symptoms, particularly night sweats and vaginal dryness. Not only does flax have estrogenic activity, studies show it is also an excellent source of essential fatty acids, necessary for metabolizing hormones. In addition, flax products have also demonstrated powerful anti-cancer effects, with just two tablespoons daily helping to reduce tumor growth in both colon and breast cancer. If you prefer to take flaxseed capsules, experts say three capsules equal the protection of one spoonful of oil.

If flax is not your thing, you can garner at least some of the protection of lignans with several other plant-based foods, including pumpkin seeds, cranberries, sunflower seeds, sesame seeds, mung bean sprouts, broccoli, carrots, grain fibers, garlic, buckwheat, and many seeds and berries.

Herbal Treatments

While soy may be among the most popular midlife remedies, it does not sit alone in Mother Nature's medicine chest. As you just read, not only are there other sources of isoflavones, and ultimately phytoestrogens, there are also some other plants and natural sources that can play a role

From the "M" File

FINDING RELIEF IN A FOUR-LEAF CLOVER

Q: I have a great deal of trouble tolerating soy, which gives me a lot of gas and causes extreme bloating, cramps, and diarrhea. A friend told me about a natural estrogen made from red clover. Does this work the same as soy—and are the benefits as great? I am forty-eight years old and flashing like crazy!

A: The product you are referring to is likely Promensil—a phytoestrogen derived from the red clover plant. Like soy, red clover is a legume and contains a number of weak plant estrogens including formononetin, bochanin A, daidzein, genistein, and coumestrol. It is, in fact, considered to be the richest source of multi-isoflavones. Although it has been less studied than soy, research on one thousand women in clinical trials worldwide has offered encouraging results. In at least four of those studies, conducted at Tufts University School of Medicine, NYU School of Medicine and Oxford University in England, Promensil was shown to have a significant impact on hot flashes and night sweats. It has also been shown not to increase breast density or increase the uterine lining, even with doses as high as 40 milligrams a day for three months. The women studied also experienced no breakthrough bleeding, clots, or weight gain. Even more encouraging was a report from the University of Cambridge in England showing Promensil could decrease the risk of bone loss by up to 50 percent in both pre- and postmenopausal women.

In terms of cardiovascular effect, red clover scored high marks again. In studies conducted at the Baker Medical Institute in Australia women treated with Promensil showed an increase in the elasticity of arteries—a good indication of heart health. According to the

in mediating menopause-related symptoms. Just as often, however, myths and half-truths abound, with many natural compounds garnering unsubstantiated and undeserved credit for working—when in fact, they don't.

manufacturer, Promensil works so well because it duplicates the natural chemicals found in the plant content of the traditional Asian diet, which normally includes soy milk, green split peas, chickpeas, and broad beans.

On the downside, a study published in October 2003 in the *Journal of the American Medical Association* compared the effects of isoflavones from red clover and a placebo on menopause-related symptoms and found both fared about the same—with a reduction in problems like hot flashes between 35 and 41 percent in both groups. That said, they also found no risk of short-term complications, so it certainly appears safe to give this compound a try, at least for a little while.

As to long-term use, no data is available on either safety or efficacy, nor is there any data on the effects of high-dose therapy, even for a short period of time. In addition, critics of red clover say that unlike soy, which has passed the test of time, this particular extract has no real history of use, particularly for menopause-related symptoms.

As to your gastrointestinal sensitivity to soy, it's fairly common, particularly in those not used to a high-soy diet. While there are no studies comparing the effects of soy to red clover head to head, it's unlikely that you will experience the same kind of bloating and gas with Promensil as you found eating soy-rich foods. However, you may also find soy supplements are easier on your system than soy foods, so you might want to try this alternative as well. If you're willing to invest a little time, and build your soy intake slowly, you may be able to "desensitize" your tummy to the effects and eventually tolerate larger amounts of soy foods without problem. The key is to start slow and build slow; when you reach your tolerance level, you'll know it.

To find additional information on Promensil, visit
www.yourmenopause.com.

To help you decide what natural treatments to try—and which ones to avoid—what follows is a rundown of the latest information, including medical studies, on some of the more popular of these remedies.

BLACK COHOSH:
THE ORIGINAL NATURAL ESTROGEN

When my neighbor Sheri first heard about the herb black cohosh, she was totally infatuated with its health claims. Reducing hot flashes, controlling mood swings, relieving night sweats—depending on the company doing the advertising, black cohosh seemed to be able to accomplish everything short of folding the wash. And, in fact, even with advertising exaggerations aside, this herb *does* appear to have some important health benefits for women.

But Sheri's fascination with this herb increased even more when she told her mother about what she was taking. Like many of us baby boomers who grew up believing we had discovered most everything for the first time, Sheri was certain that this entire herbal approach to medicine was a decidedly "Woodstock" kind of experience—unique to our generation. Her mother, however, set the record straight.

"Not only did she know about black cohosh, she claims that my grandmother actually used this herb for menopause-related symptoms," Sheri said, with some disbelief.

Well, as Sheri found out, this treatment is not "new" at all. Black cohosh is one of the oldest herbs in use—in the United States alone it has a history that dates back more than one hundred years. Meanwhile, American Indians have used the boiled root of black cohosh to treat menstrual and labor pain for even longer than that. And it wasn't always considered a "natural" treatment either. Between the years 1820 and 1926, the U.S. Pharmacopeia (the government agency that keeps track of all medications) listed black cohosh as an "official" drug.

In more recent times, this popular herb has become a mainstay of menopause-related treatment in many European countries, having been used for more than forty years on some 1.5 million women for this exact purpose. Germany's "Commission E" (their version of our FDA) heartily endorses black cohosh as a treatment for hot flashes and has approved its use at doses ranging from 40 to 200 milligrams daily.

The key compounds in this herb are known as triterpenes—chemical constituents that seem able to impact hormone activity. In fact, Commission E experts classify black cohosh as having estrogenlike activity, capable of binding to estrogen receptors. Other studies have shown it may act like an estrogen in *some* women—those whose natural levels are low—while acting as an anti-estrogen in others when their own natural levels of this hormone are too high. In this same respect, there is some evidence that black cohosh may also be physiologically selective—stimulating the vaginal lining, for example, and helping to prevent atrophy, while having no stimulating effect on uterine lining, thus preventing the potentially dangerous buildup of cells.

As with most things in life and medicine, not all experts agree. In tests conducted at three independent laboratories, black cohosh was shown not to have any estrogenic properties at all—and the suggestion was that it not even be classified as a phytoestrogen. But that isn't necessarily bad news. The herb still managed to offer some control over hot flashes. "We have no idea how it might work to relieve hot flashes," says Columbia's Dr. Fredi Kronenburg, who adds that we also have no proof of positive effects on either heart or bone health.

Other experts, however, say they know how black cohosh works. Since the symptom for which this herb is most effective is hot flashes, there is some evidence to show the link may be through the hypothalamus— that tiny area of the brain responsible for body temperature control.

"[It] works on the hypothalamus and thermo-regulating center of the brain to stimulate estrogen effects, without side effects," says Atlanta, Georgia, preventive-medicine expert Dr. Jan MacBarron.

But just the fact that black cohosh may stop hot flashes without estrogenic activity is good news for women at risk for breast or endometrial cancer. And thus far, laboratory studies *have* shown that when used for six months or less, black cohosh has no stimulating effects on breast cancer cells—a fact that has led many experts to concur that this herb is safe, even for women with a history of estrogen-sensitive diseases. This would include not only breast cancer, but also fibroid tumors, polyps, endometriosis, dysfunctional uterine bleeding, even liver and gallbladder disease, all of which have been shown to be affected by estrogen.

WILL BLACK COHOSH WORK FOR YOU?

Certainly, the studies on black cohosh—eleven published clinical trials since 1982—have offered important evidence that this herb can have at least some impact on anxiety, hot flashes, sweating, insomnia, and even vaginal atrophy. By some estimates it appears to be about 35 percent more effective than a placebo—which means that while it won't help all women, it can help some a great deal. The key to successful treatment, however, appears to lie in the product itself since the effectiveness of black cohosh is based on the total amount of triterpenoid glycosides it contains. Most of the clinical studies on black cohosh have used a specific proprietary formula sold under the brand name Remifemin, and this is also the brand that most doctors recommend. Used in Europe for over forty years, and now available in the United States, it is sold at many drug and health food stores, as well as online (see the resource section at the back of this book). Remifemin is standardized to contain 20 milligrams of root extract with 1 milligram of the triterpene glycoside 27-deoxyactein (or 26-deoxyactein) per tablet. So, if you can't find this brand, try to find a formula that duplicates these standards.

The average dose of black cohosh most effective for menopause-related symptoms ranges between 40 and 80 milligrams daily, and you may have to experiment a bit to find the dose that's right for you. While some women report relief in as little as two weeks, more often it can take anywhere from four to twelve weeks to see a real difference in how you feel. In addition, this is not a treatment you can use indefinitely. Throughout all of the studies, six months has been the longest period of time black cohosh was consistently taken. So, doctors who do recommend this herb say you should not take it longer than that length of time. Many say that if you stop for a few months, you can restart treatment for another six months. Since there is no research on the potential for estrogenic effects when used beyond six months, if you have a history of breast cancer, or any estrogen-sensitive condition, experts say check with your doctor before starting a second round of treatment.

Although side effects from black cohosh are uncommon, it has been known to cause stomach pains, intestinal discomfort, dizziness, nausea, headache, stiffness, and trembling limbs. Obviously if any of these symptoms appear, discontinue use. You should also not use black cohosh if you are taking any "designer estrogens"—drugs that need to attach to estrogen receptors in order to work. This includes tamoxifen, used in breast cancer patients, and medications like raloxifene, which is used to help protect bone health. In these instances, much like isoflavones, the black cohosh may also compete with the drug for the estrogen receptor—and if the herb gets there first, the drug may be rendered useless.

DONG QUAI: THE CONTROVERSIAL HERB IN THE MENOPAUSE GARDEN

Steeped in centuries of Chinese culture, the herb *dong quai* has been used by traditional Chinese medicine (TCM) doctors for some two thousand years in the treatment of menopause-related symptoms. And in studies conducted as early as 1963, and again in 1984, the key ingredient in this herb—a compound known as ferulic acid—was indeed shown to decrease hot flashes. More recently, however, experts have begun to debate the effectiveness of this ancient remedy. In a study published in 1997 in the journal *Fertility and Sterility,* doctors found that taking the recommended 4.5 milligrams of *dong quai* daily had no greater effect on hot flashes or vaginal atrophy than a placebo. What's more, a database search conducted by Columbia's Dr. Kronenburg found no recent clinical evidence proving the effectiveness of *dong quai* on any menopause-related problems.

So . . . could thousands of years of Chinese tradition actually be wrong? Practitioners of Chinese medicine don't believe that it is. They say *dong quai is* effective, but that it should not be used alone—or in such a low dose. Typically, they say, in Chinese medicine a much higher dosage (between 9 and 12 milligrams) is combined with at least four other herbs for an unexplained synergistic effect that allows the helpful properties of *dong quai* to come forward.

This all suggests that if you do want to give a nod to Chinese tradition and give this herb a try, purchase a formulation compounded by a Chinese medicine expert. Or, at the very least, look for a product that combines *dong quai* with other herbal ingredients. If it works, you should see results in several weeks. However, do be aware that *dong quai* increases photosensitivity, so you may experience a rash if you go out in bright sunlight. This herb should also be avoided if you are taking the blood-thinning medication Warfarin.

MORE HELP FROM MOTHER NATURE

While some plants from Mother Nature's garden are clearly geared toward the overall treatment of menopause-related symptoms, a number of other botanicals can help as well—either by treating a single symptom, such as hot flashes, or sometimes simply by improving the overall quality of your life.

Certainly, many herbal treatments contain a combination of natural ingredients designed to work synergistically to improve the way you feel. In some instances, however, you may only be suffering one or two symptoms, so it may be more beneficial for you to take only one or two of the herbs found in these products. To help get you started, here's what most doctors recommend—and what at least a few medical studies have found to be helpful during this time of life.

- **Chasteberry (Vitex):** This herb is believed to possess some hormone-regulating properties with direct action on the hypothalamus and pituitary glands. Through these centers in the brain it is believed to have some effect on progesterone production. In two German surveys of some 1,500 women, forty drops of Vitex daily for 166 days relieved symptoms of progesterone deficiency including fluid retention, bloating, breast tenderness, headache, and fatigue—with relief seen in about twenty-five days. Although some experts claim it can also help decrease hot flashes, depression, and vaginal dryness, there are no medical studies to back up these claims. The most popular form of this herb is an alcohol-based formula standardized to 100 milligrams per 9 grams of fruit extract. It is also sold in a solid form, without alcohol content. Currently the German Commission E recommends Vitex for menstrual disorders and painful breasts. The recommended dosage is 20 milligrams daily.

- **Ginseng:** Although this herb won't help you with hot flashes, it might make you feel better while you're having them! In one recent study conducted by a group of Norwegian researchers nearly four hundred menopausal women took either ginseng or a placebo for a total of sixteen weeks. At the beginning and end of the study researchers measured the women's levels of FSH (follicle-stimulating hormone) and estradiol, as well as the thickness of their endometrial lining. At the end of the study none of the women experienced any decrease in hot flashes—however, they did report less depression and an improved sense of well-being. There was also no measurable change in hormone levels or in uterine lining. Follow the directions on your product for the correct dosage.

- **St. John's Wort:** According to a number of European studies, the value of this herb is in the treatment of mild to moderate depression. While it has no effect on reproductive hormones, nor does it impact any specific menopause-related symptoms, if anxiety or depression are part of your midlife picture then this herb might help. Again, follow the product's recommended dosage.

- **Kava Kava:** If you are taking hormone replacement therapy (HRT) but find you are still experiencing significant anxiety, this herb may help. In a study published in the journal *Alternative Medicine Review* in 2001, women taking HRT who added kava kava to their regimen experienced far less anxiety than women who took HRT alone. Its mode of action is primarily as a sleep aid, and at least some experts suggest the reduction in anxiety could have been due to more restful sleep. If sleeping is a problem—whether you take HRT or not—kava kava might be worth a try.

PLANTS THAT DON'T DELIVER ON THEIR MENOPAUSE PROMISE

Among all the natural treatments for hormone-related symptoms, perhaps none has received more attention—at least in the popular press—than wild yams. A cousin to the sweet potato, this plant—and consequently treatments made from it—has long enjoyed a history as a natural source of progesterone. But experts say this is completely false. While wild yam does contain an important compound known as diosgenin, which is a precursor to progesterone, the body can't utilize it in the form found in wild yams. According to natural medicine expert Hazel A. Philp, N.D., a senior editor at the journal *Alternative Medicine Review*, "This synthesis does not occur in the human body." And while she and others say that wild yams may have some mild hormonal effects, there appears to be no proof that this plant can increase levels of progesterone.

What's more, a recent study published in the journal *Climacteric* in 2001 found that women who took wild yam supplements had no greater reduction in menopause-related symptoms than those who took a placebo. In addition, testing for progesterone in both blood and saliva found that wild yam did not alter levels at all. For more information on natural sources of progesterone that do work, see Chapter 11.

The second plant source that may not live up to its reputation is evening primrose oil. Proven to possess powerful anti-inflammatory properties—due mostly to its high content of alpha-linolenic acid (omega-3) and gamma-linolenic acid (omega-6)—it has been shown to be helpful in many conditions, including autoimmune diseases. As for its effectiveness as a treatment for menopause-related symptoms, however, don't raise your expectations too high. In one six-month study published in the *British Medical Journal* in 1994, evening oil of primrose failed to have any effect on hot flashes. However, some women reported a mild effect on night sweats. Although some natural medicine experts continue to endorse its use in the treatment of menopause-related symptoms including hot flashes, there are far more effective natural treatments you can try.

The MidLife Nutrients: What You Need

With all the attention placed on phytoestrogens and exotic plants and herbs, it's sometimes easy to forget that simple vitamins and nutrients found in everyday foods can also have a powerful effect on menopause-related symptoms. This is also true of vitamin and mineral supplements, many of which have a long history of helping to quiet symptoms and stabilize hormone activity. The B vitamins, for example, particularly vitamin B_6 and folic acid, have long been known to help in the treatment of PMS. Some experts believe they also have the ability to influence hormone production at midlife as well. At the very least they can increase your sense of well-being and help reduce fatigue—which can go a long way in helping you cope during this transitional time. In fact, there are a good deal of anecdotal reports showing that those of us who achieve a nutritional balance, via a healthy diet and supplement use, may be better able to weather all the challenges midlife throws our way. In this respect, it's important that you not only do all you can to eat a healthy diet (see Chapter 7) but also take a quality multivitamin, in a well-balanced formulation, every day.

That said, you might also want to pay a bit more attention to the following nutrients—vitamins and minerals that some studies have shown may play a small but significant role in tempering at least a few menopause-related problems.

- *Vitamin E:* While this powerful vitamin has had its ups and downs in terms of popular opinion about its health-giving powers, when it comes to menopause-related symptoms it's clearly on the upswing. While there are no modern medical studies to show it can help, there is loads of anecdotal evidence and some research conducted as early as the 1940s to show it can reduce hot flashes, control mood swings, and decrease vaginal dryness, in doses as low as 50 to 100 IUs (international units) daily. Even better news: Because vitamin E does not appear to interfere with the anti–breast cancer drug Tamoxifen, it has been successfully utilized by women using this drug to reduce hot flashes, at doses as high as 400 units daily. Currently dosage recommendations range from 50 to 400 IUs daily, although some natural health experts have advocated doses as high as 1,200 IUs.

- *Vitamin C:* This nutrient, in combination with compounds known as bioflavonoids, has been shown in at least one study to reduce the incidence of hot flashes. The key appears to be a specific bioflavonoid known as hesperidin, which is found naturally in vitamin C made from rose hips. In research published as early as the 1960s doctors found that 900 milligrams of hesperidin plus 1,200 milligrams of vitamin C daily stopped hot flashes completely for more than half the women studied, in about thirty days. More than a third reported much less severe flashes. Since there is virtually no updated research on these nutrients, and their effect seems mild at best, they are only recommended as an adjunct to other natural treatments, such as black cohosh or soy.

From the "M" File

STICKING IT TO MENOPAUSE SYMPTOMS

Q: A friend of mine used acupuncture to help her get pregnant—and it worked, even when fertility drugs didn't. I'm wondering if it could have the same kind of effects on menopause-related symptoms—particularly since they are also hormone related. I'd sure like to do something about these hot flashes and mood swings without having to take a pill. Is acupuncture worth a try?

A: As you probably already know, acupuncture is an ancient Chinese medical treatment that relies on the painless but strategic placement of tiny needles into a gridlike pattern spanning your body from head to toe. The needles are used to stimulate certain key "energy points" linked to symptoms. According to the traditional Chinese explanation, acupuncture stimulates and moves qi (pronounced "chee"), a form of life energy that ancient wisdom says must flow through the body unhampered from head to toe, 24/7, in order for us to feel healthy and well. When it doesn't, acupuncture can give our qi a gentle nudge.

"Acupuncture works to restore the flow of qi—your essence, your body energy. It has a calming, restorative effect that increases a sense of well-being," says acupuncturist Ifeoma Okoronkwo, M.D., a professor of medicine at NYU School of Medicine.

You are right to assume that it may help with menopause-related symptoms. According to the British Acupuncture Council, in one series

• *Vitamin D:* This nutrient is essential to drive calcium into bones, and taking a supplement is particularly important if you are at any risk for osteoporosis, or if you get minimal exposure to sunlight (which helps your body make vitamin D). This nutrient also helps produce a protein called osteocalcin, necessary for bones to maintain their strength. Studies also show that women who get adequate levels of vitamin D are far less likely to suffer a hip fracture than women who don't. Although the recommended daily allowance for vitamin D is

of studies conducted between 1980 and 1986 on a hundred women, acupuncture was administered twice weekly for three weeks, then once a month for a year. The result: Twenty of the women had complete remission of their hot flashes; sixty-five saw a significant improvement; and eighty-five reported an improved sense of well-being and better health. In a 1985 study doctors used acupuncture to treat twenty-five women with menopause-related anxiety and depression. The result here: Ten of the women had a complete remission of symptoms and were able to stop traditional medication; the remaining fifteen women reported a significant improvement, with a reduction in the need for medication.

An even more promising study published in 1989 found acupuncture comparable to HRT in overcoming common symptoms of menopause including hot flashes, night sweats, and mood swings. The treatments also yielded a measurable increase in estradiol and other hormones. However, monthly treatments were needed to maintain the results. More recently, studies published in 1994 by a group of Swedish researchers reported that acupuncture using low-frequency electrical stimulation twice weekly for two weeks significantly reduced hot flashes. Once weekly for an additional six weeks helped maintain the effects, which lasted up to three months after treatment was completed.

The bottom line: While the studies on acupuncture for menopause symptoms are very scarce, the evidence presented thus far lends enough credibility to the treatment to encourage giving it a try.

200 IUs, 400 IUs is frequently recommended during menopause. Still, if you get no sun exposure, many experts contend you need far more—by some accounts, up to 1,000 IUs daily may be necessary. In any event you should not exceed 2,000 units a day, which is considered toxic. By the way, even if you are outdoors a lot if you are wearing sunscreen, as you should be, your body won't be able to make the necessary amount of vitamin D. However, do be aware that because it is a fat-soluble nutrient, which means it remains in your

body, it's easy to overdose—so be sure to get your doctor's okay if you ingest levels over 400 IUs daily. And don't stop wearing sunscreen!

Follow Your Yellow Brick Road

Although the road to Menopause Oz may not be paved exclusively with flowers and herbs, they clearly grow along the way. And for some women these natural treatments may be all that's necessary to get through the hot days and sweaty nights, the bursts of anger and the flood of tears, or even the menstrual irregularities that come during this transition time. For others, however, Mother Nature may do nothing more than offer mild relief—and some of you may have difficulty finding any relief at all.

If you fall into the last two categories, don't despair. First, remember that the recommended dosages are not necessarily the right dosage for every woman. So, what works for your best friend may be too much or too little for you. Ultimately that means you have to experiment for a while until you find the right dosage. Even more important: While some of you may need only one or two of these natural treatments to find relief, others may need to add three, four, or more in combination to bring about a measurable improvement. So, also take some time to experiment with different combinations of products before you throw up your hands in despair.

The most important thing to realize is that as we pull slowly away from the use of synthetic hormone treatments, more time and energy is being devoted to studying the natural alternatives. This means that every day we are learning more about how natural treatments can help. With this in mind, I ask that you pay close attention to what you hear on the news in this regard and use whatever you learn in conjunction with what you have read here today. Indeed, in the not-too-distant future, I have a feeling that a great many of us are going to rely more on Mother Nature and less on "father pharmaceutical" to get us through this important and very "natural" time in our lives.

For the latest updates on natural therapies for menopause, visit www.yourmenopause.com.

11

HRT, Natural Hormones, and Beyond

How Your Doctor Can Help You Now

For a long time, doctors believed that HRT was the be-all and end-all way to stop menopause-related symptoms in their tracks. And then the Women's Health Initiative was born. Originally intended as a fifteen-year study of, among other things, the effects of hormone replacement therapy on women, the clinical trial was called to a premature halt when researchers began to uncover some serious problems—namely, that not only did hormone replacement therapy fail to help many women, it actually had the potential to harm us, including increasing the risk of heart attack, cancer, and stroke (see "Once Upon a Time . . ."). Or, to hear my friend Tina tell it, "We finally realized that fake progesterone and estrogen made from horse urine were not exactly what Ponce de Leon found spewing out of the Fountain of Youth." (There's nothing quite so frightening as a woman low on estrogen with a perfectly good reason to be mad as hell!)

Although the initial information released by the WHI was a "shock heard round the world," in the years since then, we have begun to temper the noise. In fact, there are now more than a few whispers of hope being uttered in the corridors of our middle years—among them, that HRT may, in fact, have some redeeming value, particularly for some women. More specifically, we now know that those of us who are prone to bone breaks are up to 24 percent less likely to have a fracture while taking hormones. This includes a 34 percent reduced risk of hip fracture—a major problem for those already diagnosed with the bone-destroying disease known as osteoporosis. In addition, hormone users can also expect a 37 percent reduction in colon cancer—a disease that is fast becoming a major health threat to women. A study of some two thousand women also taught us that up to 77 percent of those who suffer from hot flashes are likely to find relief using hormones—and believe me, if you've ever had a hot flash totally debilitate you at an important moment in your life or your career, this is certainly a statistic worth paying attention to. And in spite of the National Institutes of Health halting the estrogen-only leg of the trial in 2004 (involving women who have no uterus and could safely take estrogen without progestin), the results *still* showed a decrease in the risk of bone fracture in this group. Based on the information we have thus far, estrogen alone also does not appear to increase the risk of breast cancer—although this could change as more information from the study continues to be analyzed.

Perhaps the brightest ray of hope came not from those who participated in the WHI research, but those outside the study—doctors who began pointing out that the women who participated in the project were sixty-three years old, on average, when they began taking hormones. Why is this important? Many believe results would have been far more in favor of hormone use if the study participants had been around forty-five when they started HRT—which is the average age of most women when they begin this therapy. Indeed, because the women were older when hormone use started, it allowed for twenty years or more between the time their natural hormone production dropped off and any possible protection from HRT to kick in—clearly a window of opportunity for heart disease to take hold.

Taking the debate still further, some experts began questioning the specific hormonal formulation used in this study, wondering if it, too, may have played a significant role in the disappointing results. Speculation began as to whether or not lower doses, different combinations, or even different formulations of these same hormones might not offer a better and more helpful picture (see "Natural" Progesterone: How It Can Help and Estrogen-Only Therapy, later in this chapter).

In the summer of 2003, a researcher from the University of Pittsburgh shed an even more interesting light on why the WHI trials may have had such a dismal conclusion. According to Dr. Judith Gavaler, the threshold for hormone levels might, in fact, be so individual for every woman that in many instances study participants may have been either overtreated (leading to an increased risk of breast and ovarian cancer) or undertreated (leading to an increased risk of cardiovascular disease and stroke). In her own study, which she published in the *Journal of Women's Health*, Gavaler showed that at least 11 percent of the women on hormone therapy had blood test results indicating an estrogen overload. Statistically speaking, she says, this is more than enough of a deviation to account for the varying statistical differences seen in the WHI study, explaining why, for example, only some women experienced an increase in certain diseases—but not all.

Now if you're anything like me, you're asking, "Does this mean that hormones are not as bad as we thought? Or are they worse? Or does anybody really know—or care?" And more importantly, if this were happening with, oh, say, Viagra, wouldn't there already be a government task force working 24/7 to get us an answer?

All questions worth asking. It is, in fact, a rather shameful discovery that hormone therapy ever got to be as popular as it did without any real, solid understanding of how it worked, or even whether or not it did. Be that as it may, I like to take the positive route here. I'm thankful, first, that *somebody* finally did think enough of our gender to do the research and, second, that a number of researchers are continuing to work hard at unwinding this whole sticky ball of wax to find out what prize, if any, lies deep within the center of the controversy. And, too, we have to thank the thousands of women who helped us all by putting their health—and in some instances their lives—on the line to help us learn more, not only about hormones but about ourselves and our biology. Indeed, in mid-2004 the National Institutes of Health announced that an extension of

AT A GLANCE:
THE NEW HORMONE FINDINGS

According to the results of the WHI as well as numerous other independent studies, daily dosing with standard HRT formulations consisting of medroxyprogesterone (a synthetic progesterone known as progestin) and conjugated equine estrogen (known as Prempro) yielded the following result:

- A 26 percent increase in the risk of invasive breast cancer

- A 20 percent increase in the risk of heart attacks

- A 41 percent higher rate of stroke

- A 100 percent increase in blood clots in the lung

- A 50 percent-plus increase in incontinence

- A 25 percent increased risk of dying from breast cancer

- No protection from heart disease; no protection from Alzheimer's disease

- Possible protection from colon cancer, hip fractures, hot flashes, night sweats, insomnia, mood swings

the WHI will be ongoing through 2010, with a great many of the women in the original research group having consented to continue answering questions and providing data on their health for future analysis. No doubt, these efforts will continue to help us learn even more about a woman's body—and this important time of life—and we should all be extremely grateful to every woman who participated and continues to be a part of the research.

However, if you're anything like me—and a whole lot of my girl-friends—you're still left asking a very important question: "What do I do right now?"

For many of you the answer will clearly be to avoid HRT—at least in the form it is being offered in today. But remember how I told you early on that there are "no rules" when it comes to finding what works for your personal midlife care? This is a case in point. Because as a medical journalist who has followed and reported on this subject—*and* covered the controversy right from the very start—I can tell you with all certainty that most experts believe the book is not yet closed on HRT, even with what we know today. In fact, there are many who believe that, at least for some women, short-term hormone therapy may still be the right choice. The key, of course, is in knowing if you are one of these women—and that's what I'm going to try and help you figure out right now.

Making the Hormone Decision: How to Assess Your Personal Risks

Before you can begin to understand what, if any, risks HRT holds for you, it's important to determine if you even need hormone therapy at all. Since we now know that HRT is not going to offer much in the way of health protection for your future—at least not over and above what other, safer drugs can provide—there are few, if any reasons to take it as a source of preventive care. In fact, as of right this moment, the only real reason to consider taking HRT has to do with managing immediate menopause-related symptoms, such as hot flashes, night sweats, or vaginal complaints. The issue here is that, ideally, HRT should not be prescribed until you are officially in menopause—that is, you have not had a menstrual cycle for twelve months or more. And by this time, many of these symptoms will already have begun to wane on their own. Further, if you are still having menstrual periods, other hormone therapies may be a better, and a safer, choice (see "Birth Control Pills" and "Bioidentical Hormones," later in this chapter).

Still, if you *are* in menopause, and still experiencing symptoms—and getting no relief from other forms of treatment—then the next step would be to understand a little more about whether or not HRT can help you, and what the risks mean to you, on a very personal level. Certainly, your personal health profile as well as whatever risks are lurking in your family tree will play a role in this decision. But to help you interpret *that* data in a way that is personally meaningful to you, it's also important that you learn a little something about how the new risks associated with HRT were calculated—and how these calculations apply to your life. It all begins with understanding what doctors define as "absolute" risk, as compared to "relative" or "individual" risk.

The first term, "absolute risk," is the one that provides us with all the scary headlines—like a 50 percent increased risk or "double the risk" of illness or even death. On first glance, absolute risks always sound pretty ominous. After all, who wants to die twice as early, or suffer twice as much? And this is where the importance of "relative risk" comes into play. Because it is this statistic that calculates the likelihood of something *actually occurring in your life*. And here's an easy way to understand the important difference between the two. Let's say that a thousand people eat a red lollipop and two get sick; then a thousand people eat a green lollipop, but only one gets sick. So, the "absolute" risk of getting sick from eating a red lollipop is twice as great as if you ate a green lollipop. At the same time, however, the "relative" or "individual" risk of you getting sick when you eat a red lollipop is really only two in one thousand, as compared to one in one thousand when you eat a green one. Undoubtedly a far less scary way of looking at what is basically the same finding.

Apply this thinking to the results of the WHI hormone study, and suddenly the whole risk picture takes on a new and far less ominous look. For example, the WHI found that for every ten thousand women using HRT:

- 38 developed breast cancer, as compared to 30 who were not using hormones

- 37 had heart attacks, compared to 30 who were not using hormones

- 29 had strokes, compared to 21 who were not using hormones

- 16 developed blood clots, compared to 8 who were not using hormones

Also remember that for every ten thousand women using hormone therapy there were five fewer hip fractures, and six fewer cases of colon cancer than in those who did not use it. In terms of consequences, the actual difference between the number of HRT users who experienced these health risks was not much greater than those not using hormone therapy. So why then did the government stop the trial—and issue such stern new warnings concerning these treatments? Certainly, even one unnecessary death is one death too many. Moreover, when you multiply even these relatively small numbers by the number of women using hormones, the total number of women who *are* affected can be quite large.

At the same time, for those who may ultimately benefit from hormone therapy, and for whom no other medication or lifestyle change can do the trick, it becomes imperative to view these findings in the proper perspective—in terms of "individual," or *personal,* risk profiles. The question you need to ask yourself: "What are *my* chances for becoming one of the eight additional women who get breast cancer or one of the seven who have a heart attack?" And depending on your personal health profile—*and* whatever is lurking in your family tree—many of you may discover you are, in fact, at very *low risk* for many of the problems associated with HRT.

Please understand, I am not trying to convince you that using hormones is safe, or even okay. My personal belief is that if you can get through this time of your life without them, and there are other ways to protect your present and future health (including the natural therapies you learned about in the previous chapter and the medical treatments that are explored in the next chapter), then by all means, skip HRT. However, if you are tortured by midlife symptoms and unable to function in your personal or work life, then you should not be intimidated by media headlines that urge you to overlook a treatment option that might be right for you. Your life and particularly your good health are all about choices—and choices can and must be made on an individual basis, *one woman at a time.*

So if, for example, you have no family history of breast cancer or heart disease but a high incidence of colon cancer or osteoporosis—and you are also experiencing troubling midlife symptoms—then HRT might be worth considering, at least short term. If, however, you have even a slight increased risk of breast cancer, but also a risk for osteoporosis, then the decision becomes a bit more complex. The point here is that you have to weigh as many factors as you can to come up with the equation that is right for you.

While it is my hope that you will be discussing all of your options with your personal physician before *any* decisions are made, you may also be curious about how the experts weigh in on this subject and where they stand in regard to the hormone decision. According to statements issued by the American College of Obstetricians and Gynecologists (ACOG), "It [hormone therapy] may still play a role in the management of menopause, provided it's used at the right time and for the right reasons." Factors to consider when deciding, they say, include whether or not other medications might give you similar results without the risks.

If you are somewhat older when you are asked to make your hormone decision, ACOG also points out that the natural risk of certain diseases—such as breast cancer—increases with age.

Also worth considering, say ACOG, is the length of time you are thinking of using HRT. Some of the risks are low, they say, during the first three to five years, and rise considerably after four years or more of continuous use. Effects on the heart and blood vessels begin within the first year. Also important is the type and dosage of the treatment you are considering, with the current recommendation being to use the lowest dose of hormones for the shortest amount of time.

In addition to the recommendations of ACOG, in 2004 the North American Menopause Society (NAMS) also weighed in with an opinion. According to this group (which consists primarily of gynecologists dedicated to the study and treatment of perimenopause and menopause), while hormone therapy should always be used for the shortest amount of time possible, there should be no limits placed on the duration, provided that use is consistent with treatment goals and a patient's health is monitored regularly. NAMS and ACOG experts also recommend local estrogen therapy—in the form of cream, gels, or vaginal rings—for the treatment of vulvar and vaginal atrophy (more on this in Chapter 8).

Like ACOG, NAMS also believes no form of hormone replacement therapy should be used as either a primary or even a second line of defense against heart disease.

Ultimately, the decision as to whether or not to try HRT is up to you. At the same time, I urge you not to make this decision on your own, but instead, only after serious discussion with your doctor. First, he or she will no doubt have some very detailed knowledge of your personal health— perhaps with more information than you yourself might realize. But more important, your doctor will also be aware of what, if any, other treatments may be available to help you through this time of your life—including both natural therapies and traditional medicines. The bottom line: If you work with your doctor and trust in his or her recommendations, you should be able to make a decision that serves you now, and well into your future.

Birth Control Pills: The "Other" Hormone Therapy

While HRT may not be the panacea we had all hoped, it's important to realize that not all forms of hormone therapy are equal—or equally bad. One option that is becoming increasing popular for the management of midlife symptoms is low-dose birth control pills. How are they different from HRT? Traditional hormone replacement therapy works by adding estrogen and progesterone on top of any hormones your body is still producing naturally. Birth control pills work by first shutting down all natural hormone production and then putting back small and, more important, delicately balanced levels of estrogen and progesterone. According to NYU's Dr. Steve Goldstein, it's a subtle but important difference that can be seen and felt almost immediately, as well as in the long run: "If a woman is still making some estrogen, adding more, which is what HRT does, can cause an even bigger imbalance and possibly worsen symptoms, even if you also add progesterone." If, however, you shut down a woman's production of hormones and just add in tiny controlled amounts of estrogen and progesterone—which is what birth control pills do—then, says Goldstein, you can create a balance that can have a dramatic effect on symptoms.

HOW BIRTH CONTROL PILLS CAN HELP

As you read in Chapter 1, once you enter your forties, your ovaries no longer "hatch" eggs on the same schedule they did before. In fact, the older you get, the fewer eggs you produce, so that by the time you are a year or two away from complete menopause—in your late forties or early fifties—you are lucky to find even one or two eggs left in your "nest." However, as long as *some* egg production continues, you will also continue

From the "M" File

GETTING OFF HORMONES—WHAT SHOULD I EXPECT?

Q: I have heard that once you stop using hormones you will have the same symptoms you had when you started— meaning that eventually you're still going to have to suffer through the hot flashes and night sweats and mood swings. Is this true—and if so, then isn't it also true that hormones only delay menopause, but don't help cure it?

A: Although it's true that some women do experience menopause-related symptoms when they stop HRT, according to New York University hormone expert Dr. Steven Goldstein, a great deal of what you experience has to do with the amount of hormones you are taking, for how long, your age when you started, your age when you decide to stop, and the level of hormones your body is naturally producing at the time when you stop. Perhaps most important, he says, is whether or not you stop abruptly or taper off. Ideally, says Goldstein, if you taper your dosage very gradually, reducing the amount of hormones in your bloodstream by small amounts, you can short-circuit a great many "rebound" problems. In addition, the older you are when you stop, the less likely you are to experience symptoms once HRT is no longer being used. This is because your body's own production of hormones will have slowed to such a degree you should experience very little of the dramatic fluctuations that are behind most symptoms.

to have a supply of estrogen and, during some months, progesterone circulating through your system. How much depends on many factors, including your brain chemistry, how many times you ovulate, and your weight. Since fat cells have the ability to convert your body's natural supply of androgen (a male hormone like testosterone) into estrogen, the more extra pounds you carry, the more estrogen your body will produce— sometimes as much as triple the amount produced by a thin woman of the same age. Without *regular* egg production, however, what you fail to

Regardless of your personal profile in regard to HRT, recent research shows you are not likely to feel the "bump" of coming off hormones until about eight weeks have passed. According to a 2004 report in the journal *Obstetrics and Gynecology* hot flashes peak about the eighth week after stopping HRT. So, if you taper down over an eight-week rather than a four-week "washout," then you may experience fewer problems. Even still, remember that the worst of your problems, at least in terms of hot flashes, will probably occur somewhere between weeks seven and nine and will likely get better following that time. So, if you can get through what could be about two pretty miserable weeks, you'll likely find things are much improved shortly thereafter. Remember, the goal of any menopause-related therapy, be it HRT, birth control pills, natural hormones, or plant remedies, is to simply control symptoms, and not "cure" menopause, the way penicillin will knock out pneumonia, for example. Menopause is not a disease but rather a stage of life that all women must pass through. Remembering that can go a long way in helping you cope with whatever symptoms you do experience. The bottom line, says Goldstein, is to develop a close relationship with your doctor while withdrawing from hormone therapy and keep an accurate diary of your symptoms—including what returns, when, and with what severity. This can help when it comes time to adjust your dosage and help make withdrawal as easy and as symptom-free as possible.

produce regularly is progesterone, the hormone that is desperately needed to balance estrogen. In fact, while estrogen levels usually drop some 40 to 60 percent during the perimenopause, as ovulation fails, progesterone levels can drop to zero. The end result: Hormonally speaking, estrogen dominates—and even if levels are low, if they overshadow progesterone by any significant margin you can experience a whopping case of perimenopause symptoms, particularly PMS-type mood swings and cravings.

If that were not enough, remember that estrogen is what causes your uterine lining to build, while progesterone causes it to shed. So, when you are still making estrogen but not progesterone, your uterine lining continues to build—but doesn't shed. Over time it not only thickens but also becomes unstable, which in turn causes portions of it to break off and pull away from the uterine wall. As you read earlier, this results in the classic symptom of dysfunctional uterine bleeding, which can be quite heavy or even frightening at times (see Chapter 3).

Although HRT can sometimes contribute to all these problems (one reason doctors have always been reluctant to recommend it to women who are not yet officially in menopause), by introducing a low, but balanced level of hormones into your body, birth control pills work to alleviate many of your perimenopausal complaints, including not only mood swings but also dysfunctional bleeding. Certainly if you are also concerned about getting pregnant, it can do double duty, protecting you in this respect as well.

ARE BIRTH CONTROL PILLS RIGHT FOR YOU? HOW TO TELL

Unfortunately, for many of us who remember the first round of birth control pills that we took in the late 1960s and early to mid-1970s, even the thought of using this treatment after age forty is enough to scare the very panty liners right off your thongs. As you probably recall, the "old" Pill carried with it some *very* dramatic health risks, particularly when used after age forty—not the least of which was an increased risk of stroke and cancer. One reason is because it contained so much estrogen—up to 150 micrograms per pill. By comparison, most versions of the Pill in use today contain between 20 and 35 micrograms of estrogen. So in this respect, there is no longer a "blanket recommendation" against Pill use after the age thirty-five or even forty. In fact, these low-dose pills are frequently recommended for women over forty, not only to control perimenopausal symptoms but, as you read earlier, also as a form of midlife birth control.

Still, it's important to note that even these low-dose pills aren't without some problems. First, because the levels of estrogen and progesterone are so delicately balanced—particularly in the very low-dose pills—and because every woman's physiology is slightly different, some women experience breakthrough bleeding or spotting. While this isn't serious, it can be annoying and if it is for you, talk to your doctor. Sometimes simply increasing the hormone level with a slightly more potent Pill may be all you need to solve this problem.

If you smoke, the risks are more serious, including the risk of stroke. Although problems are far less likely to occur when using a low-dose Pill, still, if you do smoke, or if you have a history of blood clots or high blood pressure, be sure to discuss all your treatment options with your doctor before deciding if birth control pills are right for you.

If you have fibroid tumors, the experts are split as to whether or not the Pill can help you. Some doctors believe you should avoid it, since any additional estrogen might encourage these tumors to grow (see Chapter 3). Others, however, believe that the amount of estrogen in the low-dose Pill is actually *so* low, it's not likely to cause a problem. Ultimately, this is a subject for you and your doctor to discuss and decide. In addition, recent studies have shown that younger women who use birth control pills may have reduced bone density, so it makes sense to assume that the Pill won't do much to protect your bones when used during perimenopause. Depending on the result of your bone density test (see Chapter 12) you may want to skip Pill use—or, talk to your doctor about medications you can add to your regimen to help slow bone loss during this transitional time.

Finally, you may also want to skip the Pill if you are at risk for breast cancer. While any association between the Pill and breast cancer is weak at best, because the chance of developing this disease naturally increases with age, if you are already at risk, you may have to think a bit more carefully before you decide if the Pill is the right treatment for you.

If, ultimately, you decide to give the low-dose Pill a try, remember, you won't be using it indefinitely. For most women, a few years of Pill use is all that's necessary to get them over the "rough spots" of perimenopause. As hormone levels start to bottom out, some women find it's easy to go off the Pill and not suffer any major symptoms. Others, however, slide from the Pill right on over to traditional HRT—or they begin natural treatments (see Chapter 10) after Pill use subsides.

Bioidentical Hormones:
New Hope in a Bottle

While doctors aren't certain just why the WHI studies turned out as they did, one strong theory has to do with the *type* of hormones used in these clinical trials. More specifically, both the estrogen and the progesterone used in the HRT formulations were "synthetic" hormones. While you might think this simply means they were made in a laboratory, there is much more to the definition than just this. Unlike synthetic gemstones, which carry the same optical and chemical properties as the gemstones manufactured by Mother Nature, synthetic hormones (such as medroxyprogesterone acetate or norethindrone acetate, both synthetic progesterones) are *not* an exact duplicate of what is manufactured in your body. Because of this, many experts now believe that the body cannot assimilate hormone therapy the same way it can natural hormones—one reason we may not see the same benefits, such as protection from heart disease or stroke.

According to hormone expert Nisha Jackson, Ph.D., at the very least, natural and synthetic progesterone can cause entirely different biochemical reactions. As evidence she points out that only "real" progesterone and not the supplement progestin is capable of raising blood serum levels of this hormone.

While synthetic hormones were once the only choice a woman had, this is no longer the case. Another, and increasingly popular, choice is what are being called "bioidentical hormones." While many people refer to these as "natural" hormones—and even doctors themselves use this term—the label is a bit misleading. The reason is that all bioidentical hormones are made in a laboratory, in much the same way as synthetic hormones. But while a synthetic progesterone like Provera (medroxyprogesterone acetate) may tout "natural" ingredients, its molecular structure has been altered. So, the end result is *not bioidentical.* Conversely, as their name implies, bioidentical hormones have a molecular structure that is *identical* to hormones that are made by the human body. In fact, once they are in your bloodstream, your body is virtually unable to tell bioidentical hormones from what is manufactured naturally. So in this instance the term "natural" refers not to the ingredients, but to the end result. (In fashion terms, bioidentical hormones are a bit like a dress that's not just a copy of a Calvin Klein original, but an *exact*, thread-by-thread, stitch-by-stitch duplication that, once on the body, could never be told apart from the original, even by Calvin himself!)

Right now, the two most popular forms of bioidentical hormones are known as "natural" progesterone and "natural" estrogen—and many believe they may revolutionize not only the way perimenopause symptoms are treated, but also the treatment of PMS and possibly other hormone-related problems, including anxiety, panic attacks, even mood disorders including depression.

"NATURAL" PROGESTERONE: HOW IT CAN HELP

Although some doctors believe the only way to control midlife symptoms is through the use of both estrogen and progesterone together, in the last several years a new and somewhat different approach has been emerging. The theory: As long as your body is still making estrogen, skip supplementation and take only what you're missing—which in many instances is progesterone. Further, by cycling the progesterone to closely mimic a natural menstrual cycle (using it for about ten days out of every month), you can also create a kind of "artificial period" that not only helps bring the body into a "natural" balance but also works to "naturally" slough off the layers of uterine lining—much like a regular period—and reduce the cells that would otherwise continue to build. This can not only help prevent or at least control heavy, erratic dysfunctional bleeding (see Chapter 3), it can also help prevent the development of hyperplasia, an abnormal thickening of the uterine lining that can sometimes be a precursor to endometrial cancer. For all these reasons progesterone-only supplements have begun to gain popularity as a prominent line of defense, particularly when dysfunctional bleeding is a primary symptom.

In the very latest research, doctors from the Weill Cornell Medical Center in New York City found that progesterone may also have important effects on blood pressure. In their research, progesterone helped to dilate or "open up" blood vessels, as well as reduce the risk of a rise in blood pressure caused by adrenaline-like hormones secreted under stress. Progesterone also appears to help keep calcium levels in the blood high, thus working much the way some calcium channel–blocking blood pres-

From the "M" File

THE PROGESTERONE TWO-STEP

Q: I currently use a prescription oral progesterone treatment and want to switch to a nonprescription progesterone cream. Only problem is, I can't figure out how the dosages compare—and how much cream to use. Can you explain?

A: The best advice is to talk to your doctor, particularly since you are now using a prescription progesterone treatment. There may be a logical reason he or she recommended oral supplementation over other forms. That said, it's true that the different forms of progesterone contain differing amounts—but don't let that fool you. It doesn't mean that one form is more potent than another. Different forms require different concentrations in order to achieve results. To help you discuss your other treatment choices with your doctor, here's a rundown on how natural, or bioidentical, progesterone products stack up in terms of hormone concentration.

- Capsules: Doses range from 25 up to 100 milligrams—and usually require that you use a higher concentration than what is found in creams or lozenges.

sure medications do to control hypertension. This is extremely important, say researchers, since blood pressure tends to rise during the perimenopausal years and may increase the risk of stroke and even heart disease later in life.

The bottom line: If your doctor suggests progesterone-only therapy may help you, do discuss the benefits of using a natural, bioidentical product, now available in a wide variety of forms including capsules, creams, patches, and even sublingual (under the tongue) lozenges. Although many of these treatments, particularly the creams, are available without a prescription, these are usually much lower in strength and may not be sufficient for perimenopausal symptoms. In order to obtain a supplement with a high enough percentage of progesterone, you will need a prescription. Currently, the only prescription-strength bioidentical form of progesterone readily available in all pharmacies is Prometrium—a "nat-

- Drops: Typical dosing is 25 milligrams per 4 drops, with 4 to 6 drops in the evening and 2 to 4 drops in the morning a typical regimen.

- Lozenges: Available in strength of 25, 50, 75, or 100 milligrams. Since this form is quickly absorbed you can usually reduce the dosage below what is used in capsule form.

- Creams/gels: Rub between 20 and 60 milligrams of cream into the skin twice daily. (Most creams come with some type of measuring device or sometimes come in individual packettes in the correct dosage.) The cream should be applied to thin-skinned areas, such as the wrists or inner thighs. The over-the-counter preparation is a 1.5 to 3 percent solution and may require more frequent dosing than the prescription form, which is normally a 3 to 10 percent solution—with the higher dosage usually considered more effective.

ural" progesterone suspended in a peanut oil base. It's a popular supplement used not only during perimenopause but, in some instances, to treat PMS and as a pregnancy supplement to help strengthen the uterus. If, however, you are allergic to peanuts, there are other options, but you will need the cooperation of a compounding pharamacy. As mentioned earlier, these are pharmacies that make medications the "old-fashioned" way—using raw ingredients to "compound," or create, a drug to your specifications.

Most compounding pharmacies offer bioidentical progesterone in the full range of forms, (see the resource section at the back of this book). And while natural progesterone *capsules* may be the easiest to use—either from a compounding pharmacy, or in the form of Prometrium—at least some experts believe this form of progesterone is metabolized too quickly. So, in order to get the full benefits you may have to take a much higher dose than what would otherwise be considered necessary. If your doctor is not aware of how to compensate for the differences, most often the compounding pharmacy will provide a conversion table to help in prescribing the correct amount. Of course another option is to try progesterone lozenges or creams, which, by the way, many believe may be the most rapid and easily absorbed treatment (see "From the 'M' File: The Progesterone Two-Step). As a side note, you may find it interesting to know that natural, bioidentical progesterone can be compounded and blended with any of the various forms of bioidentical estrogen (see the section that follows) for what some believe may be a kinder, gentler, and ultimately safer form of HRT—something you may also want to discuss with your doctor.

In terms of side effects, almost any type of progesterone supplement you choose is likely to make you drowsy, so it's best to take them at bedtime. Another way around this is to use smaller doses and take them several times a day—a strategy that many women report offers better and more consistent symptom relief. Also note that for some women progesterone therapy can temporarily worsen symptoms for about two weeks. This may be particularly true if you have had long-standing estrogen dominance with very low progesterone. If this should occur, try to stick with it for the full two weeks. After this time you are likely to see some signs of relief. If that's not possible, lower your dosage and build up gradually. If symptoms continue to worsen, or they do not abate eventually, see your doctor.

BIOIDENTICAL PROGESTERONE: A WORD OF CAUTION

As popular as bioidentical hormones are becoming, it's important to note that some experts caution women about their use, particularly those treatments that are available without a prescription. According to ACOG experts, it's important to note that, at this point in time, no formal studies have been conducted to determine either the safety or the efficacy of natural hormones, and, they say, "many manufacturers' claims are based on studies involving synthetic progestins and not natural progesterone." They also caution that there is no evidence to date that progesterone creams can protect the uterus from overstimulation or reduce the risk of endometrial cancer.

However, a number of new studies have begun to emerge attesting to the value of natural progesterone supplements, particularly when combined with estrogen. In one study published in the *Journal of Reproductive Medicine* in 1999, when combined with estrogen supplements, natural progesterone was shown to control the overgrowth of uterine lining in postmenopausal women. Also important to note: Natural progesterone supplements have been used in Europe since 1980 in dosages of up to 300 milligrams daily, and they continue as a mainstay of hormonal treatment for everything from PMS to menopause.

Estrogen-Only Therapy: Why Everything Old Is New Again

My friend Eve is a lawyer and a staunch feminist who, bless her heart, believes everyone is created equal, including not only men and women, but also dogs, cats, birds, and, I think, certain insects. Recently she asked me why I thought a woman's body, specifically *her* body, could react so dramatically when estrogen levels started to decline.

"After all, if the only thing that is really going on here is the end of my baby-making heyday, then why should the rest of my body kick up such a fuss—or even care what my ovaries are doing or not doing," she uttered rather pragmatically one afternoon while we were sweating out a hot flash at the cosmetics counter of Bloomingdale's.

She continued: "I mean really . . . I can't honestly believe that my whole body is going nuts simply because my ovaries have stopped working—a woman is not just the total sum of her ovarian function, you know," she said as we made our way from moisturizers to anti-aging creams.

I had to admit she had made an interesting point. Still, I assured my friend that menopause is really *not* a political statement—and hormone deprivation is *not* really nature's way of gaslighting the feminist movement!

The real reason why Eve—and all the rest of us—*do* feel such a body-wide response when hormone levels fall is because they affect more than just reproductive activity. As you read earlier, there are hormone receptor sites throughout a woman's body—located in the brain, gastrointestinal tract, the breast, even in our bones and skin. These receptors act like tiny "docking stations," allowing hormones floating in your bloodstream to "park" on a cell's surface. When this occurs, the hormone sends a message to the cell's DNA, which in turn influences, to some extent, how that cell will act—in both a positive and a negative way. And in the end, this means that a lot of what is going on in all areas of your body is in some way linked to the messages being sent by your reproductive hormones to all your cells. In this respect, it's not hard to see why, when reproductive hormone levels plummet, you can feel the effects in so many different ways. It's also the reason why so many doctors came to believe that estrogen held the answer to all our problems.

And, in fact, beginning as early as the 1940s doctors were prescribing this hormone, usually in large doses, to combat the symptoms of menopause. Over the next couple of decades, however, this line of thinking took a serious turn. Studies began showing that without progesterone to counter its effects, estrogen alone caused the cells of the uterine lining to thicken, dramatically increasing the risk of uterine cancer. That discovery, in fact, is what led to the development and eventual popularity of HRT. Doctors believed that by adding a synthetic progesterone into the mix, the problems caused by estrogen alone could be squelched.

Oddly enough, however, in recent years, estrogen-only therapy emerged once again, this time prescribed for women following a hysterectomy. If there was no risk of uterine cell buildup, then, doctors reasoned, cancer would no longer be a concern. But recently, that line of thinking has also begun to change. As you read earlier, in February 2004 the final results of the WHI trials showed that estrogen-only therapy failed to protect women from heart disease, *and* it increased their risk of stroke. This finding is in perfect alignment with studies presented a few months earlier in the *Journal of the American Medical Association.* Here, researchers from the National Cancer Institute found a clear link between ovarian cancer and estrogen-only therapy. In a ten-year study of some 44,000 women— some of whom had their uterus removed but kept their ovaries, others who had both uterus and ovaries—those who used estrogen alone were found to have a 60 percent higher risk of ovarian cancer than those who took no hormones.

While it would seem as if the story should end here, surprisingly it doesn't. And the reason is the development of several new forms of estrogen—*natural, bioidentical estrogens* that some believe can offer women all the benefits of traditional therapy, without any of the risks.

WHY ALL ESTROGEN ARE NOT CREATED EQUAL

Although it's likely that you are used to hearing the word *estrogen* used to describe the female hormone made in your ovaries, in truth, this is really a very broad term used to encompass three interrelated hormones—three *types* of estrogen, each of which plays a different role in our well-being. The three types are:

- *Estradiol (E2):* Secreted by your ovaries during your reproductive years, this is the most potent estrogen and the one with the greatest impact on your overall health and well-being. From the time you reach puberty to the time you enter menopause, the majority of the estrogen circulating through your body is estradiol. Synthetic versions of estradiol make up the bulk of most estrogen replacement products.

- *Estrone (E1):* Also produced by your ovaries, this form of estrogen becomes dominant during menopause—a time when you are no longer making estradiol. In fact, unlike estradiol, which is secreted directly by the ovaries, estrone is manufactured when your ovaries convert two male hormones—testosterone and androstenedione—into this estrogen. In order for this happen, your body also creates another natural enzyme known as aromatase, which resides primarily in fat and muscle. The more fat cells you have, the more aromatase your body makes, and the easier it is to convert the male hormones into estrogen. This is one reason why overweight women appear to go into menopause at a later age—in simplest terms their fat cells help ensure a larger supply of estrogen. On the downside it's also why being overweight may increase your risk of breast and uterine cancer thanks to the excess estrogen stimulation that can encourage abnormal cell growth.

- *Estriol (E3):* This is the weakest form of estrogen and is derived from the hormone estrone. Of the three types of estrogen, only estriol does not encourage cell growth—in either the breast or the uterus. As you will learn in a few moments, this can be an extremely important fact if and when you decide to give estrogen therapy a try.

Traditionally, all estrogen therapy involved the use of synthetic estradiol. It's also the form most often found in combination estrogen-progesterone therapy. However, as bioidentical hormones move to the forefront of the treatment arsenal, other forms of estrogen are also taking center stage. In fact, there is now a growing movement among many physicians and researchers to abandon traditional estradiol treatments altogether in favor of the weaker, less potent, but seemingly much safer bioidentical estriol, or E3, estrogen—either on its own, or in combination with either estrone or estrone and estradiol. By adding estriol into the mix, doctors say the amount of the more potent and controversial estradiol can be dramatically reduced—or even eliminated—and along with it, many of the risks associated with this therapy. And studies are starting to show this may, in fact, be true.

- Reporting in *Maturitas* (the official journal of the European Menopause and Andropause Society), a group of Norwegian doctors revealed that even long-term treatment with oral estriol caused no significant increase in the lining of the uterus, when compared to women who took no hormones.

- A study published in the journal *Gerontology* in 2000 offered evidence that elderly women treated with estriol had improved blood vessel function, along with improved bone density—and no increased risk of cancer.

- The journal *Maturitas* published yet another study in 2000 comparing the effects of estriol to estradiol therapy in relation to cholesterol. The results showed that while traditional estradiol therapy continued to increase cholesterol, estriol had no such impact. In fact, estriol appeared to actually protect women against a natural age-related rise in cholesterol.

• As far back as 1980, Danish doctors were touting the benefits of estriol
when their research proved this compound actually had anti-estrogenic
effects in the breast and the uterus—latching onto estrogen receptors
in both areas and keeping the more potent estradiol from reaching those
cells. This, in turn, appeared to have a protective effect against cancer.

Add to this two Japanese studies—one published in 2000 in the journal
Maturitas, the other in the journal *Human Reproduction*—that revealed
oral estriol was safe and effective in the treatment of common
menopause-related symptoms with no increased risks to breast or endometrial tissue. In studies conducted in both Sweden and Hungary in
the 1980s and again in the late 1990s, doctors also discovered estriol had
no negative effect on urogenital symptoms, including incontinence. This
is particularly important in light of recent studies showing that the commonly used estradiol preparations *are* likely to encourage incontinence.

Other studies have also shown good results when estriol was combined with natural, bioidentical micronized progesterone in the treatment
of menopause-related symptoms, with virtually no risk of the side effects
attributed to other forms of hormone therapy.

CHOOSING YOUR ESTROGEN WISELY: WHAT TO DO

Currently, there are several types of estriol treatment in use, though almost none is considered "commercially available." That means no large
pharmaceutical company is manufacturing estriol, so you generally can't
get your prescription filled at a local pharmacy. Instead, you will have to
contact a compounding pharmacy (see the resource section at the back of
this book). Most are able to prepare either pure estriol or a two- or three-
estrogen combination product in the most common forms including capsules, gels, creams, and vaginal tablets.

The three available forms of "natural" estrogen formulations are:

• *Tri-Estrogen:* Also known as tri-est, or triple estrogen, this blend in-
corporates estriol (80 percent), estrone (10 percent), and estradiol
(10 percent). Because it is compounded specifically for each patient,
the percentages can vary according to what your doctor prescribes.

In this respect it's easy to come up with a formulation that is specific to your health profile. Tri-estrogens are also available in combination with natural, bioidentical micronized progesterone in a combined capsule that can also be custom compounded. This is a particularly good choice if you have any fears concerning the risk of endometrial cancer or if you have been diagnosed with endometrial polyps (see Chapter 3), since some studies have shown that estriol alone may increase the risk of these benign growths.

- *Bi-Estrogen:* In this treatment, estradiol is combined with estriol in a ratio of 20 percent to 80 percent, and it is often recommended when the tri-estrogen combination results in bloating or excess gas. In addition, at least some doctors also avoid the tri-estrogen formulation since there is some evidence that the estrone portion of the formula may metabolize into a cancer-causing estrogen—and leaving it out doesn't appear to make any significant difference in terms of symptom relief. Other bi-estrogen formulations include 60 percent estradiol and 40 percent estriol, which is the most potent in terms of symptom relief but obviously carries greater health risks. The other option is 70 percent estriol and 30 percent estradiol. Bi-estrogens can also be combined with natural, bioidentical micronized progesterone. The nice thing is your doctor can custom prescribe this therapy just for you.

- *Estriol Solo:* This is 100 percent pure estriol, which can be used alone or in combination with natural, bioidentical micronized progesterone. Studies have shown that 2 to 4 milligrams daily of estriol is equivalent to 0.6 to 1.25 milligrams of conjugated estrogen (estradiol) or estrone in the relief of many but not all symptoms.

Although estrogen-only therapy (even utilizing 100 percent estriol) is still reserved primarily for women who have had a hysterectomy, this is not a hard and fast rule. Depending on your symptoms and your personal risk profile, short-term therapy with any of these products may be an alternative worth discussing with your doctor. Also, don't forget that these ostensibly "safer" estrogens can also be combined with natural, bioidentical progesterone for what some believe is a kinder, gentler form of HRT.

From the "M" File

TESTERONE THERAPY—CAN MALE HORMONES HELP ME?

Q: I'm fifty-one years old and just about entering menopause—and my doctor suggested testosterone therapy that he says would help my sex life, which, quite honestly, is nonexistent these days. Is this safe to take—and will it help?

A: If, in fact, you are unhappy about your lack of sex drive and would like to reignite your intimate fire, then yes, there is some evidence that testosterone therapy can help. This hormone is present naturally in every woman's body and levels can drop, sometimes significantly, during the menopause process. Currently, many experts agree that the only safe and effective form of this treatment for women is natural, bioidentical testosterone, available at compounding pharmacies. In addition, there are also some custom-compounded hormone replacement therapies that combine "natural" estrogen and progesterone with tiny amounts of testosterone. To learn more about how testosterone may help you, see Chapter 8.

We're All Individuals—And Never Let Your Doctor Forget It!

Perhaps the most important thing that we have learned from the WHI study is not so much that hormone replacement therapy is not exactly the "glass slipper" we'd all been hoping for, but that finding the "perfect fit," regardless of the treatment, is going to be largely a matter of defining our personal needs—and finding a doctor willing to treat us in a totally individual way. While it's certainly true that the hormones that were used in the WHI trials offered disappointing, and even anger-provoking results, it's important to remember that there are many other hormone combinations as well as formulations yet to be tested. Perhaps more important, there are also a variety of other drug treatments (see Chapter 12)—and some pretty impressive natural products (see Chapter 10), which are fast proving to solve at least some of the problems previously treated by hormone therapy.

The bottom line in all of this: Every woman is different. While we all start out with a uterus and ovaries, a vagina and breasts, our individual health profiles, combined with our family history of disease, and particularly our lifestyle experiences, come together to form a uniquely different perimenopause profile for each of us. I mean, let's face it, girls, we wouldn't all wear the same pair of shoes or select the same jewelry or handbags, would we? Well, in that same way, we should also not be expected to respond identically to a single treatment or even a treatment category. And in this regard, many doctors have come to see that the otherwise traumatic results of the WHI study also have a positive side—in that it altered, dramatically and permanently, the way women and their physicians approach the treatment of menopause. No longer is the "one size fits all" mentality even a suggested line of thinking. (It doesn't even work for pantyhose, for heaven's sake—how in the world could it work for hormone therapy?) Today, the most progressive doctors—and women—know that individualized therapy is, in fact, the only possible route to successful care.

Perhaps most importantly, the WHI also taught us that time is of the essence, meaning that women should no longer be asked to "make do" with that fifteen minutes your doctor allots for an appointment—a seven-minute check of symptoms followed by a seven-minute litany of the benefits of hormone replacement therapy (with a minute left over to get on and off the table). Today, both women and their doctors must take more time to know, understand, and explore not only individual symptoms, but also individual treatment options—including those that don't need a doctor's prescription.

The information in this chapter, and in Chapters 10 and 12, can help you to know and understand more about those options. But to use this information wisely, you must open a dialogue with your own doctor and discuss the pros and cons as they apply to you. If your physician won't take the time to talk to you about choices, or if he or she is stuck in the rut of a single type of treatment (be it pro or con hormone replacement), consider finding a doctor who is willing to give you the time and individual treatment you deserve. I've made a lot of funny remarks throughout much of this book. And I hope that some of what I've written here has made you smile. But as much as I love to laugh—and hope that you do too—your health today and especially in the future is no laughing matter. There is much that can be done to soothe the savage beast of peri-menopause and menopause—and ways to ensure a happier, healthier to-morrow in the process. You owe it to yourself to find a doctor willing to be your partner in this journey—and to help you find the most enjoyable and healthy path possible.

12

Protecting Your Future Health

Becoming the Woman
You Were Meant to Be

While it may be hard to imagine now—when you're still flushing and night sweating and mood swinging from the chandeliers—at some point in the not too distant future, your life *is* going to return to normal. Or at least your biology will calm down to the point where you no longer have the desire to sit naked in the snow just to cool off. In fact, as time passes and your hormones begin to settle in, your body will become adjusted to your newer and, hopefully, improved physiology, and slowly but surely you will begin to feel more like yourself—maybe even just a little bit better.

Although getting control of hormone central may be your top priority right this very minute, it's also important to remember that there are many other aspects of your health and your health care that need attention as well. Because the truth is, we women are living longer than ever before. And while this is essentially good news, it also carries with it some important responsibilities, including an obligation to take better overall care of our health, starting right now. One important way to do that is by not waiting until a problem develops and then trying to fix it. Instead, our goal—both collectively and individually—must be to take whatever steps we can *preventively,* to ensure we are on the most solid footing possible as we step down off the menopause platform and head out into our future. The key, of course, is to work with your doctor as much as possible, identifying your personal risk factors, as well as whatever is lurking in your family tree. This can spotlight both your weak points and your strengths. Then, with just a little bit of effort—and some help from your doctor—you can begin taking whatever steps are necessary to ensure *your* future health. To help get you off on the right foot, what follows is a short, but important guide to some of the midlife medical concerns that are of prime importance to women. Certainly, not all of us will be at risk for *all* these problems—and some of us may not be at risk for any at all. Still, it's a smart idea to pay attention to what *might* affect you. With this information in hand you can work with your doctor to devise a future health maintenance plan that is perfectly suited for you.

Women and Heart Disease: What You Must Know

My friend Terry is a great lady—smart, sexy, and successful, with every intention of staying that way as long as humanly possible. That's one reason she says she made the conscious decision to begin using hormones the minute her first menopause symptom arrived.

"I don't care if they have to hook me up to a hormone IV 24/7, I'm *not* going down quiet or easy," she would say, grinning like a Cheshire cat, whenever the subject came up. But as determined as Terry was to not only preserve her youth but also protect her health, she was clearly not prepared for the hand that fate was about to deal her.

First came the WHI report—and the news that much of what she had counted on to bring her bouncing into her golden years was probably not going to help at all, and could even harm her. But clearly the bigger blow arrived when not too long afterward she found herself in a hospital emergency room, clutching her chest in what she now describes as "the most excruciating pain in the universe." Within less than an hour Terry had to face yet another sobering reality: Though just fifty-six years old, she was having a heart attack—and she needed bypass surgery to ensure her survival.

"I thought I was doing everything right," she said, still in a state of shock and disbelief. "How could this have happened to me?"

Fortunately, Terry's story has a happy ending. She recovered from her heart attack, had the bypass surgery, and she says she feels great. She also knows just how lucky she is. The harsh reality: While "heart disease," "heart attack," "high blood pressure," and "stroke" were terms once used to describe a middle-aged man's health risks, these terms now apply to women—in almost equal numbers.

Take a deep breath, now—because here's a few more eye-opening shockers:

- Sixty-three percent of women who die suddenly of heart disease have no previous symptoms.

- Each year nearly a half million American women die from heart disease—making it the leading killer of women over age fifty.

- Within six years of having a heart attack, 35 percent of all women will have another one.

- A woman is more likely to die from a heart attack than a man.

- More women die of heart disease than from *all forms of cancer combined*—with African-American women at highest risk of all.

Although heart disease may hit you later than your male partner—some ten years later by some estimates—that's only because a lot of your risk is intimately tied to your natural estrogen level. Why? Estrogen has an important positive effect on blood vessels, helping to keep them dilated and open. This, in turn, helps keep arteries free and clear of plaque deposits such as cholesterol—which in turn protects your heart. Indeed, a heart attack occurs when these deposits build up to such an extent it literally chokes off or blocks blood flow to your heart. So, the more blood that gets to your heart, the healthier your heart muscle will be, and the natural estrogen produced by your ovaries can help ensure this. This same estrogen–blood vessel link is also what helps keep your risk of hypertension and stroke under control during your reproductive years.

Perhaps more important are the links between estrogen and cholesterol. During your peak reproductive years, high levels of natural estrogen help keep levels of HDL or "good" cholesterol high as well. In general, women have much higher levels of HDL than men—and experts believe estrogen is the reason. When HDL is high, there is evidence to show that the risk of heart attack is lower. However, as estrogen levels start to plummet, HDL levels can take a dive as well, sometimes allowing levels of LDL or "bad cholesterol" to dominate. As this happens your risk of heart disease naturally increases.

What's more, we also know that the younger you are when you enter menopause—my friend Terry was just forty-two—and the sooner estrogen levels begin to fall, the sooner you start building a risk profile for heart disease, and ultimately, the faster your risk of heart attack and stroke rise.

While doctors once believed that hormone replacement therapy, specifically estrogen, would offer women the same positive, health-protecting effects as their own natural supply, we now know this is not the case. Certainly, one of the most shocking findings of the recent WHI trials was not only that estrogen therapy didn't protect women from heart disease, but that in some instances it actually increased their risk. And regardless of whether these findings will be challenged in the future, currently HRT, or even estrogen therapy alone, is not being recommended to protect a woman's heart. The good news is that there are *other* ways around the problem. In much the same way that men have taken control of their risk for heart disease, so too can women. The key to making that happen: Recognize it could happen to you, identify your personal risk factors, work with your doctor to modify those risks, and monitor your heart health at regular intervals.

EIGHT WAYS TO REDUCE YOUR RISK OF HEART DISEASE—*RIGHT NOW!*

Although part of your cardiac risk profile is linked to factors you can't control (such as your age, race, and family history of disease), fortunately, that paints only part of your health picture. Experts report that a good deal more of your risk for many illnesses, but specifically heart disease, has more to do with your *personal* risk profile—the specific health and lifestyle factors that are true for you. The good news here: Many of these factors are *under your control.*

To this end the American College of Obstetricians and Gynecologists believes that by making just a few simple changes in your life and your lifestyle, you can dramatically reduce your risk of heart disease. To help get you thinking in the right direction, what follow are some of the more important suggestions.

- *Stop smoking:* Puffing on just one to four cigarettes a day doubles your risk of having a heart attack, while smoking a pack a day quadruples that risk. Smokers who have a heart attack are more likely than nonsmokers to die, and die suddenly, often within an hour. Smoking is, in fact, a woman's single biggest risk factor for heart attack. The good news: Stop smoking today and the repair process will begin almost immediately.

- *Monitor your blood pressure:* More than half of all women over age fifty-five have high blood pressure, and most don't know it. While the condition may be symptom free, the silent damage to your blood vessels can set the stage for a heart attack, stroke, or kidney failure— all without you knowing it. Fortunately, blood pressure responds to diet and exercise. Lose just ten pounds and you could drop your pressure by ten points or more. Limit alcohol consumption and watch your salt intake, and watch your pressure fall even further. If these measures don't work, talk to your doctor about medication.

- *Eat more soy:* Consuming just 25 grams of soy protein daily (see Chapter 10) can drop your cholesterol by 10 percent. Although you may be tempted to try soy supplements, note that, so far, research has only verified the power of soy-rich *foods* to improve your health.

- *Take a drink, but just one:* One drink of red wine daily can drop your risk of a heart attack by up to 70 percent. But add just one or two more drinks to your daily agenda, and your odds reverse, increasing your blood pressure, triglycerides (blood fats), and even your risk of breast cancer.

• *Move it—or lose it!:* Sit around watching soap operas during your leisure time and watch your risk of heart disease double. But spend just thirty minutes three to five days a week watching those soaps from your exercise bike—or turn off the TV and take a walk around the neighborhood—and watch your risk drop. Exercise will also help lower your LDL (the "bad") cholesterol, and increase HDL (the "good") cholesterol.

• *Ask your doctor about aspirin:* There's good evidence to show that taking a half aspirin a day might reduce your risk of heart attack and stroke. But don't just take it on your own—let your doctor know your plan since daily aspirin use can increase the risk of other health concerns, including gastrointestinal distress.

• *Eat a bowl of oatmeal once a day:* Along with a low-fat diet and some regular exercise, oatmeal can help keep your cholesterol under control. If you already have high cholesterol, remember, for every 1 percent reduction, you reduce your risk of heart attack by up to 3 percent.

• *Watch your weight:* Your risk of heart attack, stroke, hypertension, and even diabetes goes up dramatically if you're just 30 percent over your ideal weight. But it goes down with every pound you lose! Controlling blood sugar, particularly if you are diagnosed with type 2 diabetes, can also help take some strain off your heart.

PROTECTING YOUR HEART: HOW YOUR DOCTOR CAN HELP

In addition to whatever lifestyle changes you can make, your doctor can also play an important role in ensuring your heart health. According to the American Academy of Family Physicians, your doctor should regularly perform the following screenings—and you should attempt to reach the following goals:

SCREENING: CHOLESTEROL—TOTAL, HDL, LDL, AND TRIGLYCERIDES

- Frequency: At least every two years

GOALS FOR TOTAL CHOLESTEROL:

- Desirable: under 200

- Borderline: 200 to 239

- Health risk: 240 and higher

GOALS FOR LDL (LOW-DENSITY LIPOPROTEIN)—OR THE "BAD" CHOLESTEROL:

- Fewer than two risk factors: under 160 mg/dl

- Two or more risk factors: under 130 mg/dl

- Already diagnosed with heart disease: under 100 mg/dl

GOALS FOR HDL (HIGH-DENSITY LIPOPROTEIN)—OR THE "GOOD" CHOLESTEROL:

- As high as possible, at least 45 mg/dl. A rate of 60 mg/dl or higher is known to reduce the risk of heart disease.

GOALS FOR TRIGLYCERIDES:

- Desirable levels: 200 mg/dl or less

- Optimal levels: under 150 mg/dl

SCREENING: BLOOD PRESSURE

- Frequency: At least once yearly during annual physical

GOALS FOR BLOOD PRESSURE:

- Systolic pressure (top number): under 140 mm/hg, with optimal pressure at 120 mm/hg

- Diastolic pressure (bottom number): less than 90 mm/hg, with 80 mm/hg or lower considered optimal

SCREENING: BLOOD SUGAR

- Frequency: At least once yearly during annual physical

GOALS FOR BLOOD SUGAR:

- Desirable 126 mg/dl or less

- Optimal: 110 mg/dl or less

The American College of Obstetricians and Gynecologists also suggests you talk to your doctor about a blood test known as CRP—short for C-reactive protein. This measures the level of inflammation in your bloodstream, and when the test is positive, it could suggest an increased risk of heart attack.

If your results for any of these tests are found to be outside the desirable range, very often diet and exercise may be all you need to bring your levels under control. When this doesn't work, a variety of medications can be prescribed to reduce cholesterol and control blood pressure as well as blood sugar.

Boning Up on Bone Health: What You Need to Know

If you're like many women, that midlife drop in estrogen is most strongly associated with hot flashes and mood swings, memory loss and fatigue. But while these might be the most *obvious* results, they are far from the most important. In fact, one of the most significant results of those waning estrogen levels is actually something you can't see or feel. I'm talking about the impact of estrogen on your bones. How and why are they affected?

From the time we are born a natural process called "bone remodeling" takes place. As this occurs, bone cells are continually broken down

330 YOUR PERFECTLY PAMPERED MENOPAUSE

and replaced by new ones, which are made on a regular basis. It is this re-modeling process that allows our bones to grow healthy and strong when we are young and continues to keep our skeleton strong as we get older. While calcium plays an important role in all of this, estrogen does as well—and this where the menopause connection begins. Acting much like an "escort," estrogen helps calcium and other minerals penetrate bone cells in order to keep the remodeling process going. So, when estrogen levels drop—as they do in the time period leading up to menopause—calcium can't get into bones as effectively, and the bone-*building* portion of the remodeling process slows down considerably. In fact, as early as age thirty-five, the ratio of "new bone" to "old bone" is already changing. Within the first five to seven years after we reach menopause, up to 20 percent of our bone mass can be lost—simply due to this slowdown in the bone remodeling process.

According to NYU Medical Center's Dr. Lila Nachtigall, a midlife health expert, when our bone cells are lost at a faster rate than new cells are made, our skeleton can become so weak that the risk of fracture rises dra-matically. When this occurs, we are often diagnosed with a condition known as osteoporosis—a debilitating bone disease that can have some pro-found effects on our health and our lives. The National Osteoporosis Foundation (NOF) reports that up to 1.5 million fractures occur each year due to this disease, mostly in the hip and spine. Often this leads to perma-nent disability and sometimes even early death. A woman's lifetime risk of dying from a hip fracture is the same as that from dying of breast cancer—one in every eight women are affected. Other times the disease can cause a loss in height, and the characteristic, painful, and disfiguring "dowager's hump" that develops on the top portion of the back. An even more sober-ing fact: Currently some 8 million women have osteoporosis, while another 15 million are waiting in the wings, already diagnosed with low bone mass.

TESTING YOUR BONE HEALTH: WHAT YOU NEED

Although many women believe the time to deal with bone health is after symptoms begin, nothing could be further from the truth. Most experts agree that the prime time to begin taking care of your bones is in midlife—before signs of trouble set in. The best place to begin is with a bone mineral density test—a diagnostic screening that can help determine the strength of your bones. Although there are several types of these tests available, all are painless, noninvasive, and safe. Using a very low-radiation X-ray device, the machines allow doctors to measure and calculate the thickness, or "density," of your bones.

In the past, all bone density tests relied on measurements taken in the spine, hip, or wrist. More recently, however, the FDA has approved additional testing methods that can be done on the middle finger, the heel, or the shinbone. The following are the currently accepted bone density tests, according to NOF:

- DXA (Dual Energy X-ray Absorptiometry) measures the spine, hip, or total body.

- pDXA (Peripheral Dual Energy X-ray Absorptiometry) measures the wrist, heel, or finger.

- SXA (single Energy X-ray Absorptiometry) measures the wrist or heel.

- QUS (Quantitative Ultrasound) uses sound waves to measure density at the heel, shin bone, and kneecap.

- QCT (Quantitative Computed Tomography) is most commonly used to measure the spine but can be used at other sites.

- pQCT (Peripheral Quantitative Computed Tomography) measures the wrist.

- RA (Radiographic Absorptiometry) uses an X ray of the hand and a small metal wedge to calculate bone density.

- DPA (Dual Photon Absorptiometry) measures the spine, hip, or total body (used infrequently).

- SPA (Single Photon Absorptiometry) measures the wrist (used infrequently).

While sometimes your doctor may have one or more of these machines in his or her office, more than likely you will be directed to a separate facility, often a radiologist's office or osteoporosis center.

BONE HEALTH: KNOW THE SCORE

To determine the health of your bones, a bone density scan measures your individual bone mass and compares it to two standard scores. The first score is the bone density that is considered normal for your age, sex, and size. This result is called a "Z" score. In the second comparison, your bone density is measured against that of a healthy young woman in her prime. This result is known as your "T" score. Whatever difference exists between your bones and those of a healthy young woman is known as the "standard deviation" or SD.

- If your T score is within one standard deviation of the "norm," you are considered to have normal bone density.

- If your score is between -1 and -2.5 (below the SD), you have low bone mass, or a condition known as osteopenia—frequently a forerunner to osteoporosis. For most women, a score of -1 SD equates to about a 10 to 12 percent decrease in bone density.

- If your T score is more than -2.5 below the norm, you are diagnosed with osteoporosis.

THE TREATMENTS THAT CAN HELP

In the not too distant past, any woman at serious risk for osteoporosis was automatically prescribed estrogen therapy—even if she wasn't suffering from menopause symptoms. That's because estrogen was among the best drugs to improve bone mass—and in fact it was even approved by the FDA for this purpose. However, the results of the Women's Health Initiative changed all that. While some doctors still consider estrogen a viable treatment alternative, others are inclined to suggest different, ostensibly safer approaches to bone health as the first line of defense. In addition to the exercise and dietary recommendations found in Chapter 7, there are also a number of prescription medications that can help. If your bone mineral density (BMD) is low, your risk factors high, or your T scores indicate a problem, you should talk to your doctor about whether any of the following drugs can help.

Bisphosphonates

This category includes the drugs alendronate (Fosamax) and risedronate (Actonel), both of which work by inhibiting the breakdown of bone. Studies show they can be as effective as estrogen in preventing bone loss. Research also shows both drugs may actually help the body build new bone, with an increase in bone mass most often seen in critical areas such as the spine and hip. Not surprisingly, women who used these medications were also found to have a reduced risk of spinal and hip fractures. Because both medications are absorbed through the intestines, they often cause irritation of the stomach and esophagus. However, problems can decrease if you take them on an empty stomach, first thing in the morning. Remaining upright for at least thirty minutes afterward can help even more. Most recently, Fosamax has become available as a once-weekly treatment, which dramatically confines any side effects to just one day without decreasing its effectiveness compared with once-daily dosing.

SERMS (Selective Estrogen Receptor Modulators)

You may already be familiar with these medications under the term "designer estrogens," a popular buzz phrase used to describe a class of drugs that act like estrogens in certain parts of the body while acting as anti-estrogens in others. In the case of bone health the SERM used for treatment is raloxifene (Evista). Although it acts much like estrogen in helping to strengthen the bones, it has anti-estrogenic effects in the breast and uterus, so it does not have the same cancer-causing potential as estrogen therapy. In fact, one study found raloxifene might actually protect against breast cancer, with a 76 percent reduction in the risk of invasive breast cancer in women taking this drug. Furthermore, in at least one study of nearly eight thousand postmenopausal women, those who took raloxifene, along with calcium and vitamin D supplements, reduced their risk of spinal fracture by up to 55 percent. Women who had already suffered one spinal fracture reduced their risk of subsequent breaks by up to 30 percent.

New research published in *Obstetrics and Gynecology* in 2004 found that raloxifene does not increase the risk of hot flashes, even when used directly after HRT is stopped. So if you have been taking hormone therapy for bone health and now want to stop, doctors say it's safe and effective to start raloxifene therapy immediately afterward, with no increased risk of hot flashes. The downside: There are no long-term studies on safety or efficacy of raloxifene beyond several years of use.

In the pipeline: two more medications that may soon be added to this category—lasofoxifene (Pfizer) and basedoxifene (Wyeth). Both are undergoing phase III clinical trials and could make it to market within several years. In the case of lasofoxifene, treatment thus far has shown it can increase bone density as effectively as estrogen, at the same time reducing LDL cholesterol—all without any of estrogen's negative effects on the breast or uterus. Basedoxifene, which has been shown to reduce the thickness of the lining of the uterus (thus reducing the risk of uterine cancer), is now being considered for use *with* estrogen therapy as a way to build bones without increasing the risk of uterine cancer in some women. And because estrogen would still be part of the treatment equation, there should be no increase in hot flashes.

Calcitonin

This natural hormone is manufactured by the parathyroid gland, and its job is to inhibit the breakdown of bone—something that might happen at "runaway" speed if this important biochemical were not present. Although in supplement form it appears to stop bone loss, there is no direct evidence to show it reduces the risk of fracture beyond what you would see if your bones were naturally stronger. It also appears to have the greatest influence on bones in the spine. Currently it comes in only one form—a nasal spray that must be used daily.

Fortes (Teriparatide)

This treatment is a synthetic parathyroid hormone. As a supplement it helps to stimulate bone growth at a faster rate than cells are breaking down, thus helping to maintain, or even increase, bone density. The only available form right now is a daily injection, which can make it difficult for some women to take. And because there are no long-term studies on

From the "M" File

THE BONE HEALTH WONDER DRUG

Q: I recently heard about a new class of "miracle" drugs that European women are using to control both menopause-related symptoms and bone loss. They are supposed to control symptoms like estrogen does, but without the side effects or cancer risks. Do you know anything about this? Will these drugs ever become available in the United States?

A: It seems as if you are referring to STEARs (selective tissue estrogenic activity regulator), a new classification assigned to describe just one medication, the drug Livial (tibolone), a mainstay of menopause care in Asia and Europe for more than twenty years. So far, this is the only drug in this category, but others are in the pipeline and may come to market in the future. One reason it's referred to as a "miracle drug" is because it contains properties of all three hormones produced by the ovaries—progesterone, estrogen, and testosterone. Clinical studies have confirmed that not only is it as effective as estrogen in relieving symptoms such as hot flashes, mood swings, vaginal dryness, and even sexual dysfunction, but it also helps prevent bone loss in much the same way as estrogen. (Sure meets my definition of "miracle drug"!) More good news: Tibolone does not appear to carry any of estrogen's negative effects—it does not, for example, increase breast density or thicken the endometrial lining. On the downside, there are some conflicting studies concerning a possible small increased risk of breast cancer among tibolone users, but that finding has not yet been confirmed. Additionally, there is currently no data to show that tibolone decreases the risk of fracture. However, studies are now under way, and experts anticipate that it will have a protective effect on bone. Currently, tibolone is not available in the United States. However, it is under investigation by the FDA and approval could come in the near future.

From the "M" File

IS MY BONE HEALTH AT RISK?

Q: I'm forty-seven years old and in pretty good shape. My aunt was diagnosed with osteoporosis, but my mother is fine—and I seem to be okay, so far. Can you tell me what the other risk factors for osteoporosis are—and what I should be looking out for?

A: Among the most important risk factors is a family history of the disease—but usually that risk pertains to mothers and daughters. The fact that your aunt has it is less serious, but still a caution worth paying attention to. Also, just the fact that you are female puts you at risk—with 80 percent of all cases of osteoporosis occurring in women. Other risk factors to consider are:

- Age—the older you get, the more frail your bones are.

- Race—Caucasian and Asian women are at greatest risk, but African-American and Latino women are also at significant risk.

this treatment, the FDA currently restricts its use to no longer than two years. It is normally prescribed only for women with severe osteoporosis.

ENSURING YOUR BONE HEALTH: WHAT EVERY WOMAN CAN DO

While osteoporosis remains a serious problem requiring special medical attention, ensuring stronger, healthier bones is something each and every one of us needs to address. In fact, even if your bone density test doesn't show any significant loss, it's worth taking a few extra steps to protect your skeletal health. One reason is that as we grow older, all women lose *some* bone mass—up to 3 percent per year once we pass age fifty.

The good news is, there *are* things you can do to protect the health of your bones and in some instances even slow down the natural process of

- Bone structure and body weight—the thinner and smaller you are, the greater your risks, beginning at around 127 pounds.

- Early menopause—the earlier your period stops, either due to menopause, severe dieting, or overexercising, the greater the risk to your bones.

- Cigarette smoking and excessive alcohol consumption.

- Low calcium intake.

- Sedentary lifestyle.

- The use of certain medications including thyroid hormone; anticonvulsants; antacids containing aluminum; GnRH (used for the treatment of endometriosis); methotrexate (cancer treatment); cyclosporine A (immunosuppressive drug); heparin; cholestyramine (used to control blood cholesterol levels).

If you have two or more of these risk factors, talk to your doctor about bone mineral density testing.

bone loss. Among the most important is getting enough calcium, an essential mineral. Although 99 percent of your body's calcium content is found in your teeth and bones, with the remaining 1 percent in your blood, don't let the low level in your bloodstream fool you—calcium is essential to many life functions, including the conduction of nerve impulses from brain to body, muscle contractions (including those of the heart), and the process of blood clotting. So, when your intake of calcium drops too low, and your blood level decreases, your body pulls the calcium it needs from your bones. And because calcium is essential to the bone remodeling process (remember, old bone cells continually die away and are replaced by new ones) anytime levels decrease, even just a little, bone health can suffer.

For all these reasons experts say it's imperative that you do whatever is necessary to meet your calcium requirement, particularly during this time of your life. According to the Institute of Medicine of the National Academy of Science here's what you need:

- Women aged 31–51: 1,000 milligrams per day

- Women aged 51 and older: 1,200 milligrams per day

However, bear in mind that the National Institutes of Health Consensus Conference and the National Osteoporosis Foundation support a daily intake of 1,500 milligrams per day for postmenopausal women not taking estrogen therapy, or all adults over age sixty-five.

Currently, nearly all experts agree that it's best to get your calcium from food sources, and doing so doesn't have to be difficult. Just eight ounces of low-fat milk or yogurt, for example, will net you up to 450 milligrams of calcium, while three ounces of low-fat cheese gets you about the same (see Chapter 7 for more calcium-rich menopause-friendly foods).

To help ensure that the calcium gets to your bones, ensure you are getting enough vitamin D. In fact, without vitamin D calcium would simply pass through your digestive system unused. If you take a multivitamin, chances are your vitamin D requirements *are* being met. You can also drink milk that is fortified with vitamin D to be extra sure. You should not, however, exceed 2,000 units of vitamin D a day, since anything over that amount may be toxic to your body.

To ensure optimum calcium absorption many experts recommend that you spread your intake out over the course of your day. Since the body is less efficient at absorbing calcium when levels are very high, limiting consumption to 500 milligrams at a time will ensure that your system is not so overloaded that you miss the opportunity to absorb what you take. If you choose to get your calcium via supplements, you should also try to spread them out over the course of a day, taking no more than 500 milligrams at any one time.

Can you take too much calcium? While it's less likely to harm you in the dietary form, anything over 2,000 milligrams daily, particularly in supplement form, could cause you problems, including an increased risk of severe constipation and calcium-rich kidney stones. Iron and zinc levels can also drop when calcium rises too high.

CHOOSING A CALCIUM SUPPLEMENT:
WHAT YOU MUST KNOW

Although getting your calcium from foods is the safest and best way, sometimes this is not possible. When this is the case, taking supplements is essential. But if you're anything like me, just one trip down the supplement aisle at the local grocery store or pharmacy, and your head spins! The wide variety of calcium supplements—including the many brands and types to choose from—can make finding the right product a daunting task. But making an effort to do so is important because not all calcium supplements are alike. Among the most important differences: factors that influence how much of the calcium in your supplement actually gets inside your body *and* is available for use by your bones. For the most part, a lot of that has to do with how much "elemental" or "pure" calcium is present in the supplement. Indeed, all calcium—both in foods and in supplement form—is part of a compound, usually mixed with a variety of other substances. During the digestion process, the compound portion dissolves and the elemental, or pure, calcium remains—and that's what is available for your body to use. Depending on the type of calcium compound you take, you could end up with vastly different amounts of the pure mineral in your bloodstream. Here's how some of the most popular types break down in respect to levels of elemental calcium:

- Calcium carbonate: yields 40 percent elemental calcium

- Calcium citrate: yields 21 percent elemental calcium

- Calcium lactate: yields 13 percent elemental calcium

- Calcium gluconate: yields 9 percent elemental calcium

This means that if you take a supplement containing 1,000 milligrams of calcium carbonate, typically, 40 percent of that—or 400 milligrams— will be elemental calcium. So that's what is considered "bioavailable" and ready for use by your body. The remaining 60 percent or 600 milligrams would be carbonate—which has little value.

The most popular form of calcium supplementation *is* the carbonate compound—not only because it contains the most elemental calcium, but also because it does not require a great deal of stomach acid to digest. The second most popular form is calcium citrate—which is the type found in most antacid or heartburn treatments, such as Tums. Because this form does require extra stomach acid to digest, it is best taken with meals.

Regardless of the type of calcium you choose, the source—where it comes from—also makes a difference. According to nutrition specialist Linda Houtkooper, Ph.D., of the University of Arizona College of Agriculture, the calcium supplements you want to avoid are those derived from dolomite, bone meal, or oyster shells. The reason is the possibility of contamination with lead.

While the FDA has set limits on the amount of lead a calcium supplement can contain (7.5 micrograms of lead per 1,000 milligrams of calcium) there is currently no regulatory agency looking over manufacturers' shoulders, so it's anybody's guess as to who is obeying the rules and who is not. Houtkooper says avoiding these potentially dangerous sources is your best guarantee of safety. In addition, she also points out that certain forms of calcium—including calcium phosphate, calcium lactate, and calcium gluconate—contain such a small amount of elemental calcium that you would have to consume very large amounts in order to meet your daily requirements. For this reason she suggests you also avoid these supplements.

DOWN THE HATCH: HOW TO GET THE MOST FROM YOUR CALCIUM SUPPLEMENT

No matter how potent your calcium supplement, if it doesn't dissolve quickly enough in your stomach, you'll get few if any benefits. To test what is known as the "dissolution factor" of your supplement, place one tablet it in a glass of warm water. If it doesn't dissolve completely within thirty minutes then it's not likely to dissolve in your stomach quickly enough to do you any good. One way to ensure that your product is likely to dissolve quickly is to check the label for the term "USP Approved." This means it was tested by the United States Pharmacopeia, a government agency that tests, among other things, a supplement's ability to dissolve quickly. Although submission to the USP by manufacturers is totally voluntary, when the label carries the seal of approval you know it passed the test. At the same time not having the USP label doesn't mean the product "flunked"—it could also mean it simply wasn't submitted for review.

What you eat around the time you take your supplement can also make a difference in terms of how much of the calcium you actually absorb. That's because certain foods can bind to calcium and decrease absorption into your bloodstream. This is true, by the way, whether you are getting your calcium from foods or from a supplement. So, you should avoid foods containing the following compounds for at least several hours before and after you ingest calcium:

- *Oxalic acid*—found in chocolate, raspberries, strawberries, peanuts, baked beans, spinach, kale, pecans, and beer.

- *Phytates*—found primarily in some cereals, legumes, and nuts.

- *Insoluble dietary fiber*—including whole-wheat and other whole-grain products and wheat bran.

- *Tea*—it's the tannins or acids that can decrease absorption, plus it also contains oxalic acid.

SIX FAST AND EASY BONE BOOSTERS

With the help of the National Osteoporosis Foundation and the American College of Obstetricians and Gynecologists, here are six fast and easy ways to ensure your skeletal health and make certain you remain strong from head to toe.

BONE BOOSTER #1: ADD POW WITH POWDERED MILK

Just one tablespoon of powdered milk contains 50 milligrams of calcium. You can use it to increase the calcium level of any food, adding it to puddings, milk, yogurt, baked goods, even soups or stews.

BONE BOOSTER #2: SNACK ON NUTS AND SEEDS

We often don't think of these goodies as being good for our health, but depending on which ones you choose, they can contain a powerhouse of nutrients that are important to your bones. For the best bone-bang for your snacking buck, reach for dry-roasted almonds, brazil, macadamia, soy, and pistachio nuts, and sesame and sunflower seeds.

BONE BOOSTER #3: INCREASE SOY INTAKE

The key nutrients here are isoflavones the same phytoestrogens that can reduce some menopause-related symptoms such as hot flashes (see Chapter 10). Although there remains some controversy over whether or not other components of soy, including phytates, may disrupt calcium metabolism, overall the evidence indicates that increasing dietary soy can have positive effects on bone health.

BONE BOOSTER #4: TAKE A HIKE

Weight-bearing exercise—the kind that causes your lower body to work against gravity—is a great way to encourage the production of new bone cells and keep the bone remodeling process going. If you walk just ten minutes at a time, three times a day, three days a week, you'll be doing your bones a world of good.

BONE BOOSTER #5: SIT IN THE SUN

Just fifteen minutes of sun exposure daily will ensure you get all the vitamin D you need to absorb and utilize calcium. If you are wearing a sunscreen your skin can still make vitamin D, but you'll need to sit outdoors a little longer—up to thirty minutes daily.

BONE BOOSTER #6: DRINK TEA

In studies on more than 1,200 women, researchers from the University of Cambridge School of Medicine found those who drank at least one cup of tea every day—or more—had 5 percent more bone mineral density in their lumbar spine as well as in other key areas where bones are measured. The finding remained true even after compounding factors were eliminated—like smoking, hormone therapy, coffee drinking, or milk consumption. They speculate that the weak estrogenic effects of the isoflavonoids in tea may have some bone-sparing effects.

Protection from Cancer:
You Can Make a Difference

"I can't stand it," my friend Natalie said one day, throwing up her hands in exasperation as the waiter at Tavern on the Green handed us a pair of luncheon menus.

"I beg your pardon, madam, is there something wrong?" That was the waiter. Natalie gave out a disgusted "Achhh" sound, while I just shook my head and muttered under my breath, "She doesn't get out often," as I watched the waiter back off quietly, a decidedly alarmed look on his face.

"Are you *crazy*?" I whispered in a hushed but animated tone once he was out of earshot. "You're going to get us tossed out of the nicest restaurant in NYC," I said, even though her reaction was not new to me. In fact, it happens pretty much every time we sit down to have lunch. Natalie looks at the menu and suddenly the sum total of every news report she has heard about cancer risks comes rushing into her brain all at once.

"I can't help it," she said, annoyed that I was annoyed. "But I just give up, because no matter what I eat, or wear or breathe or drink or smoke or drive, it's going to give me cancer," she said, slamming the menu closed.

"Drive?" I questioned. "Natalie, you can't get cancer from driving," I said, hoping to give her some shred of hope that life in the new millennium wasn't all *that* bad.

"Well . . . maybe not from driving," she conceded, "but I'll bet it's only because they haven't looked at the possibility yet!"

The truth is, I understand exactly how my friend feels. As a medical reporter, I sort through dozens of new studies and reports on cancer nearly every day. And yes, I must admit that on some days it seems as if simply getting out of bed in the morning increases our risk of some form of this disease. And what's more, those risks loom larger with every birthday that passes. According to the American Cancer Society, up to age thirty-nine a woman's risk of getting any kind of invasive cancer is 1 in 52. But by the time she crosses the line to age forty, the all-cancer risk jumps to 1 in 11. When age sixty rolls around it's 1 in 4. And while breast cancer remains a leading health concern for women, it doesn't stand alone. Today, lung, colon, skin, uterine, and cervical cancer are giving us gals a run for our lives as well.

On the other hand, my medical experience has also taught me that although the list of risk factors for this disease seems to grow longer every day, so too does the list of important, positive moves we can all make toward better health. In fact, I think if there's any really bright side to the world we live in today, it's that as we go forward to discover more about what can harm us, we can't help but also find ways to stop that harm from occurring. And while *sometimes* it can seem as if there are dangers lurking everywhere—in our food, our water, even in the air we breathe—at the same time there can be solace in much of our world as well, if we just know where to look. The really good news: With a little bit of knowledge and minimal effort, all of us, but especially we women, have the power to control our health destiny in ways never before possible.

UNDERSTANDING CANCER PREVENTION: WHAT YOU NEED TO KNOW

When I first began my career in medical journalism, I was fortunate enough to interview a very wise and learned physician. His name was Dr. Hugh Barber, and he was a true pioneer in the field of women's cancer research. I can remember talking to him one day in the hospital and discussing the idea of preventive cancer care—in particular some new advances in mammography. I told him how I thought this new technology could have a tremendous impact on breast cancer rates. And I can remember how shocked I was when he disagreed.

"Getting a mammogram is important," he told me, "but it's not going to prevent cancer." In fact, he went on to say that there was almost nothing that he, or any doctor, could do for me or any other woman to prevent cancer.

"That's pretty much all in your own hands," he said.

As I opened my mouth to argue with him, suddenly a light went on in my brain. It was at that moment I realized that even the best diagnostic tools were just that—*diagnostic* tools, ways to discover what is already present, and not strategies for stopping a disease from occurring. It was also at that same moment I began to fully understand and appreciate not only the true meaning of disease prevention, but the vital role that each of us can play in the protection of our own health. In truth, preventing disease has very little, if anything, to do with what your doctor does—because at the point where he or she intervenes with a test or a screening, you are, at best, finding your problem early. And while this too has a place in helping to keep us healthy (and I'll get to that in a few minutes), it's not going to *prevent* us from getting sick. As hopeless as this sounds, it is really quite a positive revelation. Because it means that a good deal of what *can* help us avoid disease—even catastrophic illnesses like cancer—is, as Dr. Barber said, really in our own hands.

And while sometimes our options can seem, as they did for Natalie, so overwhelming we just throw up our hands and scare the bowties off waiters, when you clear away all the smoke and mirrors and just concentrate on the research, the concepts that can protect us are not all that vast or complicated.

Do we know everything there is to know about cancer prevention? Certainly not. And will some of what we view as helpful today turn out to be less than perfect tomorrow? Probably. But I can tell you with some certainty that at least some of what we know today can make a difference in our health and our lives right now, and will continue to be part of the "bigger picture" as time goes on.

THE FOUR CANCER SCREENINGS YOU MUST HAVE

As you read just a few moments ago, there is no physical exam—and no laboratory test—that can protect you from cancer. Once this disease is diagnosed, there is only treatment. However, what we now know is that the stage at which that cancer is diagnosed—essentially how early in the game the disease is found—can make all the difference when it comes to surviving, and thriving for many years after.

For this reason it's imperative that you participate in at least some basic cancer screenings on a regular basis. If you are already at risk for certain diseases—if they run in your family, for example, or if you have certain other risk factors present in your current life—these exams should be conducted more frequently, and you should rely on your doctor's suggested schedule. In other instances you may be able to skip a year or more between screenings and still be well protected. Again, your doctor should be the one to advise you on what's best.

However, to help get you started, here are some suggestions based on the guidelines of the American Cancer Society and the American College of Obstetricians and Gynecologists concerning four of the most important cancer screenings for women—and the suggested time frame for testing.

1. BREAST CANCER SCREENING

Although there has been some controversy over the need for breast cancer screening in younger women, once you enter your middle years, there is no mistaking the need for regular breast exams—both those you do monthly on your own and those your doctor or other health-care professional performs. To ensure your breast health, here are the accepted guidelines to heed:

- *Mammogram:* Yearly beginning at age forty.

- *Clinical breast exam (CBE):* A regular part of your periodic health exam, every year beginning at age forty.

- *Self breast exam:* Monthly beginning in your twenties, but definitely starting no later than age forty (see "How to Do a Self-Exam" following this section).

- *Exceptions:* If you are at increased risk (a strong family history, genetic tendency, a history of breast cancer) talk to your doctor about adding additional tests to your annual screening, including a breast ultrasound or MRI.

2. PAP SMEAR

While it is likely you have been having this test from the time you became sexually active (it's that quick exam where your doctor swabs the inside of your vagina with a specially treated swab), midlife is no time to stop, even if your sex life has. The reason: This test is also an important way to check for HPV—the human papillomavirus, a precursor to cervical cancer. Although most women routinely receive a Pap test once a year, here are the latest guidelines from ACOG as to when your midlife Pap smear exam should be done:

- *Traditional Pap smear:* If you have three consecutive annual tests with negative results, then you can wait two to three years for your next screening.

- *Traditional Pap smear/High-risk HPV test:* Under this option you will receive a Pap smear and a genetic test for the human papillomavirus. Once you test negative on both tests, they only need be repeated every three years. If only one test is negative, your doctor will likely suggest more frequent screenings.

- *Exceptions:* If you are HIV positive, have low immune function due to disease or organ transplant, were exposed to DES in utero, or if you were previously diagnosed with cervical cancer, more frequent screenings will be necessary—as often as once a year.

You no longer need a Pap smear if you have had a hysterectomy, and your cervix was removed for benign (noncancerous) reasons *and* you have no history of abnormal or cancerous cell growth. If you have had a hysterectomy and have experienced abnormal cell growth, an annual Pap smear is still necessary until you have three consecutive normal Pap smears—at which point testing can be discontinued.

Although the American Cancer Society suggests discontinuing Pap smear screening in all non-risk women over age seventy, the American College of Obstetricians and Gynecologists says that due to a lack of studies on older women and cervical cancer, it does not suggest any set age to stop routine testing, but rather encourage individual decisions based on personal health history.

Important: Whether or not you require a Pap smear, ACOG recommends you continue to have annual gynecological exams, including pelvic exams, regardless of your age. It is particularly important to maintain these exams during perimenopause and in the first several years after you enter menopause.

3. COLON/RECTAL CANCER TESTING

Beginning at age fifty, women are advised to follow one of these five testing schedules:

- *Yearly fecal occult blood test (FOBT)* Try to avoid the following prior to testing: nonsteroidal anti-inflammatory drugs such as Advil, Aleve, or aspirin for seven days; vitamin C in excess of 250 milligrams daily from either supplements or fruits, all juices for three days; all red meat for three days. If you are unable to do so, consult with your doctor.

- *Flexible sigmoidoscopy every five years* (a test that internally examines the lower colon through the use of a flexible, hollow, lighted tube inserted through the rectum).

- *Yearly fecal occult blood test (FOBT) plus sigmoidoscopy every five years.*

- *Double-contrast barium enema every five years* (a special X ray of the colon utilizing a contrast dye that is infused into the intestines via the rectum using enema-like tubing).

- *Colonoscopy every ten years* (this test involves a longer version of the sigmoidoscopy tubing, allowing doctors to look inside your entire colon and remove any growths or other tissue abnormalities).

If any of the first four tests are positive, they should be immediately followed by a colonoscopy.

- *Exceptions:* You may need to undergo testing earlier or more frequently if you are at increased for colon cancer, including having a personal history of andenomatous polyps, a strong family history of colorectal cancer or polyps before age sixty, a personal history of chronic inflammatory bowel disease, or a family history of hereditary colorectal cancer syndrome (familial adenomous polyposis or hereditary non-polyposis colon cancer).

PROTECTING YOUR FUTURE HEALTH 349

4. SKIN CANCER SCREENING

This professional, medical once-over should be conducted by your doctor during every annual physical, regardless of your age. It is especially important *not* to skip this exam in perimenopause and the years that follow since this is the time when many skin cancers are diagnosed. You should also examine your own skin monthly—not just the moles and markings that are present, but your entire body complexion. Use a mirror to see your back, plus the backs of your legs and arms, and do check the soles of your feet. Should you notice any of the following warning signs bring them to your doctor's attention as soon as possible:

- One half of a mole or birthmark does not match the other in color, shape, or size.

- The edges of your mole or birthmark are irregular, ragged, notched, or blurred.

- The color is not consistent—particularly if you see shades of blue, red, or white mixed with brown or black.

- The area is larger than a quarter inch or growing rapidly.

Other things to look out for include a sore that does not heal; a new growth; spread of pigment from the border of a spot to surrounding skin; redness or a new swelling beyond the border; change in sensation including itchiness, tenderness, or pain; change in the surface of a mole including scaling, oozing, bleeding, or the appearance of a bump or nodule.

CANCER PREVENTION: SEVEN IMPORTANT STRATEGIES THAT CAN SAVE YOUR LIFE

When it comes to preventing cancer, no one has more control over your life than you do! Studies show that simple changes in things like diet, exercise routines, and lifestyle habits can go a long way in reducing your risks. The following seven strategies—based on guidelines from the American Cancer Society and ACOG—will help get you started on a

THE BREAST SELF-EXAM OR (BSE)

Although many women get in the (good) habit of examining their breasts once a month after each menstrual cycle ends, when periods become erratic or disappear altogether, too often so does the monthly breast self-exam. If you count yourself among those who have let this vital life-saving strategy slip by the wayside, it's time to get back to business!

The truth is, more breast lumps and abnormalities are found by women during a self-exam than are discovered by doctors or mammograms. The really good news is that when they are found early—during a self-exam—you have the very best chance for a highly favorable outcome. Even better news: Most breast abnormalities found during a self-exam are *not cancer*. But if you find one that is, you have very likely just saved your own life.

To do a monthly breast self-exam follow these six easy steps from the American Cancer Society:

- Begin by lying down with a pillow under your right shoulder, and place your right arm behind your head.

- Using the finger pad tips of the three middle fingers on your left hand, lightly touch your right breast.

- Press just firmly enough to feel your breast underneath your fingertips—try to mimic the way the pressure feels on your breast when your doctor is doing the exam.

- To examine the entire breast you can go clockwise in a circular motion, or up and down—just be certain to examine the entire breast, and to use the same method each month.

midlife prevention program and put you on the right path to the ultimate in preventive health care.

STRATEGY #1: EAT PROACTIVELY

While a good deal of the information linking food and health focuses on what we *shouldn't* eat, cancer prevention strategies put the spotlight on

- Repeat the procedure on the left breast, placing a pillow under your left shoulder and raising your left arm, while using the fingers on your right hand to do the exam.

- Repeat the entire exam—both breasts—while standing, with one arm behind your head as you examine the corresponding breast. Be certain to go all the way under each armpit in the standing exam. To make it easier to do the standing exam, you may want to try it in the shower, when your skin is wet and soapy.

WHAT ARE YOU LOOKING FOR: Any abnormalities, areas that are hard or painful or where there is a lump—usually the size of a pea or smaller. You should also take a moment to examine your nipples and areola (the darkened skin around each one), looking for any discharge (you can squeeze each nipple lightly), blood, thickened skin, or a crepe or "orange peel" texture. If you do find any of these signs, don't panic—remember, most breast abnormalities are not cancer. Do, however, contact your doctor as soon as possible and have your breast health verified.

If you have not been regularly doing breast self-exams and aren't sure what feels "normal," do your first exam after a doctor's appointment where your physician has examined your breasts. Certain that you have no abnormalities, you'll then be able to know exactly how a normal breast should feel—which means you'll be better at detecting any abnormalities, if and when they occur.

the foods that are good for us. In some instances, adding health-wise foods to our diet can compensate for the times when our other lifestyle choices are less than perfect. Studies show the most important cancer-fighting foods for women are fresh fruits and vegetables (particularly cruciferous vegetables like broccoli, cauliflower, and cabbage); whole grains; foods rich in omega-3 essential fatty acids such as fish and flaxseeds; green or black tea; fiber-rich foods such as brown rice, wheat bran, and oatmeal; calcium in any form but especially low-fat dairy foods.

How much do you need? Experts say five servings of fruits and veg-etables a day is a good number to shoot for, along with 20 grams or more of fiber. Two to three cups of tea a day are excellent, while fish should be consumed about three days a week. Calcium *every day* is a must. That said, three servings are better than two and one is better than none—so do what you can to incorporate as many of these foods into your diet as you can, as often as possible.

STRATEGY #2: EXERCISE MORE

While it's hard to believe that something as simple as taking a walk could protect you from cancer, evidence shows that it can. In one study of 25,000 Harvard University graduates, researchers discovered that those who exercised regularly were less likely to develop cancer than those who spent their free time as couch potatoes. Studies elsewhere have shown that active women have a lower incidence of breast cancer, as well as cancer of the reproductive tract. While doctors aren't certain what the link is, some say physical activity—even something as simple as walking—can increase the release of cancer-fighting enzymes, compounds that work to neutral-ize the cancer-causing factors we all face every day.

STRATEGY #3: REDUCE ALCOHOL INTAKE

Possibly one of the more confusing set of findings in disease prevention came along when some researchers announced that drinking alcohol could be good for the heart—around the same time that others found it might increase the risk of cancer, particularly in the breast. But experts say the key to making the most of both recommendations lies in our per-sonal health history, as well as the *amount* of alcohol we consume. According to registered dietician Karen Collins of the American Cancer Research Institute, "Alcohol does not pose equal risks for all women." For example, studies show that women who don't get enough of the B vita-min folate—or its derivative, folic acid (see Strategy #5) are at much greater risk for breast cancer—so alcohol is likely to affect these women more. In other instances, certain genetic factors can make drinking any amount of alcohol on a regular basis a risky activity. Another example: If you are at high risk for breast cancer (particularly if you, your mother, or your sister has had this disease), then according to the American Cancer Society, even one drink a day may increase your risks further. But let's say breast cancer is nonexistent in your family but there *is* a history of heart disease. Then clearly, taking that one drink a day is going to help more than harm you.

If you are like most women, then you'll probably fall somewhere in the middle—or maybe circumstances are such that you aren't even certain what your family health risks are. When this is the case, experts say let moderation be your guide. Instead of one drink a day, cut back to three or four drinks per week—enough, perhaps, to give your heart some protection, but hopefully not so much as to increase your risk of breast cancer. If you think your risks of breast cancer are going up—if, for example, you have decided to use hormone therapy—then cut back even further, to just two or three drinks per week maximum. Remember, too, that not only does drinking too much alcohol raise cancer risks, the benefits of cardiac protection are lost as well when you overdo it.

STRATEGY #4: CONTROL YOUR WEIGHT

There is no question that obesity can increase your risk of a number of diseases—and now cancer may be among them. According to the National Cancer Institute (NCI) obesity can play a role in the risk of breast, colon, endometrial (uterine), cervical, ovarian, kidney, and gallbladder cancer in women. Some studies also link weight with cancer of the liver, pancreas, rectum, and esophagus, though these diseases are far more rare. Although the association may be clear, the reason behind the link is not. And because obesity is often associated with other negative lifestyle factors—such as lack of exercise, high alcohol intake, and poor diet—it's difficult for researchers to separate out whether the level of body fat is the precise problem, or the factors that lead to the obesity increase the cancer risks. In either case, controlling your weight is going to have a positive effect on many areas of your health—be it reducing your risk of cancer or helping you to avoid other catastrophic illnesses. The really good news: Losing weight, no matter your age, can reduce your risks.

STRATEGY #5: INCREASE YOUR INTAKE OF FOLIC ACID

Although doctors have long praised the B vitamin folate and the deriva-tive, folic acid, as a must-have during pregnancy (just 400 micrograms a day can dramatically reduce the risk of birth defects), today researchers know that these are also powerful anticancer nutrients, dramatically re-ducing the risk of breast cancer at any age.

Among women who drink alcohol—a risk factor for breast cancer—studies show high levels of dietary folate can offer even greater protective effects. The supplements are thought to work by partially reversing some of the cancer-causing DNA damage that occurs in cells when alcohol is consumed, particularly in large amounts. In further studies, a combined intake of 600 micrograms daily, from food and supplements, yielded a 43 percent reduced risk of breast cancer in women who drank 1.5 drinks per day—compared to women who drank the same amount but did not take folic acid supplements. The bottom line: Whether you drink alcohol or not, ensuring you get at least 400 micrograms of folic acid daily can save your life. At the same time, don't go megadosing—at least not yet. In amounts greater than 1,000 micrograms daily, folic acid could cover up a B_{12} deficiency—which, left undiagnosed for any significant length of time, could lead to permanent nerve damage. High levels of folate can be found naturally in dried beans, pasta, and leafy green vegetables. As of several years ago, all grain products sold in the United States—including bread, pasta, and cereal—were mandated by law to be fortified with a de-rivative of folate known as folic acid. According to the American Cancer Society, it's actually about twice as easy for your body to absorb folic acid than the folate that occurs naturally in foods.

STRATEGY #6: DON'T SMOKE

Yes, I know, you've heard it a thousand times before—maybe two thou-sand by now. Not only can smoking increase menopause-related symp-toms, it's horrendous for your heart, your bones, your lungs, even your *complexion.* But did you know that in addition to increasing the risk of lung cancer it's also behind many other forms of this disease? According to the latest report from the U.S. surgeon general, women who smoke have a much higher risk of developing cancer of the throat, bladder, esophagus, and liver, as well as colorectal and, especially, cervical cancer. Several new studies also suggest an association between exposure to secondhand smoke and breast cancer. And, the more you smoke, the higher your risks go.

STRATEGY #7: LEARN TO RELAX—AND GET ENOUGH SLEEP!

While stress has always been linked to heart disease, and even stroke, it's only recently that doctors have come to see it may also increase the risk of cancer. In a Swedish study of some 1,400 women, doctors found that those who reported being under stress for significant periods of time had a higher risk of breast cancer. Moreover, studies now show that sleep deprivation, a strong indicator of stress, may play a role in cancer as well. In a report featured in a 2003 issue of the journal *Brain, Behavior and Immunity* researchers drew interesting connections between stress, lack of sleep, and the production of hormones linked to cancer progression, including the effects of the "sleep" hormone melatonin on estrogen-related breast cancers. In studies presented elsewhere it was learned that women whose production of the classic stress hormone cortisol was elevated for extended periods were also at much higher risk for breast cancer.

The bottom line: In addition to providing possible cancer protection, reducing your stress levels *and* getting adequate rest may also lower your risk of cardiovascular disease and help keep blood pressure under control, and it may even help you get through your menopause symptoms with greater ease. And how often can you beat disease by simply staying in bed an hour longer—and relaxing? How lucky can you get!

You . . . Only Better: Some Final Thoughts for Your Future

Among the legendary quotes made famous by actresses popular in Hollywood's golden age, the one that always stands out the most for me is an off-the-cuff quip uttered by the glorious Bette Davis in her golden years. That quote: "Getting old ain't for sissies!" In fact, no matter what your starting point—age forty, forty-five, fifty, or beyond—as years go by, life can get tougher: tougher on the body, tougher on the mind, even tougher on the spirit. In fact, another one of my favorite, albeit anonymous, quotes has always been: "Want to make God laugh? Just tell Him your plans for the future."

Indeed, it seems no matter how well we think we are set for the days ahead, something *always* manages to come along and screw things up! Be it disease, divorce, a daughter-in-law who's driving you crazy, or a son who is putting you in an "early grave," life in the second half of your life is never going be as calm or serene as you hoped it would be.

But the other side of the coin is the knowing that as the years go by we are not just older, but infinitely wiser and more able to cope—and perhaps more ready to enjoy some of the little gifts of life that we may have had to bypass when we were raising our children, building our careers, or sometimes just struggling daily to make ends meet. Still one more of my favorite quotes: "It's such a shame that youth is wasted on the young." Indeed, as we round the bend past forty, fifty, and beyond, life definitely takes on a new and greater meaning. It *can* also become sweeter, richer, and fuller, and love can be warmer and even more passionate than ever before.

The key to getting the best of it all now, and in the future, is to take good care of yourself. "I will guard my health—both body and mind" should become the mantra by which you live your life in the days and years to come. But perhaps the greatest advice I ever received—and what I'd like to pass on to you now—is to hold on to your spirit, come what may. If just one thought from this book remains with you, let it be that no matter what has happened in the past, no matter what you are facing right now—hot flashes, night sweats, and mood swings galore—no matter what stresses or challenges you face in the future, you must hang on to your spirit and be true to the woman you are deep down inside, the woman you always knew you could be. Live your life with as much enthusiasm as if it were just beginning, and as much joie de vivre as if it could all disappear tomorrow. To this end, I leave you with just one more quote—one that I hope will take you through today, tonight, and all the years to come:

Dance as if no one were watching;

Sing as if no one were listening;

And live every day of your life as if it were your last.

Thank you for making me a part of your life—and for letting me share part of my life with you. I hope I have made the experience worth while—and I hope you have found a few laughs along the way as well. If you'd like to share your midlife experiences with me, and the ways in which you've coped with the challenges we all face, please feel free to write me. And certainly if you ever have a question about anything covered in this book, please don't hesitate to let me know.

COLETTE BOUCHEZ

E-mail: Colette@yourmenopause.com

Resources

Menopause Organizations/ Information

North American Menopause Society
P.O. Box 94527
Cleveland, OH 44101
800–774–5342
www.menopause.org

Menopause (Journal of the North American Menopause Society)
www.menopausejournal.com

Menopause Online
www.menopause-online.com

Minnie Pauz
www.minniepauz.com

Power-Surge.com
www.power-surge.com

Women's Health Information

American Academy of Dermatology (AAD)
1350 I St. NW, Suite 870
Washington, DC 20005
202–842–3555
www.aad.org

Aging Skin Net (of the AAD)
www.skincarephysicians.com/
agingskinnet/index.html

American College of Obstetricians and Gynecologists
409 12th St. SW
Box 96920
Washington, DC 20090
202–863–2518
www.acog.org

American Society of Plastic Surgeons
444 E. Algonquin Rd.
Arlington Heights, IL 60005
(Plastic surgeon referral service)
1–888–4–PLASTIC
(1–888–475–2784)
www.plasticsurgery.org

HERS Foundation (Hysterectomy Educational Resources and Services)
422 Bryn Mawr Ave.
Bala Cynwyd, PA 19004
610–667–7757
Toll free: 888–750–HERS

www.hersfoundation.org
e-mail: hersfdn@earthlink.net

National Osteoporosis Foundation
1232 22nd St. NW
Washington, DC 20037
202–223–2226
www.NOF.org

National Uterine Fibroids
Foundation
1132 Lucerno St.
Camarillo, CA 93010
805–482–2698 or 877–553–NUFF
www.nuff.org

National Women's Health
Information Center
800–994–9662
www.4women.gov

National Women's Health Resource
Center
120 Albany St., Suite 820
New Brunswick, NJ 08901
877–986–9472
www.healthywoman.org

Uterine Balloon Therapy
Gynecare, P.O. Box 151
Sumerville, NJ 08876
888–496–2273
www.gynecare.com

The Women's Sexual Health
Foundation
www.twshf.org

Incontinence Information

American Urogynecologic Society
2025 M Street SW, Suite 800
Washington, DC 20036
202–857–5329
www.aug.org

National Association for Continence
Box 8310
Spartanburg, SC 29305
800–BLADDER
www.nafc.org

The Simon Foundation
www.simonfoundation.org

Incontinence Product Information

Bruce Medical Supplies
(mail-order supplier of incontinence
products)
www.brucemedical.com/incontinent.
html

DesChutes Medical Products, Inc.
(medical products for urinary
incontinence, including the
FriaSystem for women, a handheld
Kegel trainer)
800–383–2588
www.deschutesmed.com

Kegel exercises (information)
www.kegel-exercises.com

Kimberly Clark Corporation
(manufactures Depends)
800–558–6423
www.depend.com

UroSurge, Inc. (manufactures both
AcuTrainer, a device that aids bladder
retraining by signaling and tracking
voiding times, and the PerQ SANS
System, a sacral nerve stimulation
device)
800–658–5965
www.urosurge.com

Compounding Pharmacies

Martin Avenue Pharmacy
10 West Martin Ave.
Naperville, IL 60540
630–355–6400
www.martinavenue.com

University Compounding Pharmacy
1875 Third Avenue
San Diego, CA 92101
800–985–8065
www.ucprx.com

Women's International Pharmacy
2 Marsh Court
Madison, WI 53718
608–221–7800
Toll free: 800–279–5708
Fax: 800–279–8011
www.womensinternational.com

Women's International Pharmacy
12012 N. 111th Ave.
Youngtown, AZ 85363
623–214–4700

Midlife Products and Services

Suppliers

As We Change
For: Natural vitamin E suppositories;
soy supplements; flaxseed
supplements; feminine products
6255 Ferris Square Suite F
San Diego, CA 92121
858–456–8333
800–203–5585 (to shop by phone or
call for catalog)
www.aswechange.com

Transitions for Health
For: Natural Personal
Lubricant/Vitamin E; Pro-Gest
Natural Progesterone Cream
800–888–6814 (to shop by phone or
call for catalog)
621 SW Alder St. Suite 900
Portland, OR 97205
www.emerita.com

Index

human papillomavirus, 346–47
hyaluronan, 154
hyaluronic acid, 154
hydroquinone, 141
hyoscyamine, 90
hypermenorrhea, 46
hyperplasia. *See* endometrial hyperplasia
hypomenorrhea, 47
hypothalamus, 22, 24
hysterectomy, 54–55, 59, 60–61, 64, 347
  deciding whether to have, 68–74
  estrogen therapy after, 4, 314–18

imipramine, 91
incontinence, 72, 75–103, 204
  hormone therapy and, 3, 80, 92, 298, 317
  medications for, 90–92
  normal bladder function, 77–78
  perimenopausal changes, 78–80
  seeing a doctor, 87–90, 93
  self-help techniques, 83–86, 98
  surgical treatments, 97–99
  types, 80–82
  urine collection devices, 93–97
infections
  urinary tract, 81, 94–95
  vaginal, 40–41, 42
insomnia. *See* sleep and sleep problems
insulin metabolism, 182–87, 191–92
intercourse. *See* sex and sexual dysfunction
interferon, 65–66
iron, 173, 338
irregular periods, 11–12, 44–45. *See also* DUB
isoflavones, 274
  in soy foods, 278–80
  supplements, 275–76, 278, 282–83
itching, 152–53
IUDs, 49

kava kava, 289
kava root, 264
Kegel exercises, 83, 85
kinetin, 120
kojic acid, 141

lactic acid, 40, 111
lactobionic acid, 113
laparoscopy, 64
L-ascorbic acid, 115–16
lasofoxifene, 334
lead, in calcium supplements, 340
lentigines. *See* liver spots

leptin, 182
LH, 10
libido. *See* sex and sexual dysfunction
licorice, 43, 178, 234
lignans, 274, 281
liposuction, 151–52
liver spots, 140–41
lotus blossom, 118
low-dose birth control pills, 242, 303–7
low-glycemic diet, 186, 190–93
lupus, 165, 170
luteinizing hormone, 10
lysine, 56

magnesium, 195
magnesium ascorbyl phosphate, 115
makeup. *See* cosmetics
malic acid, 111
mammography, 344, 346
Mandelic acid, 141
meditation, 257–58
mefenamic acid, 53, 56
melatonin, 264, 355
memory loss, 72, 252–53
menometrorrhagia, 47
menopause, defined, 8. *See also* perimenopause
menorrhagia, 46–47
menstrual cycle, 10–12, 44–46. *See also* DUB
metabolism changes, 181–87, 188
methylsulfonylmethane, 175
metrorrhagia, 47
mifepristine, 65
migraine headaches, 25
minoxidil, 166–67, 173
miscarriage, 49
monosodium glutamate, 25
mood swings, 18–19, 245–47
  acupuncture for, 293
  causes, 247–50
  exercise and, 200–201
  HRT and, 298
  medications for, 335
  plant estrogens for, 234
  sleep and, 25
  vitamins for, 291
MRI scans, 55, 63
MSG, 25
MSM, 175
muira puama, 233–34

About the Author

~~~~~~

An award-winning medical writer and former reporter for the *New York Daily News,* Colette Bouchez has more than twenty years of journalism and medical research experience. Her weekly consumer health articles are syndicated by the *New York Times,* and she is a feature beauty and health writer for WebMD. Her previous books include *Your Perfectly Pampered Pregnancy* (Broadway 2004), *The V Zone—A Woman's Guide to Intimate Health,* and *Getting Pregnant.* She lives in New York City. For more information, visit her Web sites at: www.Colette Bouchez.com and www.yourmenopause.com